HEARING AIDS
A MANUAL FOR CLINICIANS

HEARING AIDS
A MANUAL FOR CLINICIANS

Editor

Robert A. Goldenberg, M.D.
Department of Otolaryngology
Wright State University
Dayton, Ohio

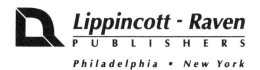

Lippincott - Raven
P U B L I S H E R S
Philadelphia • New York

Printed in the United States of America

9   8   7   6   5   4   3   2   1

Library of Congress Cataloging-in Publication Data

Hearing aids : a manual for clinicians / [edited by] Robert A.
Goldenberg.
     p.   cm.
   ISBN 0-397-51687-8
   1. Hearing aids — Handbooks, manuals, etc. I. Goldenberg, Robert
A.
   [DNLM: 1. Hearing Aids. WV 274 H433 1996]
RF300.H39   1996
617.8'9 — dc20
DNLM/DLC
for Library of Congress   96-23365
                                    CIP

Care has been taken to confirm the accuracy of the information presented and to describe generally accepted practices. However, the authors, editors, and publisher are not responsible for errors or omissions or for any consequences from application of the information in this book and make no warranty, express or implied, with respect to the contents of the publication.

The authors, editors, and publisher have exerted every effort to ensure that drug selection and dosage set forth in this text are in accordance with current recommendations and practice at the time of publication. However, in view of ongoing research, changes in government regulations, and the constant flow of information relating to drug therapy and drug reactions, the reader is urged to check the package insert for each drug for any change in indications and dosage and for added warnings and precautions. This is particularly important when the recommended agent is a new or infrequently employed drug.

Some drugs and medical devices presented in this publicaiton have Food and Drug Administration (FDA) clearance for limited use in restricted research settings. It is the responsibility of the health care provider to ascertain the FDA status of each drug or device planned for use in their clinical practice.

To Debby and Ted
for their love and understanding
all these years

Contents

Contributors

Patricia A. Chase, M.S.   *Department of Hearing and Speech Sciences, Vanderbilt University, 1114 19th Avenue South, Nashville, Tennessee 37212*

Richard E. Cole, BPE   *Island Acoustics Hearing Services, 645 Fort Street, #309, Victoria, British Columbia, Canada V8W 1G2*

Linda L. Donaldson, M.A.   *Beltone-Apple Creek Hearing Aids and Audiological, 9206 Haddix Road, Fairborn, Ohio 45324*

Judith S. Gravel, Ph.D.   *Associate Professor of Otolaryngology and Pediatrics, Albert Einstein College of Medicine, Montefiore Medical Center, 1300 Morris Park Avenue, Kennedy Center Room 842, Bronx, New York 10461*

C. Marke Hambley, BC-HIS   *Island Acoustics Hearing Services, 645 Fort Street, #309 Victoria, British Columbia, Canada V8W 1G2*

Ed W. Johnson, Ph.D.   *Consultant, 4151 Colbath Avenue, Sherman Oaks, California 91423-4207*

Patricia K. Lambert, Ph.D.   *Division of Audiology, University ENT Specialists, 222 Piedmont, Suite 5200, Cincinnati, Ohio 45267*

Richard T. Miyamoto, M.D.   *Indiana University Medical School, Riley Hospital, 702 Barnhill Drive, Suite 0860, Indianapolis, Indiana 46202*

Joel M. Mynders, A.B.   *Board Certified Hearing Aid Specialist, 129 North Church Street, West Chester, Pennsylvania 19380*

Richard H. Nodar, Ph.D.   *Senior Staff Audiologist, Department of Oiolarnygology and Communication Disorders, The Cleveland Clinic, 9500 Euclid Avenue, Cleveland, Ohio 44195-5034*

Daniel J. Orchik, Ph.D.   *Chief of Audiology, Shea Clinic, and Hearing Services of Memphis, 6133 Poplar Avenue, Memphis, Tennessee 38119*

Wayne J. Staab, Ph.D.   *Dr. Wayne J. Staab & Associates, 512 East Canterbury Lane, Phoenix, Arizona 85022*

Robert W. Sweetow, Ph.D.   *Director, Department of Audiology, and Associate Clinical Professor of Otolaryngology, University of California, 400 Parnassus, A-705, San Francisco, California 94113-0340*

Donna S. Wayner, Ph.D.   *Associate Clinical Professor of Surgery, The Hearing Center, Albany Medical Center, 43 New Scotland Avenue, Albany, New York 12208*

Preface 1

Hearing aids have come a long way since they were first invented in the late 1800s. The early aids were large body instruments with battery packs that had to be strapped to the leg or waist. They were nothing more than crude, weak amplifiers using carbon microphones. In the ensuing 100 years hearing aids have evolved into extremely sophisticated instruments capable of amplifying and processing sounds in such ways as to compensate for most degrees and types of hearing loss. Many of us in clinical medicine may not be aware of the degree of assistance that hearing aids provide for our hearing-impaired patients. In our practice we have found that we are able to recommend hearing aids for patients with even a mild hearing loss, whereas years ago we reserved amplification only for those with severe hearing impairments or those with a conductive hearing loss.

This book is particularly helpful for all clinicians whose patients have hearing difficulty. We physicians are in a unique and vital position of being able to influence the patient to accept hearing aids as a way to improve their communication ability. The patient who comes to see his or her physician for a hearing problem may be told that there is no medical or surgical treatment and that "nothing can be done." The opposite is true. The physician is in an essential position in that he or she can recommend the patient be evaluated for a hearing aid. On the other hand, if the physician does not strongly endorse this option, the patient may not be motivated to pursue a hearing aid. We have found that many of these patients will gradually withdraw from many activities because of their hearing difficulties.

With the knowledge gained by reading this book the clinician will gain a working knowledge of hearing aids, the fitting process, and the many advances in new hearing devices. He or she will be in a much better position to advise and council their patients who are seeking help for their communication difficulty.

John W. House, M.D.
President
House Ear Clinic

Preface 2

Family physicians and other primary care providers encounter patients with hearing loss on a daily basis. The patient is often less aware of the problem than are family members who have been compensating for some time. Often in a quiet examination room where we speak directly to the patient we may not detect a hearing loss at a routine office visit. People fail to self-report the loss either because they do not recognize it or because they wish not to recognize it. We have all heard complaints that "people are not speaking clearly anymore" and that "too many people are mumbling and talking at the same time." These are sure signs that a personal hearing loss has not been considered. Another group of patients recognize that their hearing has deteriorated but have known someone, often years ago, who could not be helped.

About the only people who recognize the magnitude of the problem are television advertisers, who make sure that anyone in the near vicinity can hear the ad. In fact, there are approximately 22 million people in the United States who have some degree of hearing deficit. These deficits range from minor inconveniences to true disabilities. Only 5% to 10% of this hearing-impaired group use any type of hearing aid on a routine basis. What a shame that so many miss the sounds of our great world such as music, conversation, and signs of danger. The elderly, who make up a fair portion of the hearing-impaired population, may have other areas of diminished senses such as sight, taste, and tactile integrity. Maximizing each sense is important for continued independence.

Hearing Aids: A Manual for Clinicians will help every clinician who attempts to help a hearing-impaired patient. Up-to-date information is included that will make the clinician better able to make a successful referral for hearing aid services and better able to counsel the patient on an ongoing basis. This manual contains practical information for the clinician and for the patient. Patient education may improve after the clinician has read this book. New and up-to-date information about cochlear implants will help the reader decide which patients are candidates. This book is a comprehensive guide for the caregiver who cares about hearing disability. Comprehensive care includes the goals of maximizing the motor groups, mental competence, and the special senses. Hearing can be improved for millions of Americans.

Edward T. Bope, M.D.
President, American Board of Family Practice
Director, Riverside Methodist Hospital Family Practice Residency

Preface 3

Hearing Aids: A Manual for Clinicians may be one of the most important texts that family physicians and primary care specialists reference in the next few years. The importance of the subject—hearing loss and hearing aids—is reinforced by the growing trend for delivering health-care services in a managed-care environment in which a primary care referral is a necessity, and well-documented evidence that individuals with hearing problems most readily seek and accept treatment when it is recommended by a physician. This book will help clinicians provide a service that their patients expect from them.

Hearing loss is the third most prevalent chronic condition in older Americans. Although estimates vary, it is indisputable that well over 25 million people in the United States experience some degree of problem with hearing and the vast majority of those people are adults over 50 years of age. Millions more Americans will move into the 50+ age bracket as the baby boomers "come of age" and these baby boomers were exposed to more frequent and louder rock music, environmental noise, and a host of other auditory assaults than any other generation in history. As they continue to work to a later age, their untreated hearing loss may become not only a quality-of-life issue but also a productivity problem in America.

Hearing Aids: A Manual for Clinicians provides good news for physicians and their patients. As you will discover in these chapters, audiologic assessment of hearing loss is more accurate and sophisticated than ever before. Additionally, this trend in evaluation is mirrored in the advances in hearing aid technology over the past 5 years. Smaller, more comfortable, and more selective amplification is available, leading to high rates of satisfaction with hearing aids by new owners. Because hearing aids are the only treatment available for most individuals with hearing loss, this is indeed good news.

This text will enhance hearing health care in the United States even if it accomplishes just one goal—increasing hearing screening as a routine element in physical examinations. Currently, less than 20% of physical examinations include hearing screening. If every practitioner who reads this book increases that frequency, we will all benefit.

Carole M. Rogin, M.A.
President, Hearing Industries Association

Preface 4

For many years there has been an increasing need for an authoritative overview on the subject of amplification for the hearing impaired. Years of clinical experience have shown that successful hearing-aid fitting requires much more than the simple recommendation of a device. In addition, recent advances in hearing aids provide long-awaited possibilities for improving the hearing and, therefore, the lives of persons with hearing impairment. These improvements in hearing aids, along with developing philosophies of education, and rehabilitation of persons with hearing impairment, are subjects with which clinicians must be familiar.

The information contained in this book covers a broad range of subjects of interest to clinicians who deal with persons who have hearing impairment. To present this information, Dr. Goldenberg has done an excellent job of bringing together a group of authors who are nationally known for their previous contributions to the fields of otology, audiology, and hearing aid dispensing. The contributions of this multidisciplinary group will be helpful for clinicians in practice and in training to become the clinicians of the future. It is my hope that this book will contribute to improved services to the millions of persons with hearing impairment served by the clinicians for whom this book is intended.

Robert W. Keith, Ph.D.
Professor and Director
Division of Audiology
Department of Otolaryngology/Head and Neck Surgery
University of Cincinnati Medical Center
Cincinnati, Ohio
Past President, American Academy of Audiology

Acknowledgments

I wish to personally thank each author for their diligence and hard work in writing the excellent chapters contained in this book. These professionals have responded positively to a rather heavy editing pen in order to achieve the major objectives of this book. It has been most exciting for me to bring all this information together.

I also sincerely thank Wendy Weiser for her valued administrative and secretarial role; I gratefully acknowledge the direction and support of Kathey Alexander, Editor-in-Chief at Lippincott–Raven Publishers, and Rhoda Dunn, the Developmental Editor, for making my job as editor extremely easy and pleasurable.

Today, those who evaluate and dispense hearing instruments are fortified with an increased sense of professionalism. Research and development is rapidly creating advances in miniaturization, programming capabilities, and digital technology. Each of us who cares for the hearing impaired is invigorated with the exciting opportunities for treatment in the future.

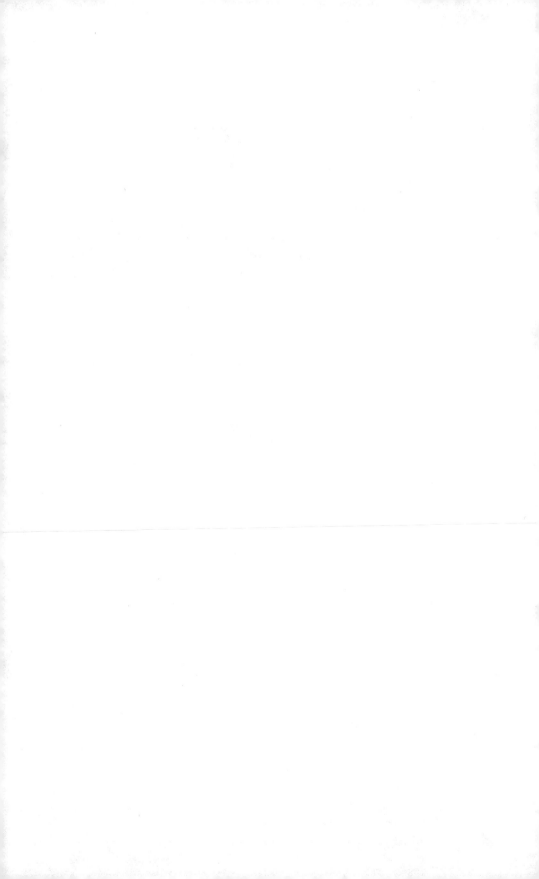

How to Use This Book

This book is a practical manual for busy clinicians. At the beginning of each chapter key points emphasize the chapter's contents. The introductory synopsis for each chapter is found in a separate section at the front of the book. These synopses provide a brief, easily readable condensation that may be all the information required by some readers. The chapter text itself is a thorough and detailed explanation of the various aspects of hearing aid dispensing.

Although originally conceived to educate the otolaryngologist, this manual has just as much importance for the primary care physician, who is often the point of entry for the hearing impaired. Because of its condensed format and intentionally easy readability, it also may benefit the audiology student or practicing audiologist who is just beginning to learn about hearing aid dispensing.

I hope this manual is as enjoyable and beneficial to you as it was for me to put together.

R.A.G.

SECTION ✦ *I* ✦

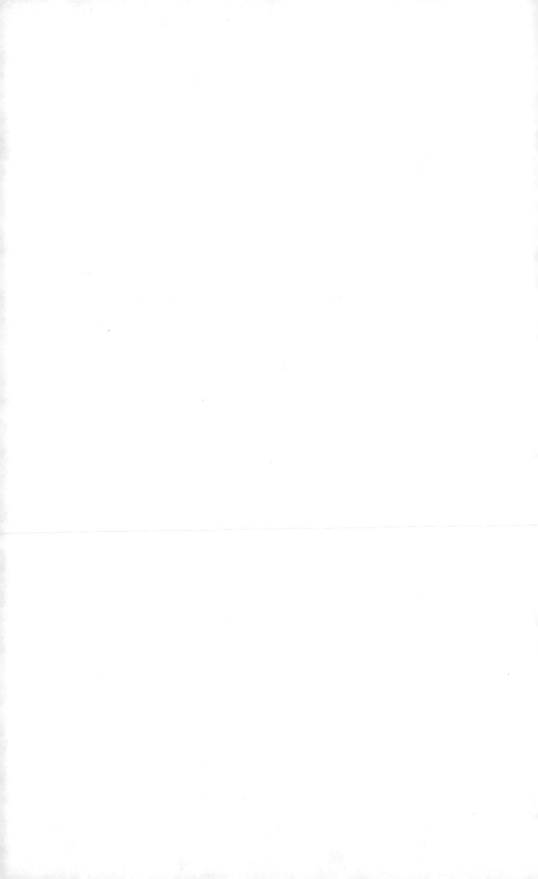

Synopses

CHAPTER 1: ADVISING A NEW HEARING AID CANDIDATE

Patients often rely on information and advice from their physicians to determine whether hearing aid use is appropriate or necessary. This chapter offers practical suggestions for counseling patients about hearing aids. The issues addressed are divided into eight general categories.

Criteria for Candidacy Candidacy should be based on the patient's subjective needs rather than on the audiometric test results. A poorly motivated patient is a poor candidate regardless of the degree of hearing loss.

Determination of Style Hearing aids are available in a variety of size, shapes, and models. Regrettably, many patients choose the style of hearing aids strictly on the basis of cosmetics. Although cosmetic considerations cannot be ignored, decisions regarding which style of aid is most appropriate for a specific patient should be based on physical and audiological factors, including age, general physical and mental health of the patient, the patient's (as opposed to only the family's) motivation, finances, cosmetic preferences, and communication needs.

Determination of Number of Hearing Aids Unless there are medical contraindications or significant differences between the ears, two hearing aids afford better hearing than one. Two aids are particularly better for hearing in noise, enhancing signal-to-noise ratio by optimizing position, improving localization ability, and preventing central deterioration of the unaided ear.

Selection of Hearing Aid Model The introduction of digitally programmable devices has greatly improved hearing aid effectiveness. This new generation of aids offers greater flexibility, multiple programs, and advanced compression circuitry. Finances, cosmetic considerations, and, most importantly, communication needs help determine the appropriate model.

Advantages and Limitations of Hearing Aids Despite marketing claims, no hearing aids eliminate background noise. Modern compression technology allows for adequate gain for soft sounds and minimal (or no) amplification of loud input signals. With regard to clarity, even the most sophisticated hearing aid's ability to clarify speech may be limited because of inner ear and/or central auditory nervous system distortion.

What the New User Can Expect   Because the main goal of amplification is to facilitate the ease of communication, some patients may be disappointed when they experience only minimal benefit during the initial evaluation of amplification. Proper counseling can alleviate this difficulty. Patients must be educated that several weeks may be required before they adjust to the new pattern of sound and learn new "recognition" cues.

Cost of Hearing Aids   The reasons that hearing aids cost so much are that (a) they are sold in relatively low volume; (b) the amount of time and money spent by manufacturers on research and development is considerable; and (c) the amount of time spent by the audiologist with a patient is significant.

How to Find a Reputable Dispenser   Patients should be discouraged from selecting a dispenser from an advertisement in the newspaper or the yellow pages. Physicians should ally themselves with local professionals who have demonstrated the scientific knowledge and moral integrity to provide their patients with quality care. A trial period is essential.

CHAPTER 2: THE PERCEPTION OF SOUND BY NORMAL LISTENERS

Listening involves subjective sensations, and as such, the results are often variable. This is different from the physical characteristics of sound, which are consistent under identical conditions and are measured easily.

It becomes important to understand the relationship between the physical stimulus and the sensation it elicits. This is better understood by first understanding the fundamental psychoacoustic issues of the perception of sound.

Sound   Four items are necessary for sound to be created and heard: (a) a vibrator, (b) a force to set the vibrator in motion, (c) a medium to carry the forced vibrations, and (d) a system to hear the vibrations. Although sound can be transmitted through a variety of media that include light, solids, liquids, and gas (air), it is the latter that is of interest to the listener. Sound waves become a movement (propagation) of a vibratory disturbance through the air medium without permanent displacement of the air molecules themselves.

The physical and psychological correlates include frequency (pitch), intensity (loudness), and spectrum (quality). Frequency is measured in the number of vibrations (cycles) that occur each second (cycles per second) and is identified in Hertz (Hz). A higher Hertz tone has more cycles per second than does a low-frequency tone. The psychological correlate is pitch and is measured in mels. There is an indirect relationship between the two in that as frequency is doubled, the psychological pitch increases an octave, or one complete range in the singing scale. An approximate number of pitch changes detectable is 1,400.

The intensity of sound is measured in decibels (dB), and is the pressure or power of a sound. The human ear loudness function follows a logarithmic scale; at low-intensity levels very little intensity increase is required to notice a difference in loudness. However, at high-intensity levels, substantial increases in intensity are required to notice a loudness change. When measured in sound pressure, the difference between the threshold of pain to the softest sound heard is a ratio of 10 million to 1. Loudness is the subjective correlate and depends on the intensity of the sound source. Generally, as intensity changes, the subjective sensation of loudness changes in a corresponding but not identical manner. The unit of measurement in loudness is the sone. About 280 perceptually different loudness levels are perceived.

The spectrum of sound is what distinguishes between individuals saying the same word or musical instruments playing the same note. Quality is the subjective correlate and is related to the overtones of the basic sound.

Sound ranges along a continuum with pure tones (consisting of one frequency), through complex tones (consisting of multiple frequencies, such as speech), to noise (consisting of irregular frequencies and intensities).

Hearing Acuity   The softest sounds the human ear can detect across frequencies identifies the threshold. At the other extreme are the thresholds of tolerance, with the threshold of discomfort being an important measure. Between the two thresholds is identified the dynamic range of hearing. The frequency range of human hearing is from a low of about 20 Hz to a high of about 20,000 Hz. With respect to an understanding of the levels of sounds, the following are used as references: barely perceptible (0 dB); whisper threshold (20 dB at 5 feet from the speaker); normal conversational speech (65 dB at about 3 feet); a pneumatic drill (90 dB at 10 feet); and discomfort at 100 dB.

Pitch perception is distributed to selected places along the basilar membrane of the cochlea and has led to a generalized place theory of pitch perception. Loudness perception is dependent on the number of nerve fibers in the cochlea activated by the stimulus.

Hearing acuity is also affected by masking, the condition in which one sound interferes with the ability to hear another sound. Some sounds are better maskers than are others. Upward spread of masking is identified as the condition in which low-frequency sounds have a tendency to interfere with high-frequency sounds.

Binaural Hearing Effects   "Binaural" refers to the use of both ears. "Diotic" refers to the use of both ears but with identical sound presented to each ear. "Dichotic" describes the condition in which different sound waves are presented to each ear and is the preferred type of listening. "Monotic" indicates the condition in which sound is presented to one ear only. Binaural hearing allows the listener to localize sound and hear at a more sensitive level and allows for improved listening in noise and the ability to separate primary sounds from background or unwanted sounds.

Speech Recognition Normal conversational speech varies in intensity over a 30-dB range. Most energy is in the lower frequencies, peaking at about 400 to 500 Hz. Vowel sounds tend to be lower in frequency and have most of the energy. Consonants are higher in frequency and, although they contain much less energy, contribute substantially more to speech recognition. A signal-to-noise ratio of about 20 dB is required for good intelligibility for normal listeners. Additionally, speech recognition can be affected by filtering (cutting) low frequencies or by filtering high frequencies. However, when the bandwidth is narrowed, an increase in intensity must take place to maintain speech recognition at a consistent level. Although distorted speech is not recommended, under certain conditions even drastic distortion can have little affect on speech recognition. Speech stimuli are more readily understood when they contain redundancy or more clues.

Effect of Aging The prevalence of hearing loss increases with age. Individuals over 57 years of age can expect approximately a 31% prevalence of hearing loss, and it is significantly greater in men (33%) than in women (27%). Most significant changes in hearing acuity begin between 40 and 50 years of age and continue into the 80s. Hearing levels in men are slightly inferior to those in women, especially in the high frequencies. Also, when listening tasks are made more difficult, speech perception tends to decline with age.

CHAPTER 3: EFFECTIVE LISTENING

This chapter addresses several listening strategies that have applications for the hearing impaired as well as any listener exposed to difficult listening situations. The difference between hearing and listening is defined: hearing refers to the broad spectrum of a person's interaction with sound, whereas listening involves active participation of that person with a sound or sounds.

Any attempt to assist individuals with hearing loss falls under the broad umbrella of aural rehabilitation, which has been defined as addressing "the total communication function of the hearing impaired individual." It may include hearing instruments, training, and speech conservation. Children are dependent on their families and hearing professionals, who constitute a support team; adults are encouraged to acknowledge their hearing problems and take responsibility for helping themselves along with support from family and professionals.

"Speechreading" is a term preferred to "lipreading" because it is more descriptive of the process of understanding spoken language by synthesizing lip movements, facial expressions, context, environment, time of day and year, body language, and gestures. Speechreading lessons should be recommended for any person who cannot understand conversation even with a hearing aid. Auditory training consists of a seven-step process that begins in infancy and progresses through childhood and adulthood. A profoundly deafened child will never progress beyond the first several steps without help.

Most individuals with hearing impairment appreciate the enormous spectrum of listening environments. "Quiet" is rarely silent and "noisy" may vary from two people speaking to 80,000 voices cheering. There are good and bad listening environments. Bad environments should not necessarily be avoided but must be dealt with. Preferential seating refers to the best seat in the house: up front, centered, better ear toward the speaker and away from extraneous noise.

The approach to counseling may vary greatly depending on the counselor's personality and the personality of the patient and patient's family. The patient should remember the keys to effective listening, should not hesitate to tell the speaker that there is a hearing problem, should be observant and attentive to the speaker and surroundings, should be aware of the topic or subject matter, and, lastly, should try to relax and avoid tension. The family should be aware of three watchwords: *Assistance* suggests methods to facilitate communication; *Compassion* means trying to understand the individual's distress and alleviate it; and *Tolerance* is critical (*ACT*).

Although you may choose to delegate any or all of the counseling methods presented, it is imperative to understand this subject to be able to exchange information with your patients.

CHAPTER 4: EVALUATING THE PATIENT

Audiological tests are building blocks to measure hearing function for each patient. Every hearing evaluation is a series of individual tests (blocks) that when put together build a reliable, defensible, and valid assessment that is specific for an individual with comparison with known standards. Variability for auditory sensitivity is either extrinsic (related to equipment calibration and testing methodology) or intrinsic (related to intelligence, attention level, motivation, and task orientation). These variables noted in the testing environment may impact the hearing aid fitting process itself.

Every audiological test must be performed in a standardized manner that can be easily replicated and understood. Otoscopy should reveal any obvious abnormalities of the outer ear or tympanic membrane. Collapsed canals (which create a conductive hearing loss during a test procedure with earphones) are common in the very young and very old. Audiometers measure the intensity of sound presented to the ear in decibels. A decibel is simply a measurement of loudness intensity, but different equipment measures this intensity to different references; it is important to know which reference level is being used and what the conversion factor is.

Testing may be conducted by air conduction pathways or bone conduction pathways. Interaural attenuation is the amount of energy needed for the test signal presented to the poorer ear to cross the skull and stimulate the better ear. This value is 40 dB or greater, which will require masking the better ear. Most audiometric tests are best performed in sound-isolated, sound-treated, or sound-reducing rooms. Audiograms may present data in graphic or tabular form. The former is a simpler method to visualize the type and degree of loss; the latter is more precise and practical for multiple tests. The actual method of presenting auditory signals to the patient may vary from examiner to examiner but must be consistent and uniform from test to test.

The type of hearing impairment is based on the relationship between air and bone thresholds and the level of intensity. There are five primary categories of hearing impairment: none (normal), conductive, sensorineural, mixed, and central auditory. There are also five levels of hearing loss: none (normal), mild, moderate, severe, and profound. Although air and bone thresholds are good determinants of the level and type of impairment, speech audiometry allows for better determination of a patient's specific hearing needs. Speech may be presented in the form of spondee words, phonetically balanced words, and continuous discourse. The most comfortable loudness level verifies the level of listening comfort. The uncomfortable loudness level is the hearing level at which sound is harsh or annoying. Both are important in fitting hearing aids and define the patient's practical dynamic range of hearing.

Impedance audiometry measures the compliance and movement of the tympanic membrane as well as the contraction of the stapedius muscle but is not a measure of hearing thresholds. The articulation index establishes speech energy for a patient and is useful in determining hearing aid candidacy. A master hearing instrument is used by many hearing aid dispensers as a means of fitting hearing aids. Real ear measurement (REM) uses a probe microphone in the ear to measure the sound-pressure levels at the tympanic membrane. Used with and without a hearing aid, REM is an objective method of measuring hearing levels and validating hearing aid use. Sound-field audiometry places signals into a room environment by using speakers rather than earphones; it is often used for behavioral testing of infants or small children and for testing patients with and without hearing aids. The term "hearing aid evaluation" may refer to the entire test battery from the first examination to postfitting testing or simply to the process of validating hearing aid effectiveness.

CHAPTER 5: HOW HEARING AIDS WORK

In the most basic terms, hearing aids collect sound from the environment and electronically boost these collected sounds. An input signal enters the microphone, which transduces the mechanical vibration to an electrical current. This current passes through an amplifier circuit, which increases in energy and then enters the receiver (speaker), which transduces the electrical current back into sound waves. A power source (battery) is required.

Components of hearing aids include microphones, telecoils, receivers (speakers), batteries, preamplifiers, amplifiers, and circuit limiters. There can be signal processing, monitoring, filtering, and programming circuits. Variable resistors allow for adjustment by the dispenser, and patient controls allow for adjustment by the patient; the latter include volume controls, tone switches, directional microphone switches, telephone switches, on/off switches, and remote controls.

There are several styles of hearing aids. The most common style is the in-the-ear (ITE) type, followed by behind-the-ear (BTE), in-the-canal (ITC), and completely-in-the-canal (CIC). Body aids and eyeglass aids are not commonly used any more. At the present time there are about 60 companies manufacturing over 600 styles and models of hearing instruments.

This vast array of technology underscores the need for a simplified categorization of hearing aid circuits. Some of the basic circuitry is described herein.

A linear circuit is one that amplifies sound, which enters the microphone with no alteration except an increase in loudness. One problem with this circuitry is distortion of sound above the maximum output level. A traditional compression circuit modifies this problem by compressing or softening selected sounds. Signals are automatically triggered at the input level, output level, or a combination of both. This circuitry is not standardized and varies among manufacturers. Adaptive compression circuits differentiate between the incoming sounds and compress these sounds selectively.

One of the newest types of circuitry is the digital programmable circuit. The digital function is to program responses and not to perform signal processing, which is still an analog function. (There are a few totally digital hearing aids commercially available and this new technology is making rapid advances.) The advantage of digital programming is in allowing the patient and dispenser together to set several different circuits for the aid. These circuits are then programmed into the hearing instrument. The patient can select at will one circuit for watching TV, another for business conferences, another for restaurant environments, etc.

CHAPTER 6: SELECTING A HEARING AID

Efforts to improve the ability of humans to hear may be traced back to early recorded history. Cupping the hand behind the ear or placing an animal horn in the ear were typical of early attempts to enhance hearing. The ultimate refinement in mechanical-type hearing aids may be credited to musical instrument manufacturers. They used metal, shells, and finally plastic to produce trumpets, horns, tubes, and ear scoops.

The first electrical hearing aids are attributed to Alexander Graham Bell's invention of the telephone. He adapted his telephone device to a simple hearing aid to help his hearing-impaired wife.

Progress in hearing aid development since the turn of the century has been phenomenal. Carbon granule aids with magnetic receivers were the first step. The invention of the vacuum tube led to hearing aids using crystal microphones and receivers. The power source requiring separate battery packs evolved into very small batteries that could be contained within the aid itself.

The next leap forward resulted from the invention of the transistor. This provided for a significant reduction in circuit size and the need for only one battery. The design of aids progressed from body-worn instruments to head-worn aids. The head-worn appliances changed from eyeglass to postauricular, to all-in-the-ear, to canal, and finally to the deep-canal instrument.

Concomitant with style and design changes were significant changes in circuitry. Miniaturization resulted in the acceptance of hearing aids by many more hearing-impaired individuals.

Most of the aids currently manufactured use an analog system. However, there are an increasing number of analog–digital instruments. There are some fully digitalized aids, but they are limited by the size of the power source currently available.

Adjustable hearing aids have been available for many years. Changes could be made in frequency response patterns and in volume limiting to assure that amplification stayed within the tolerance limits of the user. These adjustments were made with a small screwdriver or by means of a mechanical switch. The most recent advance in adjustability is the electronically adjustable programmable hearing aid. Multichannel, multimemory aids provide the largest number of programmable acoustic parameters ever devised for the hearing impaired.

Some individuals with special hearing problems cannot be fitted with conventional aids. Hearing-impaired individuals with marked unilateral loss, with intolerance to earmolds in the canal, or with constantly draining ears must be fitted in special ways. Different aids have been developed for these special problems.

Many of the hearing impaired have great difficulty understanding in theaters, churches, and auditoriums. This problem is addressed through the use of group hearing aids. The newest development is infrared listening systems. Speech is picked up by microphones and transmitted via infrared rays to the listener's binaural receivers.

All hearing-impaired individuals should be considered candidates for amplification in both ears. Fitting a patient monaurally may increase difficulty in understanding in group situations and in background noise. Unless there are specific contraindications for fitting both ears, every candidate for hearing aids should be considered a candidate for binaural amplification.

CHAPTER 7: FITTING THE HEARING AID

Selecting and fitting hearing instruments involves a fine balance between art and science, as well as an understanding of the theory of selecting and fitting hearing instruments. Today's dispenser requires a solid background in the anatomy and physiology of the ear, hearing disorders, the physics of sound, audiometric testing protocols, electronics, the psychology of the hearing impaired, and counseling.

A perfect protocol for fitting hearing instruments does not yet exist. Until one does, dispensers must follow fitting strategies that they find work best.

Each patient needs to undergo an accurate hearing test. Based on the results, an appropriate hearing instrument is ordered. Once received, the hearing instrument must be checked by the dispenser, using both a subjective listening test and an electroacoustical test to ensure that it is performing up to the manufacturer's specifications.

The first step in fitting the patient is to establish a prescriptive target. Prescriptive methods state that for a given hearing loss at a given frequency, a given amount of gain is required to achieve maximum understanding. Because there are many prescriptive methods, choosing the most effective method for a particular patient is often difficult.

Next the dispenser must work closely with the patient to fine tune the instrument, ensuring that the hearing instrument is delivering the amount of gain specified by the prescriptive target. The two most common methods for measuring hearing instrument gain in the ear are functional-gain and insertion-gain measurements. Both these measurements attempt to determine how much gain a hearing instrument provides across a range of frequencies.

Functional gain is a psychoacoustic measure of the difference between unaided thresholds (patient not wearing a hearing instrument) and aided thresholds (patient wearing a hearing instrument) as measured in a sound booth with speakers. Functional-gain measurements are based on behavioral responses, where the participation of a patient can greatly affect the accuracy of the test results.

Insertion gain is an electroacoustic measurement of the difference in decibels between sound pressure levels measured in the ear canal with and without a hearing instrument in the ear. Insertion gain is measured using computerized probe microphone equipment. Unlike functional-gain measurements, insertion-gain measurements are based on quantifiable physical measurements obtained in the ear canal.

Insertion-gain measurements are best for verifying most hearing instrument fittings. However, functional-gain measurements have an advantage over insertion-gain measurements for patients who require tight or deep-fitting ear pieces.

Although insertion-gain measurements give an objective measure of hearing-instrument performance, they tell us nothing of what the patient thinks of the hearing instrument. Because the ultimate determination of hearing instrument satisfaction rests with the patient, it is helpful for the dispenser to have the patient complete a questionnaire that rates the effectiveness of the hearing instrument. For patients, participation in such an evaluation process allows them to see for themselves how much they are benefiting from amplification. Another useful tool for measuring the effectiveness of amplification is the articulation index, which expresses the proportion of the average range of speech cues audible to a patient. Both these methods give patients greater confidence in the fitting.

Hearing instrument technology makes it easy for dispensers to forget that they are dealing with a patient, not an ear. No matter how technically sound a fitting is, the patient who does not like the hearing instrument will return it or, worse, keep it and not wear it. For a successful fitting, both dispenser and patient must work closely. The dispenser must show that everything possible is being done to take care of the patient needs; the patient must work with the dispenser to achieve the best results possible.

In the future, successful dispensers will need support from many different areas. Manufacturers and distributors of hearing-related products will most likely provide the bulk of the support. However, cooperation between other members of the hearing health team (the family physician, otolaryngologist, audiologist, and hearing instrument specialist) will be a key element in the future dispenser's success.

The potential of hearing instrument technology staggers the imagination. Today's new circuits are multiprogrammable, multichanneled, and often are small enough to be hidden within the ear canal. Multiband compression and remote control are also available. The hearing instrument of tomorrow will press the limits of our present paradigm. This industry has never seen such exciting times.

CHAPTER 8: USING THE HEARING AID

Having a hearing loss means much more than just not being able to hear well. It can bring many experiences that change how a person interacts with family, friends, and fellow workers. It can affect how an individual feels about himself or herself.

Some may consider the hearing aid as the end process in coping with a hearing loss. However, it is just the beginning. Experience indicates that those persons who follow a guided gradual adjustment and training program to hearing aid use realize a smoother more satisfactory transition to better hearing.

The Orientation to Hearing Aids Program has been designed to help the clinician assist patients in using hearing aids more effectively. Patients are actually learning to hear again, this time somewhat differently. There must be a gradual but steadily increasing adjustment to amplification. Safety information should be renewed. Proper cleaning, care, troubleshooting, earwax removal, battery checking procedures, and telephone use should be practiced under supervision.

Hearing instruments should be worn at home initially, where the noise level is low. The instruments should be set at a comfortable volume in order to rediscover familiar sounds and the user's own voice. Wearing time should start at 2 to 3 hours per day and gradually increase over several weeks. Patience is essential.

Often a patient questionnaire on communication performance assessment is helpful in allowing a patient and his or her family to identify feelings and areas of ignorance or misunderstanding, as well as to provide topics for further discussion.

A schedule should be presented for regular care, cleaning, and maintenance. Listening experiences vary. Each patient should try the instrument in a variety of environments: quiet living room, kitchen, watching television, quiet dinner table, noisy restaurant, back yard, street, church, lecture, theater, driving, and shopping malls. Certain listening tips will be helpful: using concentration skills, asking people to repeat, using speechreading skills, using good lighting, obtaining good seating, keeping alert for key words, and maintaining a sense of humor. Tips for others are helpful in communicating with the hearing impaired: speaking slowly and distinctly, allowing your face and mouth to be seen in a good light, moving away from background noise, and asking what might improve the situation for the hearing aid user.

Telephone use is a specialized situation that can be mastered with instruction and practice. Television usage and public address systems with or without assistive listening devices also can be improved through practice and education. Local and national self-help groups, listed at the end of this chapter, are excellent resources for the hearing aid user.

CHAPTER 9: HEARING AIDS FOR CHILDREN

Infants and young children with hearing loss must hear speech comfortably and consistently in order to develop spoken communication. Today, children with all degrees of permanent bilateral sensorineural hearing loss, and even those with unilateral hearing loss (one normally hearing ear and one with hearing loss), high-frequency hearing loss (with normal hearing in low and midfrequency regions), and hearing loss associated with early persistent and recurrent otitis media, may all be candidates for some form of amplification for at least part of their day. In addition to the commonly recognized forms of personal hearing aids, amplification technology options also include frequency-modulating (FM) systems, frequency transposition hearing aids, cochlear implants, and other types of assistive listening devices.

By virtue of academic and clinical training, the audiologist is the professional best qualified to select, evaluate, and manage amplification for infants and young children with hearing loss. Interdisciplinary collaboration and a family-centered approach are essential for optimizing outcomes for infants and young children with hearing loss and their families. Primary caregivers, otolaryngologists, pediatricians, family practitioners, speech–language pathologists, day-care providers, and educators are essential team members and provide critical medical and developmental input.

The comprehensive audiologic assessment of young children is an ongoing process. Audiologic test results acquired from behavioral, electrophysiologic/physiologic, and acoustic immittance assessments are considered together. No single test should be used to determine a young child's hearing status; rather, information gathered through a battery of test procedures should be used to delineate hearing function. In order to avoid habilitation delays that negatively impact the child's ultimate function, intervention sometimes must be initiated before precise audiologic information is completely available. Thus, it is important that hearing aids selected for young children be flexible in tone, gain, and output-limiting characteristics so that the appropriate adjustments can be made as new information is procured.

Today, carefully formulated pediatric prescriptive selection and evaluation procedures are preferred for the fitting of hearing aids to infants and young children. These methods have been developed specifically to meet the acoustical and practical needs of infants and children with sensorineural hearing loss. For example, one procedure requires only that the audiologist obtain an audiogram from the child. With current behavioral and electrophysiologic test methods, frequency-specific responses can be obtained reliably from infants and young children at any age. These threshold values are entered into a program (an optional computerized version is available) and an individual prescription generated. The prescription provides hearing aid gain and output target parameters appropriate for that child according to his or her particular age and hearing loss. In addition, current technology allows further individualization and verification of the hearing aid settings through direct measurement of the acoustic parameters (termed "real-ear microphone measurements"). In the majority of cases, binaural behind-the-ear hearing aids with tamper-resistant battery and volume controls are appropriate for infants and young children with bilateral hearing loss.

It is stressed that the information gathered over time by all members of the team is critical to the success of the hearing aid selection and evaluation process. Because this is a dynamic process continually impacted by development, the input of the team ensures that the child's outcome will be optimized. Ultimately, however, parents and primary caregivers are the best advocates for their child. Thus, it is important to foster their active and informed participation throughout the hearing aid selection, evaluation, and management process. In this manner, children with hearing loss learn the importance of accepting responsibility for their amplification and, in turn, become their own best hearing health advocates.

CHAPTER 10: COCHLEAR IMPLANTS

A cochlear implant is an electronic device that consists of an electrode array surgically implanted into the cochlea, an external unit consisting of a microphone that picks up sound energy and converts it to an electrical signal, and a signal processor that modifies the signal, depending on the processing scheme in use. The critical residual neural elements stimulated appear to be the spiral ganglion cells or axons of the auditory nerve; damaged hair cells of the cochlea are bypassed. The most widely used signal processor selects key features of speech to be presented to the central auditory system through the electrode array; a later coding scheme processes amplitude, voice pitch, and first and second formant information via the implant. New processing technology analyzes acoustic input in terms of the relative amplitude of 16 different filters; another allows programming in either digital or analog mode and is extremely flexible.

Profound hearing loss poses a monumental obstacle to the acquisition and maintenance of effective communication skills. Early identification in infants is key to the development of speech and language. Current selection criteria are as follows: 2 years of age and older, profound nerve deafness, little or no benefit from hearing aids, no medical contraindications, high motivation and appropriate expectations, and (for children) enrollment in an educational program that emphasizes auditory skills.

Implant benefit in adults is measured using a battery of audiological tests that assess sound, speech detection, and speech reception with the implant compared with the patient's preoperative performance with hearing aids. In children, similar testing parameters are used, but they must be interpreted on an absolute scale of progress over time (in years) rather than compared with previous hearing aid use. New testing procedures are being developed to assess acquisition to new perceptual skills.

Among the most important factors affecting performance is auditory nerve survival; however, there is no effective way to determine this before implantation. In children, age at onset of deafness seems to make little difference in performance, unless the subjects were deafened postlingually (after 5 years of age), in which case much higher speech reception scores are achieved. Speech perception performance improves gradually in prelingually implanted children.

Although the primary role of a cochlear implant is to make speech sounds accessible auditorily, cochlear implants also serve as aids to speech production. Multichannel cochlear implants with constantly improving speech processing technology permit electrically transmitted information to even more effectively transcend the deafened peripheral auditory system.

CHAPTER 11: ASSISTIVE TECHNOLOGY FOR THE HEARING IMPAIRED

Assistive technology is defined as any device, other than a hearing aid, that enhances the hearing-impaired individual's ability to hear and understand speech or be aware of environmental signals. Thus, assistive devices may provide auditory, visual, or tactile information.

Assistive technology may be used either in addition to or instead of a hearing aid. Whether an assistive device is used alone or in addition to a hearing aid depends on several factors, including degree of hearing loss, speech understanding ability, and motivation to use a hearing aid.

Assistive technology can be subdivided into auditory devices, telecommunication devices, and alerting devices. The most common auditory systems use infrared and frequency modulating (FM) transmission. Infrared systems use light waves to transmit sound, whereas FM systems use radio waves for the same purpose. Both types of systems offer maximum flexibility while providing outstanding sound quality.

Devices are available to improve telephone usage by providing either auditory or visual enhancement. Auditory enhancement is provided by a number of telephone amplifiers. Amplifiers may be added to an existing telephone in several ways, or an amplified telephone may be acquired as a total replacement. Finally, a telephone device for the deaf can provide a visual image by allowing the hearing-impaired individual to communicate using a typewriter keyboard over the telephone line.

Alerting devices may use either a visual or tactile signal. Devices are available to make the hearing-impaired individual aware of any signal in the home and work environment, including alarm clocks, telephones, and smoke alarms, among others. The selection of a specific device depends on several factors, including the type of sound to be monitored and the environment in which it is located.

Assistive technology adds a dimension to the help that the clinician can offer to hearing-impaired patients and their families, thus enhancing the image of both the clinician and his or her practice.

CHAPTER 12: THE PROBLEM PATIENT

The fitting of hearing aids to patients with hearing loss is not an exact science. There are many variables to contend with during the hearing aid selection and fitting process. There is a wide range of audiometric patterns among the hearing-impaired population as well as significant anatomical differences in this group. It is not simply a matter of obtaining an audiogram and selecting a hearing aid that will amplify sound in the frequency range of the hearing impairment.

Patients with hearing loss in the high-pitch range (high-frequency sensorineural hearing loss) are particularly difficult to fit with amplification if they have normal hearing in the lower pitch range (low frequencies). Some of the problems encountered in this group are overamplification in the low-frequency range, whistling or squealing (feedback), and an unnatural voice quality for the user. Modifications are available for many styles of hearing aids to reduce these problems. Some of the newer styles of hearing aids that fit completely in the ear canal show promise for the patient with high-frequency sensorineural hearing loss. Digitally programmable hearing aids are well suited for these difficult hearing losses because of their enormous fitting flexibility. Precise and quick modifications can be made to the amplified sound to achieve patient satisfaction by reprogramming the hearing aid(s).

Some patients demonstrate a poor ability to understand speech even with sophisticated amplification systems. This is a challenging problem, and there are no clearcut solutions. Sometimes the ability to understand speech improves over time once hearing aid use begins. Other times the use of amplification does not prove to be beneficial for understanding speech, but may provide information about environmental sounds.

Certain congenital or postsurgical conditions may result in anatomically abnormal outer ears. These ears will pose some difficulty in the hearing aid fitting process because of retention problems and, possibly, feedback problems. With perseverance, obstacles can usually be overcome. Not all styles of hearing aids are compatible with anatomically abnormal ears.

One of the main objectives in fitting hearing aids is to provide the patient with better hearing for speech in as comfortable an instrument as possible. Comfort is based on the sound quality as well as on the physical coupling of the instrument to the ear. With some audiometric patterns, the goal is fairly easy to achieve. The patient with a 40-dB conductive hearing loss and anatomically normal outer ears should be simple to fit with a variety of hearing aid styles. These patients do not generally show tolerance problems related to the intensity of the amplified signal. Therefore, it is easy to provide adequate amplification without discomfort. Unfortunately, patients with sensorineural hearing loss usually report discomfort when sounds reach intensity levels not far above their threshold for hearing. There are new hearing aid circuits that do a good job of addressing this problem by limiting the amount of amplification for loud sounds.

In patients with one normal or nearly normal hearing ear and one "dead" ear, there are fairly specific choices for amplification. It is possible to fit hearing aids that take the signal from the poor ear and transmit the incoming signal to the better hearing ear. The dead ear does not receive the information. It is routed to the other ear by means of a frequency-modulating (FM) signal or through a wire crossing the back of the head at the hairline. In some instances, the signal may even be transmitted through the bones of the skull by means of a high-powered hearing aid in the poor ear.

Introduction

Which is worse—loss of sight or loss of hearing? What a terrible choice to have to make, much less to be affected by both.

As a Fellow at the House Ear Institute in 1973, I heard this dilemma discussed among eminent ear and hearing specialists on many occasions; no conclusion was ever reached. It has been my personal observation over the past 25 years that some-one who has not lost either sense will usually say that blindness would be more disabling. Someone who has already experienced profound deafness, however, will almost always choose loss of sight as the lesser of the two problems.

Loss of hearing is an invisible handicap. It creates a sense of isolation, dependence, and frustration. Pleasures such as the appreciation of music and familiar environmental sounds are gone. There can be a severe loss of communication with family, friends, and even the world at large. It is a handicap often unrecognized by the speaker (and in some cases by the listener). Often the patient suffers alone, in silence.

For those profoundly hearing impaired persons who are part of the very vibrant and outspoken deaf community, the term "handicapped" may not be viewed as politically correct. For those who choose to live in a hearing world, however, help is needed to survive—much less thrive—despite a hearing loss. Hearing-impaired patients are often unaware of how much they are missing and of the burden that this loss can place on family and close friends.

Among the elderly, admission of a hearing impairment is often viewed as an acknowledgment of advancing age and can consequently be met with stubborn opposition. Young children and adolescents who are hearing impaired are often subjected to negative reactions stemming from peer pressure and even ridicule from those of their own age who view them as different. Hearsay—one person's unsuccessful experience related to yet another and another—often creates a lack of confidence in hearing devices, even before the patient has sought help for the problem or investigated possible solutions. In any of these instances, the suggestions of hearing devices can be met with skepticism. Is it any wonder, then, that fewer than 25% of the patients who could potentially be helped with hearing aids actually wear them?

Knowledge and education—combined with gentle, understanding care by the health-care professional—can resolve many medical dilemmas; the treatment of sensorineural deafness is no exception. Realistic acceptance by the elderly patient of the normal aging process can be reinforced by compassionate encouragement to seek treatment. With young patients, early diagnosis and intervention is critical. One must not simply tell patients to wait and see if a child will outgrow a delay in speech and language development.

Knowledge and education concerning hearing loss also should extend to the services available today to assist the hearing-impaired patient. While the traveling salesperson is still suspect, there may be a need for in-home dispensing of hearing aid devices, particularly with increasing emphasis on home health care.

As hearing professionals have increased their efforts in research and development, they have decreased their employment of certain questionable marketing efforts that might appear misleading to the public. In other words, there is much less emphasis on "selling" and much more emphasis on "fitting"—a critical change in philosophy that represents a truly professional attitude.

Those professionals who dispense hearing aids—be they audiologists, hearing aids specialists, or physicians—are increasingly better trained and knowledgeable in their art. Accurate audiometry, made possible by more sophisticated advances, makes hearing aid fitting both an art and a more exact science than it once was.

A primary care physician, who is often the first point of contact, is in a unique position to have a major influence on the patient who could benefit from a hearing aid. If this physician minimizes or debunks a need for treatment, any subsequent professional who might attempt to fit that patient with a hearing aid will be swimming upstream.

Conversely, if that same physician were to encourage treatment, the hearing professional would encounter the patient in calmer waters and, thus, have more of an opportunity to provide care that could very likely be successful. How sad it is when a clinician's lack of knowledge and understanding compounds the patient's ignorance of facts. *The initial response of the first clinician who encounters the patient will likely determine whether the patient will undertake effective treatment for his or her hearing loss.*

Dealing effectively with the stubborn or resistant patient, dispelling the negative effects of adolescent peer pressure, and reinforcing the need for effective treatment in someone who truly needs it comprise the art of medicine. These are the challenges and responsibilities of today's caregiver.

The purpose of this book is to present the clinician with the most current facts available regarding the effective fitting and use of hearing aids today.

Twelve experts in the field of hearing aids were selected, not only for their knowledge of the subject, but also for their ability to write in a way that can be clearly understood by those unfamiliar with this very specialized area. Although sections of this book are necessarily technical and might appear formidable, the reader who perseveres will be rewarded with a comprehensive understanding of the evaluation of sensorineural deafness and the subsequent methods available today to treat this problem with effective hearing instruments and devices.

The excellent chapters in this book present a number of major concepts:

In Chapter 1, Robert Sweetow discusses how hearing aid candidacy should be based on a patient's subjective needs and not solely on audiometric test criteria. An artful clinician can motivate a patient who is not aware of a problem. The cost of hearing aids and the need for binaural amplification also are addressed.

In Chapter 2, Wayne Staab discusses the perception of sound and describes the elements necessary for sound to be created and heard. He writes about the range of human hearing acuity, emphasizes the need for binaural hearing, presents the requirements for speech recognition, and describes the effects of aging on hearing.

In Chapter 3, Rich Nodar covers effective listening. He reminds us that the acceptance of hearing loss by a patient is based on several factors and that listening strategies and aural rehabilitation can help this process. A physician or other practitioner can set a positive tone.

In Chapter 4, Linda Donaldson describes the battery of audiometric tests that are used to allow for proper evaluation and fitting of hearing devices. As the clinical skills of an audiologist become intertwined with the dispensing skills of a hearing specialist, the patient will benefit from improved hearing instrument fittings.

In Chapter 5, Joel Mynders explains how hearing aids collect sound from the environment, amplify it, and present it to the ear. No matter how sophisticated the device, there is a limitation on its performance because of the underlying disease process of the inner ear.

In Chapter 6, Ed Johnson describes how the selection and fitting of hearing aids represent a fine balance between art and science, for both the practitioner and the patient. Despite the many sophisticated methods used today, successful fitting often comes down to what sounds best to the individual ear.

In Chapter 7, Marke Hambley and Richard Cole describe the process of testing hearing. They emphasize the importance of cooperation among all members of the hearing health team treating the patient.

In Chapter 8, Donna Wayner postulates that listening is as important as hearing. It is therefore incumbent on the hearing-impaired patient to develop keen listening skills to supplement the hearing instrument.

In Chapter 9, Pat Chase and Judy Gravel describe the special situation of hearing aids for children. Early identification and management, often by an audiologist specializing in pediatrics, is necessary to maximize speech and language development. This initial assessment is often part of an ongoing assessment that may require the expertise of many other members of a professional team.

In Chapter 10, Rich Miyamoto explains how cochlear implants provide help for the profoundly deaf and reminds us that cochlear implant technology and testing procedures have improved the quality of conventional hearing aids and should continue to do so into the future.

In Chapter 11, Dan Orchik describes how assistive listening devices may be used instead of hearing aids for selected minor impairments or, in certain situations, to supplement the use of hearing aids.

In Chapter 12, Pat Lambert discusses how some patients are more challenging to treat because of the characteristics of the hearing loss. In these cases, the results of treatment might not be ideal; so the patient must balance realistic expectations with the motivation and desire to achieve satisfactory outcomes.

"There are none so blind as those who will not see." Let not the same thing be said about hearing and about those clinicians who, through increased education and knowledge, can truly make a positive difference for the hearing impaired.

Robert A. Goldenberg, M.D.
Editor

SECTION ✦ II ✦

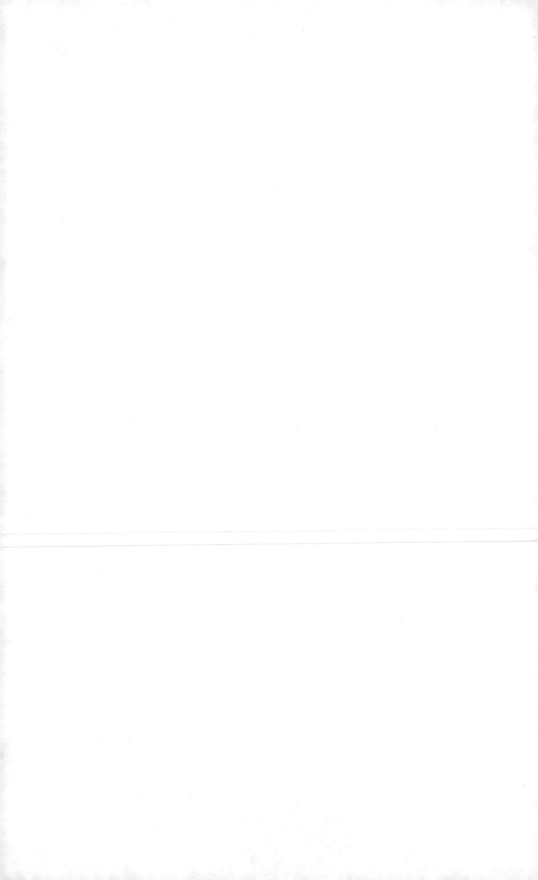

HEARING AIDS: A MANUAL FOR CLINICIANS,
edited by Robert A. Goldenberg
Lippincott–Raven Publishers, Philadelphia © 1996

C H A P T E R ✦ *1* ✦

Advising a New Hearing Aid Candidate

Robert W. Sweetow

Department of Audiology, University of California, San Francisco, California

Key Points

Criteria for hearing aid candidates • determination of style • advantages of binaural fitting • limitations of hearing aids • what the new user can expect • cost of hearing aids • finding a reputable dispenser

Patients often rely on the information and advice received from their physicians to determine whether hearing aid use is appropriate or necessary for them. The information the physician has to offer is frequently obtained via communication from the media or manufacturers with vested interest. Thus, the objective of this chapter is to prepare the physician with accurate, up-to-date information that can be used when advising patients for whom the recommendation of hearing aids is warranted.

Certain questions and comments regarding hearing aids recur frequently. These issues can be divided into eight general categories: criteria for candidacy; determination of style; determination of number of hearing aids; selection of hearing aid model; advantages and limitations of hearing aids; what the new user can expect; cost of hearing aids; and how to find a reputable dispenser.

CRITERIA FOR CANDIDACY

As technology advances and as societal and occupational demands change, so do the modern criteria for candidacy for amplification. Through the mid-1960s, the common belief among audiologists and physicians alike was that hearing aids were beneficial to individuals with conductive hearing losses but were not helpful for sensorineurally impaired listeners. Patients were informed that hearing aids could make sounds louder but would not make sounds clearer. The rationale behind this thinking was that because conductively impaired listeners could process speech "normally" once the decrease in audibility was overcome, hearing aids would provide benefit simply by amplifying incoming sound in a linear manner. Generally, this was true. However, it was erroneously believed that sensorineurally impaired listeners could not use hearing aids effectively because increasing volume would not necessarily overcome the decrease in clarity or diminished speech discrimination ability exhibited by these patients. This attitude was reinforced by reports of unfavorable results from those sensorineurally impaired patients who did try hearing aids. Of course, it is now recognized that early attempts at fitting sensorineurally impaired listeners with hearing aids were seriously hampered by (a) the limited choice of electroacoustic variations obtainable with wearable amplification systems of 25 years ago, (b) the use of fitting strategies that are now known to be flawed, and (c) limitations in the electronic and acoustic capabilities of the earlier instruments (1).

The days of applying a single standard as a determinant of candidacy are over. Clearly, measures such as the Speech Reception Threshold (the faintest intensity level at which a patient can correctly identify words) or the Pure Tone Average (the threshold mean of three frequencies: 500, 1,000, and 2,000 Hz) fail to distinguish candidates for modern amplification. Classifications used two decades ago (hearing better than 25 dB is normal; 26–50 dB is a mild loss; 51–70 dB is a moderate loss; 71–90 dB is a severe loss; and 91 dB and poorer is a profound loss) are insufficient to describe the complexity of the subjective term "handicap." Instead, candidacy should be based on the patient's subjective needs. Occupational and social demands vary greatly among individuals. A judge who has a mild hearing loss may desperately need amplification, whereas the retired elderly patient living alone who has the exact same degree of hearing loss may not.

Patients must ask whether they find themselves stressed or fatigued after a day of straining to listen. They must ask themselves whether the ability to hear, but not understand, is adequate for their needs. They must unselfishly examine whether they are becoming a burden to others, even if they do not personally recognize difficulty hearing. They need to be reminded that wearing a hearing aid is not necessarily a mark of infirmity; rather it is a mark of courtesy to others.

Even patients with relatively mild hearing losses are often now considered candidates, thanks to technological improvements in hearing aids. In reality, it has only been in the past several years that hearing aid technology has advanced to the point where the issue of candidacy is based on the patient's communicative needs rather than on the patient's audiometric characteristics. As stated, 20 years ago professionals believed that patients with sensorineural hearing losses were not suitable candidates for hearing aid use. More recently, it was believed that patients with normal hearing through 1,500 or 2,000 Hz, or patients with unilateral hearing losses, were not reasonable candidates. Similar beliefs were held for patients whose word recognition abilities and loudness tolerance levels were low. Advances in technology now allow for good fitting of most of these patients. The critical variable is whether the patient experiences difficulty hearing or increased stress and strain in daily function (2). Amplification may simply relieve the strain of hearing, as opposed to improving word recognition or making sounds louder.

However, this alone can be a significant benefit. Thus, it is often advisable to go through the free trial period to determine whether the benefit warrants the expense.

Unfortunately, despite the need, many patients resist trying hearing aids. There are two axioms characterizing patients who have been told that they should wear amplification. The first is that practically no one wants to wear hearing aids; the second is that no one wants to spend money or waste time solving a problem unless they perceive that one exists.

Opposition to wearing hearing aids arises for three main reasons: hearsay, social stigmata, and cost. Most everyone has friends or relatives who have purchased hearing aids that currently reside in their dresser drawers. These unsuccessful wearers of amplification are more than happy to spread the gospel on the limitations (some accurate, some not) of hearing aids. Second, despite the fact that people of all ages have hearing impairment and use amplification, there is an undeniable social stigma attached to wearing hearing aids (3). The issue of vanity is being addressed, in part, by the continuing trend toward miniaturization of hearing devices. However, not all hearing-impaired listeners are candidates for the very tiny new hearing aids. Thus, societal stigma is likely to remain a difficult hurdle to overcome. It is regrettable that hearing aids are often dispensed to patients who lack motivation toward amplification. A poorly motivated patient is a poor candidate for amplification regardless of the degree of hearing loss. Vanity, combined with perceived adequate hearing in ideal acoustic environments, produce hearing-impaired listeners who are resistant to hearing aids. These potential candidates for amplification may have heard stories that hearing aids make sounds uncomfortably loud, but not any clearer. Third is the relatively high cost of hearing aids (an issue addressed later in this chapter). One must consider the cost-to-benefit ratio, i.e. the expense associated with hearing aids may be unacceptable to a potential user who denies having anything more than a slight problem.

Thus, the answer to the question of whether a vehemently reluctant patient should be forced into trying a hearing aid is probably no. It is difficult to undo the damage that may be done if the borderline candidate prematurely tries, and then fails, with amplification. For these patients it may be advisable to wait until next year when they may clearly perceive the need. However, encouraging patients to put forth the effort toward a free trial period with the understanding that it is possible that they may be pleasantly surprised is certainly worthwhile. These guidelines are not meant to imply that just because patients have the need for amplification, that they will be successful users. There are numerous factors, in addition to poor motivation, that mitigate against success. For example, speech discrimination ability becomes diminished because of four main factors: (a) reduced audibility, (b) cochlear distortions, (c) abnormal central auditory processing, and (d) impaired cognitive function. Modern technology allows the audiologist to correct for reduced audibility. However, the other three factors may not be subject to correction by amplification, so they can, in fact, render a poor prognosis for success with amplification.

DETERMINATION OF STYLE OF HEARING AIDS

In the early 1950s, listeners were limited to a choice of two styles of hearing instruments: body-worn aids or eyeglass aids. Neither of these styles are in common use today. Now there are a great number of options regarding hearing aid style. Hearing aids that fit inside of the ear are available in a variety of size, shapes, and models. They include the fully occluding custom all-in-the-ear model, the thinner low profile, the partially occluding half concha, the even less occluding helix model for high-frequency losses, and the tiniest of styles, the canal, mini-canal, and completely-in-the-canal aids. Illustrations of these hearing aids are provided in other chapters.

It is highly regrettable that many patients choose the style of hearing aids strictly on the basis of cosmetic factors. Although cosmetic considerations cannot be ignored, decisions regarding which style of aid is most appropriate for a specific patient should be based on both physical and audiological factors. The physical factors are as follows:

1. Deformity or variations of pinna
2. Depth of concha
3. Size of external canal
4. Manual dexterity of user
5. Excessive ear wax
6. Draining ears

Anatomical characteristics may dictate the style. Certain deformed pinnae are not conducive to behind-the-ear (BTE) hearing aids. The depth of the concha may determine the appropriateness of certain in-the-ear (ITE) model instruments; and in order to be able to wear the in-the-canal (ITC) or the smallest of hearing aids, the completely in the canal (CIC) types of hearing aids, the meatus must be of sufficient diameter and must have a sharp enough contour to retain the aid, but not so tortuous that it precludes easy insertion and removal.

Not only is the removal and insertion of canal hearing aids difficult for certain patients, particularly the elderly, but the ability to manipulate the volume control and battery must be considered and tested before such aids are prescribed. In addition, the patient whose external auditory meatae produce excessive cerumen, or require adequate ventilation, may be ill advised to wear ITC or even certain full concha ITE aids. Draining ears or ears otherwise having medical contraindications to the use of an earmold imply the need for open, nonoccluding earmolds or possibly bone conduction type systems that do not enter the ears at all.

Audiological factors include:

1. Degree of hearing loss
2. Configuration of hearing loss
3. Need for special features
4. Acoustic feedback

Individuals demonstrating regions of normal hearing, particularly in the low frequencies, are best served by systems that do not occlude the ear canal. Currently, severe and profound hearing losses are best served by BTE style aids.

The need for special features such as directional microphones and/or the inclusion of a telecoil (a magnetic induction loop) also determine the style of aid. Telecoils allow the hearing aid to bypass its microphone and amplify signals presented electromagnetically (by law, nearly all telephones produce electromagnetic leakage for this very purpose). In addition, telecoils interface with a variety of assistive listening devices.

Feedback results from leakage of amplified sound from the earmold back into the hearing aid's microphone and is an important consideration in the selection and fitting of amplification. Generally, acoustic feedback is more likely to occur the closer the microphone is to the receiver. Therefore, BTE aids have an advantage over smaller ITE or ITC aids. Many manufacturers provide feedback controls, which at present are little more than a potentiometer that reduces high-frequency amplification. Although this does indeed accomplish the desired effect of reducing feedback, it does so at the expense of reducing the audibility of vitally important high-frequency consonants. Thus, this is often not an acceptable trade-off.

Probably the most common inquiry from patients today relates to whether they can use one of the really small, "invisible" hearing aids. Hearing aids keep getting smaller and smaller, but small does not necessarily mean better. A canal-type hearing aid implies that no part of the hearing aid extends into the concha area. There are two types of canal hearing aids. The ITC aid fills the cartilaginous portion (outer half) of the ear canal, whereas the CIC is inserted several millimeters into the canal and extends into the osseous portion of the meatus, terminating within 5 mm of the tympanic membrane. The hearing aid is removed by a monofilament that lies in the tragal notch. The advantages of ITC hearing aids are as follows (4):

1. Most "invisible" systems
2. Baffle effect of outer ear used
3. Lower distortion levels
4. Less acoustic feedback

Because the receiver (or loudspeaker) of the hearing aid is located closer to the eardrum, the volume of air trapped in the meatus that needs to be displaced is less than for conventional fittings. Therefore, less hearing aid amplification is needed to produce the same sound pressure at the tympanic membrane as with BTE hearing aids. Less gain (the difference between the sound pressure at the microphone of the hearing aid and the sound pressure emanating from the loudspeaker, or receiver, of the hearing aid) often means lower distortion levels and a lower likelihood of acoustic feedback. Any ITE or ITC aid that terminates within 5 mm of the eardrum will achieve this effect; these are termed "deep canal fittings."

The disadvantages of ITC or CIC fittings are:

1. Increased blockage with wax
2. Possible occlusion effect on user's voice
3. Uncomfortable
4. Manual dexterity required
5. Can't use with severe/profound loss

If the receiver terminates in the cartilaginous portion of the canal, there are often mechanical problems due to cerumen blockage. If the receiver terminates in the cartilaginous portion of the canal, patients often complain of the occlusion or "barrel effect" in which their voices sound hollow, as if they were in a tunnel. The deep canal placement may be uncomfortable. Because the aid is so small, there is no room to vent the aid to relieve pressure buildup or to release unwanted low-frequency amplification.

It is not unusual to find that the most important factors determining success or failure of a fitting are those unrelated to audiometric findings. In particular, one must take into consideration all of the following factors: the age and general physical and mental health of the patient; the patient's (as opposed to only the family's) motivation; finances; cosmetic considerations; and communication needs. It is interesting to note that in a recent survey finances and cosmetics were listed by only a small percentage of respondents as primary reasons for rejections of aids and that the most commonly cited reasons for patient rejection were difficulty hearing with background noise and discomfort from loud sounds (5). Problems presented by the latter reason need not occur if proper, modern-day fitting techniques are followed; the magnitude of the first mentioned shortcoming has been somewhat reduced but remains a significant problem.

Preconceptions aside, there is much to be said cosmetically for fitting a patient with a small or mini-BTE aid coupled to the ear with an open earmold. Many, including this author, believe that a mini-BTE aid coupled to the ear with an open earmold is less conspicuous than most ITE and many ITC aids.

A critically important advantage of BTE aids and some ITE (although currently not ITC) aids is the inclusion of a telecoil (magnetic induction loop). As mentioned earlier, this feature allows the hearing aid to bypass its microphone and amplify signals presented electromagnetically.

There are certain distinct advantages of ITE aids over BTE aids, as well. Because of the placement of the microphone, ITE aids take advantage of the pinna effect as well as the concha resonance. These effects can enhance the signal entering the canal by as much as 2 to 5 dB compared with a BTE microphone placement. As much as a 5-dB enhancement has been demonstrated for ITC hearing aids (6). It also can be justifiably argued that the pinna provides a natural directional effect for ITE aids similar to that provided electronically for directional microphone type BTE aids.

It has been stated in the past that BTE aids provide greater electroacoustic variability to the fitter than ITE aids because of their greater space to include potentiometers. Currently, however, many ITE aids contain as many as three variable active potentiometers for electroacoustic parameters such as gain, frequency response, output, resonant peak control, and compression characteristics. Furthermore, the use of digitally programmable aids allows for maximum flexibility in all styles.

DETERMINATION OF THE NUMBER OF HEARING AIDS REQUIRED

Many patients inquire about the necessity of wearing two hearing aids as opposed to one. This question may arise due to financial or psychological (vanity) considerations. Over 60% of hearing aid fittings in the United States are binaural. Typically, word recognition scores measured in quiet, sound-treated rooms often are not sensitive enough to prove or disprove the notion of binaural superiority with regard to hearing aid use. Even so, preference investigations and anecdotal reports of enhanced laterality and more comfortable listening through binaural systems abound. Laboratory generated psychoacoustic data clearly demonstrate a number of binaural listening advantages (7). Of these, perhaps the most important are:

1. Better hearing in noise
2. Enhanced signal-to-noise ratio
3. Improved localization ability
4. Possible deterioration of unaided ear
5. Binaural summation

Better Hearing in Noise: Release from Masking (or Binaural Squelch Effect)

Numerous studies show that an individual's threshold in noise can be improved if the signal reaching each ear has a different phase. When the brain receives different audible signals at the two ears (dichotic listening), it has the ability to cross-correlate and process the primary signal better than if the signal is monaurally received or diotically (exactly the same signal at both ears) received.

Enhanced Signal-to-Noise Ratio by Virtue of Optimizing Position

The presence of the head produces a shadow of approximately 6.5 dB (less in the low frequencies, as much as 18 dB in the high frequencies, those most responsible for comprehending consonant sounds). Theoretically, then, in situations where there is noise originating from one location and speech originating from a second location, the overall signal-to-noise difference between a monaural direct signal (sound source closest to the aided ear) versus a monaurally indirect signal (sound source closest to the unaided ear) could be 13 to 36 dB. Because of the fluctuating nature of our acoustic environment, listeners find themselves in these adverse positions (wherein the "good" ear is closer to the unwanted background noise and the "bad" ear is closer to the desired sound source, i.e., speech) nearly 50% of the time.

Improved Localization Ability

Humans determine the location of an externally generated sound by means of (a) interaural differences in intensity, (b) interaural differences in phase or relative time of arrival, and (c) interaural differences in spectral cues.

Possible Deterioration of the Unaided Ear

The ultimate goal of aural rehabilitation is not just rehabilitating the impaired peripheral system. It is also essential to retrain the central auditory system. Although it is debatable whether disuse of an ear will produce further reduction in peripheral loss (i.e., pure tone thresholds), there is ample evidence of neurological degeneration.

Binaural Summation

Absolute binaural thresholds are 2 to 3 dB better than monaural thresholds. At suprathreshold levels, where listeners receive amplified sound, summation increases by as much as 6 to 10 dB. Thus, a hearing aid user can achieve the same loudness perception from binaural hearing aids set at a lower volume control setting than with a monaural aid. This may greatly reduce feedback problems. In addition, one might reason that if binaural stimulation sounds louder than monaural stimulation, it would be necessary to limit the maximum power of a hearing aid to keep it from exceeding the patient's loudness discomfort level. However, when patients match the loudness of binaural and monaural stimuli, this summation effect occurs for soft sounds, but there is no reduction in binaural loudness discomfort levels versus monaural loudness discomfort levels. In fact, most indicate that the binaural stimuli can be more intense than the monaural stimuli before it produces discomfort. Thus, it follows that the dynamic range of listening is greater for binaural listening than for monaural listening.

Therefore, the general rule is that unless a significant asymmetry exists between the ears in either sensitivity, loudness tolerance, or word recognition ability, the standard should be trial with binaural amplification. Of course, there are patients for whom one ear is clearly unaidable either because of a total lack of auditory sensitivity (i.e., after certain destructive surgeries), extremely poor word recognition ability, vastly reduced loudness tolerance, or medical conditions precluding the insertion of anything into the external auditory meatus. For these patients, CROS (contralateral routing of signal) aids are available (some in wireless FM form).

SELECTION OF THE APPROPRIATE HEARING AID MODEL

Hearing aid technology probably has changed more in the past 5 years than it has in the previous 20 years. Perhaps the greatest improvement has come about because of the understanding that there are two basic rules that must be followed if a hearing aid fitting is to be successful: soft sounds must be made audible, and loud sounds must not be uncomfortable. In the past, many users indicated that in order to hear soft sounds they had to turn the volume control of their hearing aids up high. This did accomplish the objective of hearing soft sounds, but it produced the undesired effect of making loud sounds uncomfortable. The reason this occurred was because there was the same amount of gain produced by the hearing aid, regardless of the intensity of the sound entering it. This is referred to as linear technology. A better way of controlling loudness while still providing sufficient gain for soft sounds is with compression. With compression hearing aids, there is more gain for soft inputs than there is for higher inputs. In other words, when the sound entering (or in some cases, exiting) the hearing aid reaches a certain level, the gain of the hearing aid is reduced.

Another great improvement in hearing aids has been the introduction of digitally programmable devices. Not all hearing-impaired listeners require the use of these computer-programmable hearing aids. Furthermore, programmability, per se, does not imply superior listening performance. The advantages of digitally programmable hearing aids are as follows:

1. Flexibility
2. Multiple memories
3. Advanced compression circuitry

Flexibility

Changes in hearing can easily be accommodated, as can unusual audiometric configurations and fluctuating hearing losses.

Multiple Memories

It is often useful to be able to change the hearing aid characteristics (gain, frequency response, loudness-limiting compression, etc.) depending on the environment one encounters. The use of multiple memories (multimemory programmable hearing aids may have as few as two and as many as eight) allows the user to change program memories with the touch of a button.

Advanced Compression Circuitry

At present, certain programmable hearing aids allow for advanced capabilities such as full dynamic range compression and multiple channel compression. The disadvantages of programmable aids are that they are more expensive than conventional systems and that they are not universally available.

Some patients wonder whether all programmable hearing aids are basically alike. Of the 30 or so models produced by about 20 manufacturers, there are two levels of digitally programmable aids. The first consists of systems that essentially operate as "electronic screwdrivers." They have enormous flexibility in programming electroacoustic parameters such as frequency response, compression, and maximum output. The second consists of systems that not only include this flexibility in programming, but also divide the incoming signal into two or more bands that each have their own unique set of programming instructions. In addition, some systems contain multiple memories so that the user can, at the touch of a button or a remote control, alter the system to produce a different, preprogrammed response. Perhaps the most significant feature available in programmable hearing aids is the multiple-channel (or multiple-band) compression capability. Now that audiologists have a better understanding of the importance of providing adequate gain without exceeding the physical saturation limit of the aid and the individual's loudness discomfort level at each frequency, the accurate measurement of these features has become an essential part of the fitting process. As a result of these enhanced procedures, it has become abundantly clear that significant differences exist not only among individuals with nearly identical audiograms, but also among the loudness growth of specific frequencies for a given individual. In other words, a patient can demonstrate loudness tolerance problems for certain frequencies but not for others. Therefore, the electroacoustic characteristics programmed into the hearing aid should differ for the various frequencies. Through the use of multiple channels (some systems have two, some have three) a completely unique set of signal-processing instructions can be provided for different frequencies. As such, a certain acoustic environment can trigger a response that, for example, produces additional high-frequency gain while simultaneously reducing low-frequency gain. This is especially useful in that if the offending loud noise is comprised only of low frequencies, for example, the aid would lower the gain for the low frequencies without changing the gain for the high frequencies (as will occur with aids that have single-channel compression).

Given the changes in hearing aids, and the plethora of available options, it is helpful to discuss how hearing aid selection procedures have changed. No longer are audiologists choosing the "best" system on the basis of which preselected hearing aid provides the highest monosyllabic word recognition score during a hearing aid evaluation. It is now acknowledged that this comparative approach was flawed in a number of respects. For example, monosyllabic words presented in a quiet, nonreverberant environment are not representative of reality. Furthermore, it is now believed that a period of time is needed to acclimate to various amplified systems. Perhaps most important, however, is the current thinking concerning the importance of restoring normal loudness relations. The comparative approach largely ignored this factor. Current hearing aid selection procedures begin with the establishment of targets for gain and maximum output. These computer-generated targets are based on an individual's threshold data, loudness tolerance levels, rate of loudness growth, and ear canal resonance. Aided and unaided (real ear) measurements are performed using probe microphones inserted to within a few millimeters of the eardrum (8). Attempts are made to approximate target levels, but these are only starting points. Once the audiologist is "in the ballpark," fine tuning adjustments are made based on the individual's preferences. Recent formulas are now being tested to help establish proper targets for the most recently introduced technology, incorporating nonlinear, multiband compression circuits. Once the hearing aid characteristics are set based on these procedures, further validation is performed by assessing listening performance in a variety of acoustic conditions.

ADVANTAGES AND LIMITATIONS OF HEARING AIDS

Hearing aids are not new ears. Despite marketing claims, no hearing aid eliminates background noise. Indeed, normal listeners experience background noise daily. Even so, the most frequent complaints voiced by hearing aid users are that noise is amplified too much, certain sounds become too loud for the user to bear, and some speech still is not clear. Attempts are made to minimize amplification of background noise, however, because noise is composed of many of the same frequencies as speech, and it is impossible to shut out noise without also adversely affecting the quality of the speech signal. There is better news regarding the problem of sounds becoming too loud. The proper use of modern compression technology should provide adequate gain for soft sounds while minimally (or not at all) amplifying loud input signals. With regard to clarity, even the most sophisticated hearing aid's ability to clarify speech is limited by the degree of inner ear and/or central auditory nervous system distortion.

Patients with certain audiometric configurations (i.e., normal hearing through 2,000 Hz with a high-frequency loss above) should be informed that there may be no measurable improvement in speech discrimination performance, even if the hearing aid seems beneficial to the listener. This occurs because the hearing aid evaluation process may be reflected rather than show the benefit from the hearing aid itself. The patient may not be able to improve upon recognition scores for laboratory tasks void of extraneous demands on attention. Word recognition testing in quiet environments is an example of such a low-demand task. Subjects in this situation might prefer amplified speech because it is easier to process; however, performance may not be improved because the hearing aid is not providing enough new information to the patient that could not be accessed simply by applying full attention. In other words, the hearing aid helps in quiet by allowing the subject to work less hard, but recognition scores, which were near the maximum (even unaided), are not significantly improved. The true test comes in noisy or "high demand" environments, where attention is resource limited. In these conditions, the information provided by the hearing aid may no longer be redundant with processes the listener could have accessed on his or her own by paying full attention, so now the device may be shown to be of value. Thus, testing must be conducted in high-demand conditions, such as created by sufficiently poor signal-to-noise ratios (9). Aside from the actual testing situation, however, the new user needs to be reminded that hearing aids are not ideal in all situations. They are called aids because they aid in hearing; they do not make hearing perfect. If they improve the listener's daily listening skills, they are successful.

Another frequently mentioned concern of patients is that their own voices sound odd when wearing hearing aids. The reason this occurs is that when an ear is open and an individual speaks, he hears himself mostly by air conduction (the more sensitive pathway through the outer and middle ear), as well as by bone conduction (through the inner ear). When the ear is occluded, however, air conduction transmission is reduced and bone conduction perception is enhanced. Also, the normal, unoccluded ear canal produces nearly a 20-dB resonance centered around 2,700 Hz. When an ear is occluded, for example with a hearing aid or closed earmold, this resonance is eliminated. Furthermore, an unoccluded ear allows for an escape of long-wavelength, low-frequency sounds, but when the ear is occluded, these low-frequency sounds are trapped in the ear canal and cannot escape. These factors account for enhanced bone conduction perception in the low frequencies. To the listener, it sounds as if he is talking in a barrel or experiencing an echo. This occlusion effect can be minimized by (a) keeping the ear as open as possible, (b) reducing low-frequency gain, and (c) using a coupling configuration that contacts with the osseous rather than the cartilaginous portion of the meatus, thus reducing vibration.

As mentioned earlier, a common occurrence that may discourage certain patients is the presence of feedback, or an annoying whistling sound emanating from their hearing aids. Many assume incorrectly that feedback means that the hearing aid is malfunctioning. There are two types of acoustic feedback: that produced internally from the hearing aid (indicating an aid in need of repair) and the more common external feedback produced by a leakage of amplified sound out of the ear canal and back into the microphone of the hearing aid. Usually, external feedback can be corrected by (a) reinserting, or possibly remaking, the earmold (or ITE shell); (b) plugging, or reducing the diameter of any vents in the coupling system; (c) reducing the amount of high-frequency gain (this is typically an unacceptable trade-off because of the resultant loss of high-frequency audibility); or (d) altering the resonant peak of the hearing aid with acoustic dampers, filters, or potentiometers.

Another limitation of hearing aids is that listeners have increased difficulty hearing when the source is physically located at a distance from the listener. This occurs, for example, in large conference rooms or auditoriums. Intensity decreases as physical distance increases. Unfortunately, most background noise surrounds the listener, so although the intensity of the speech decreases with distance, the intensity of the noise may not. This is one reason why hearing aids transmit sound so well if the speaker talks right into the microphone, but at longer, more realistic, distances, reception diminishes. It would be ideal to have the sound produced at the source transferred directly to the listener without losing any intensity. It is obviously impractical, however, to ask the speaker to move closer to the listener's ear. One way of achieving this effect is with direct audio input, in which the speaker holds a microphone that is hard wired to the hearing aid itself near his mouth. Many hearing aid wearers are reluctant to ask the speaker to do this, however. An alternative approach is available through infrared transmission, FM transmission, or inductance loop transmission (10). These systems are currently used by many theaters, concert halls, houses of worship, and households. One of the best uses is for television listening. The portable transmitter, usually a box smaller than most cable boxes, and microphone are located near the television loudspeaker. The sound picked up by the microphone is then transmitted to a receiver, worn by the listener without any decrease in intensity. These devices can transmit with minimal distortion over a considerable distance (up to 50 feet). Assistive listening devices such as these are becoming increasingly apparent in public places due to the recent legislative enactment of the Americans with Disabilities Act.

WHAT THE NEW USER CAN EXPECT

Because many patients with sensorineural hearing loss deny the presence of a hearing impairment or lack sufficient motivation, they often demand to be convinced concerning the improvement that a hearing aid can provide. Because the main goal of amplification is to facilitate the ease of communication, some patients may be disappointed when they experience only minimal benefit during the initial evaluation of amplification. Proper counseling can alleviate this difficulty. Patients must be educated that prediction of long-term benefit from amplification is tenuous at best because of the initial adjustment and learning process that takes place. Most hearing aid wearers require several weeks before they adjust to the new pattern of sound and learn new recognition cues.

It is essential to assist the patient in establishing realistic expectations. Patients must be informed that factors such as cochlear distortions, central auditory nervous system deficiencies, deficits in cognitive processing, degree of loss, and shape of audiometric configuration, noisy environments, large rooms, and certain talkers will create serious obstacles that even the most suitable amplification system may not overcome. It is important to differentiate peripheral from central pathology as the cause for reduction of hearing because only peripheral dysfunctions (reduced audibility and cochlear distortion) are subject to benefit from amplification.

The new user needs to be oriented to the world of amplification. Some require a gradual "break-in" wearing schedule, whereas others need to be encouraged to wear the hearing aid immediately during all waking hours. Many require additional aural rehabilitation, either individually or in groups with other hearing impaired individuals and family members.

Patients must accept that time is required for adapting to hearing aids. Recent studies suggest that aided speech discrimination ability can grow as much as 3 months after the use of a new hearing aid (11). Most dispensing audiologists currently allow for a 1-month trial period with new hearing aids. If market conditions allow, trial periods may be extended to further accommodate this acclimatization.

COST OF HEARING AIDS

Patients justifiably ask why hearing aids cost so much. They cite the often lower cost of a higher fidelity stereo system and wonder why these imperfect hearing instruments cost what they do. Some of the reasons that hearing aids cost so much are listed as follows:

1. They are sold in relatively low volume (i.e., approximately 1. 7 million hearing aids for some 30 million hearing impaired are sold in a year compared with several millions of stereos).
2. The amount of time and money spent by manufacturers on research and development is considerable. One manufacturer claims to have spent over $20 million developing a single model.
3. The amount of time spent by the audiologist with a patient is significant. An average of five direct contact hours is spent during the first year that a patient receives a hearing aid(s). This time spent is critical for new users, particularly to assist the acclimatization process.

Mail order, or budget clubs can afford to sell hearing aids inexpensively because the electronic components of hearing aids are inexpensive and the hearing aids are often placed on the user with minimal (or in the case of mail order) no instructions or fine tuning adjustments. Furthermore, the patient may be charged for every return visit, including minor tubing change and adjustments. Thus, in the long run, the patient is likely to pay as much or even more. In addition, the minimal training required for a dispensing audiologist is a Masters degree, whereas mail order or discount centers are often staffed by sales people having minimal training. When a patient receives a hearing aid from nonprofessionals in this manner, the hearing health-care professionals, otolaryngologists, or audiologists, may be "taken out of the loop."

HOW TO CHOOSE A REPUTABLE DISPENSER

The delivery system of hearing aids in the United States has changed dramatically in the past two decades. Most states require licensure with continuing education requirements, which are essential to keep up with the rapidly changing technology. Twenty years ago, audiologists were not allowed to dispense hearing aids because it was considered a conflict of interest. Fortunately, it is now normal for audiologists to assess the hearing loss, prescribe the amplification, and provide fitting and follow-up care. This is not to say that a dispenser must be a licensed audiologist to dispense hearing aids. There are numerous examples of experienced traditional dispensers who have been in the business for many years and who either chose, or were unable through circumstances, to obtain an educational degree. For these individuals, the experience they have gained from years of practice has been invaluable.

Patients should be discouraged from selecting a dispenser from an advertisement in the newspaper or the yellow pages. Physicians should ally themselves with local professionals who have demonstrated the scientific knowledge and moral integrity to provide their patients with quality care. General physicians might obtain information from local otolaryngologists or from local university settings. In addition, there is much to be learned from the personal experience of other patients. Perhaps most important, however, is that the selected dispenser should offer a trial period of at least 1 month.

CONCLUSIONS

In this chapter, some of the truths and myths of hearing aids have been explored. The physician must be honest with the patient and present a realistic outlook about the advantages and limitations to be derived from amplification. Even though dramatic improvements have been made, hearing aids remain imperfect devices. The physician best serves the patient's needs by being informed, recognizing and admitting when answers are not readily available, and, above all, being a good listener in order to determine the needs of the individual.

REFERENCES

1. Killion MC. A high fidelity hearing aid. *Hear Instrum* 1990;41:38–39.
2. Sweetow R. Hearing aids and assistive listening devices. In: Jackler RJ, Brackmann DE, eds. *Textbook of Neurotology.* St. Louis, MO: Mosby Year Book; 1994:1345–1359.
3. Surr R, Hawkins DB. New hearing aid users' perception of the "hearing aid effect." *Ear Hearing* 1988;9:113–118.
4. Staab W, Finlay B. A fitting rationale for deep fitting canal hearing instruments. *Hear Instrum* 1991;42:6–10.
5. Berger K, Hagberg E. Hearing aid users attitudes and hearing aid usage. *Monogr Contemp Audiol* 1982;3:24.

6. Gartrell E, Church GT. Effect of microphone location in ITE vs. BTE hearing aids. *J Am Acad Audiol* 1990;1:151–153.
7. Carhart RC. The usefulness of binaural hearing aids. *J Speech Hear Disord* 1958;23:42–51.
8. Hawkins DB. Clinical ear canal probe tube measurements. *Ear Hear* 1987;8(suppl):74–81.
9. Beck L. Issues in the assesment and use of hearing aid technology. *Ear Hear* 1991;12 (suppl): 93–99.
10. Compton CL. Assistive devices. *Semin Hear* 1989;10:104–120.
11. Gatehouse S, Killion M. HABRAT: Hearing aid brain rewiring accomodation time. *Hear Instrum* 1993;44:29–32.

HEARING AIDS: A MANUAL FOR CLINICIANS,
edited by Robert A. Goldenberg
Lippincott–Raven Publishers, Philadelphia © 1996

C H A P T E R ✦*2*✦

The Perception of Sound by Normal Listeners

Wayne J. Staab

Dr. Wayne J. Staab & Associates, Phoenix, Arizona

Key Points

How sound is perceived • how hearing acuity is affected • effects of binaural hearing • aspects of speech recognition and understanding • effect of aging.

What do we hear when we listen? This involves the nature of our sensations when we listen to auditory stimuli and is a part of the fields of psychophysics and psychoacoustics. These experiences are subjective; therefore, the results obtained are often variable, even within the same individual under different circumstances or different occasions. As a result, the information related to what we hear when we listen has much greater variability than what is obtained by purely physical measurements, which are consistent under identical conditions. From this it would appear that physical quantities would be most desirable to reference as indications of how normal listeners hear sounds. Unfortunately, physical measures do not reflect the subjective properties of sound, properties that provide a true indication of how a listener responds to sound. Psychoacoustic (subjective) experiences are the only true indications of how the overall hearing mechanism responds to sound. Nevertheless, to understand the psychoacoustic experiences, it is helpful to relate them to physical (measurable) acoustical properties of sound. Many current hearing tests and hearing aid fittings can be better understood from a careful consideration of these principles.

PSYCHOPHYSICAL METHODS

To study the relationship between the physical stimulus and the sensation it elicits, methods must be identified to quantify both the stimulus and the sensation. When used for threshold determination, physical stimulus measurement is straightforward. Measurement of the threshold sensation elicited is more difficult, however, and is performed by indirect methods. Procedures to measure both these thresholds were developed by Fechner (1) and have come to be known as (a) the method of limits, (b) the method of adjustment, and (c) the method of constant stimuli. It is important to note that these procedures can be used to measure functions other than absolute thresholds. For a more detailed discussion of these methods, the reader is referred to Hirsh (2).

In the method of limits, the experimenter controls the intensity of the stimulus and its presentation. This is very close to the procedure used to obtain thresholds in pure-tone audiometry. In the method of adjustment, the listener plays an active role in the control of the stimulus. The patient has control of the stimulus and adjusts its magnitude to satisfy his or her criteria of detectability; an example would be the task involved in Békésy audiometry. In the method of constant stimuli, the listener assumes a passive role in the manipulation of stimulus intensity. Known also as the "method of right and wrong cases," the attempt is to obtain a percentage or ratio measure of judgments of right and wrong, or equal and greater, etc. Variations of these, identified as adaptive, scaling, and matching procedures, are discussed by Humes (3).

SOUND

Before we can discuss how we hear as normal listeners, it is important to understand something about sound waves in general and sound waves in air specifically. The discussion is limited to those characteristics of sound that aid in conveying the fundamental psychoacoustic issues of the perception of sound.

Sound can travel through a variety of media, including light, solids, liquids, and gas (air). We are most interested in sound waves in air because these are what we are normally exposed to. Air consists of small particles (molecules) that are constantly in random (but generally gentle) motion around an average "stable" position. These molecules are bumping into each other continuously but have a level and range insufficient for the normal human ear to detect. However, when an external vibratory source is applied to them, the magnitude of the particle displacement increases and is identified as sound by the listener. A chain of events occurs, represented by air particles being closer together at times (compression) and rebounding to be further apart at other times (rarefaction). The sound wave becomes a movement (propagation) of a vibratory disturbance through the air medium, without permanent displacement of the molecules themselves. Figure 2-1 illustrates this effect of sound propagation for a tuning fork, but can be generalized to other sound sources as well.

Physical Properties of Sound

Three parameters used to describe this propagation of vibrations of air molecules are frequency, intensity of sound, and the spectrum. A number of other significant characteristics of sound are identified later in this chapter.

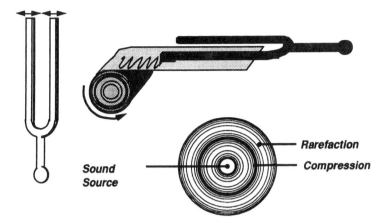

FIG. 2-1. Simple harmonic motion illustrated with a tuning fork as the sound source (vibrator). Compressions and rarefactions of air molecules are shown below, indicating that it is the wave propagation and not the air molecules themselves moving from the vibrating source to the listener.

Frequency is the rate at which air particles vibrate, or undergo a complete compression and rarefaction. One successive compression and rarefaction is called one cycle (Fig. 2-2). The number of cycles that occurs in 1 second is the frequency and is expressed in Hertz (Hz). For example, 10 successive compressions and rarefactions within 1 second is 10 cycles per second, or 10 Hz. Five hundred successive compressions and rarefactions within 1 second is 500 Hz. The description of this type of simple wave motion is simple harmonic motion (SHM), also called a sine wave. Pure tones are examples of SHM.

Intensity and amplitude are terms used to describe the energy delivered at a given point during a sound. Specifically, this can be expressed in terms of power, pressure, or energy. It is important to understand that there is a tremendous energy

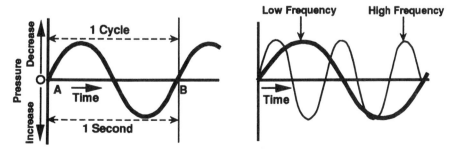

FIG. 2-2. The frequency relates to the number of complete compressions and rarefactions that occur during a 1-second time period (left graph). The right graph illustrates a sine wave (simple harmonic motion) of two different frequencies.

difference between sounds at threshold versus those at upper levels of discomfort. If measured as sound pressure, the difference between the threshold of pain to the softest sound heard is 10 million to one; however, if expressed in the intensity (power) of sound, the difference is a ratio of 100 trillion to one (Fig. 2-3). The decibel (dB) is used as the unit of measure to express the energy of a sound. It is a number that expresses the ratio between two sound intensities or pressures, whether they be to one another or of a sound relative to a reference sound. When the energy of a sound wave is measured in all directions from the source, it is identified as power. We are not interested generally in the total power emanating from a sound source but that measured through a defined area at right angles to the direction of the propagation of the wave. This is referred to as the intensity of the sound wave and is measured in decibels relative to 10^{-16} Watts/cm^2. (In electronics, voltage is measured, and it calculates the same as power). On the other hand, the pres-

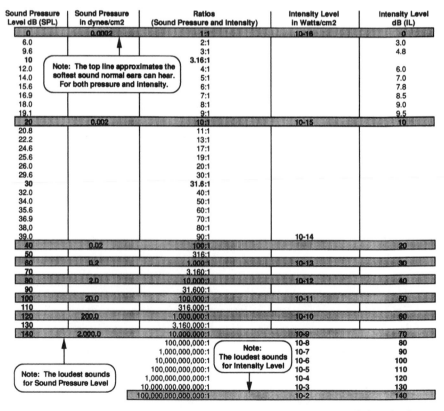

FIG. 2-3. The relationships of sound pressure and intensity ratios to the decibels and reference equivalents. The logarithmic nature of hearing is easily visualized. It takes substantially more increases in sound pressure and intensity as sounds become louder for a person to notice a difference.

sure of a sound wave identifies the force exerted over an identified area of surface, much as what happens when a microphone responds to sound pressure waves. Measurements made this way are referred to as pressure measurements and are expressed in decibels relative to 0.0002 dynes/cm² (today, decibels re 20 μPa). All decibel references to sound pressure level (SPL) use 0.0002 dynes/cm² (or its equivalent) as the reference sound pressure. In both cases the reference levels of 10^{-16} Watts/cm² and 0.0002 dynes/cm² have been chosen arbitrarily and tend to be near (but are not) the softest sounds the human ear can detect.

The spectrum of a sound is a diagram that shows the relative amplitudes of the frequency components of a sound. Whereas pure tones can be described adequately by frequency and intensity, most sounds (including speech) are complex and do not lend themselves to this simple description. Complex sounds consist of a number of frequencies existing at the same time and with varying intensities. It is differences in their spectra that allow for distinguishing between individuals saying the same word or musical instruments playing the same note.

The continuum of sounds ranges from pure tones to complex tones. A tuning fork produces a pure tone; it consists of only one frequency. Complex tones, on

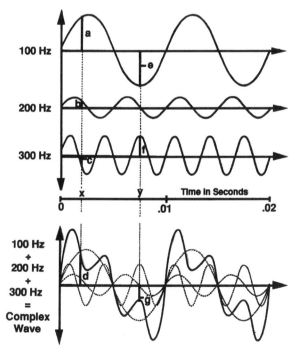

FIG. 2-4. An example of how a complex wave (bottom curve, solid line) can be analyzed into its individual frequencies. The mathematical process is called Fourier analysis.

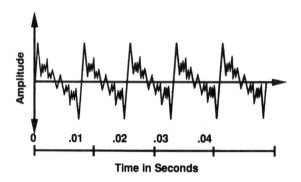

Time in Seconds

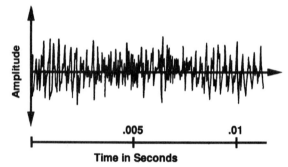

Time in Seconds

FIG. 2-5. Complex sounds can range from musical tones (*top*) that have a periodic wave (the waveform repeats itself and the signal can be analyzed by Fourier analysis) to noise (*bottom*). Noise is aperiodic, which means that it has no distinguishable repetitive waveform and cannot be analyzed into individual frequencies.

the other hand, can be analyzed into a number of sinusoidal waves having different frequencies, amplitudes, and phases by a mathematical procedure called Fourier analysis. An example of this is illustrated in Fig. 2-4. The lowest frequency of a complex tone is called the fundamental frequency. For speech, the fundamental frequency for men is about 120 to 150 Hz and for women about 210 to 240 Hz. Speech and other musical sounds have another commonality: even though the waveform is complicated, it clearly shows repetitions of the same shape; it has periodicity, meaning that the wave shape can be repeated (called a periodic wave). Noise, on the other hand, consists of irregular frequencies and intensities, has no clear fundamental frequency, and has an aperiodic wave shape (Fig 2-5).

HEARING ACUITY

Sound waves that reach the ear are simply mechanical vibrations of air particles. Still, to be perceptible, they must be within a certain range of frequencies and intensities.

Thresholds of Audibility

Absolute Hearing Threshold

This is the intensity at which a sound is just distinguishable from silence, where the presence of sound is detected 50% of the time. The lower curves of Fig. 2-6 illustrate the absolute auditory threshold to pure tones under earphones (MAP, minimum audible pressure) and in the sound field through loudspeakers (MAF, minimum audible field) by a variety of investigators (curves 1, 2, 3, 4, and 6). Frequency is shown on the horizontal axis, whereas the vertical axis refers to sound pressure level (dB re 0.0002 dynes/cm^2 = dB re 20 μbar). The differences in the absolute hearing thresholds represent a variety of patient selections and threshold measurement methods.

Tolerance Thresholds

The upper curves of Fig. 2-6 (curves 7–12) identify the intensity levels at which listeners begin to hear sound uncomfortably as well as feel it. Between about 120

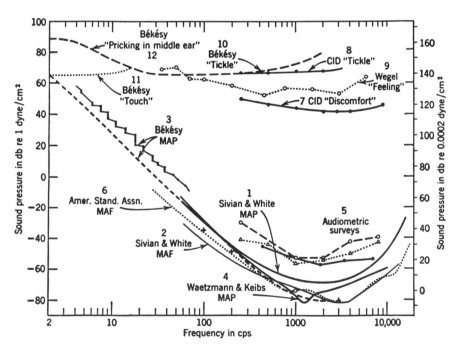

FIG. 2-6. Attempts at determining the thresholds of audibility and the thresholds of feeling. Shown are auditory absolute thresholds (curves 1–6), and the upper tolerance boundaries of the auditory comfort range (curves 7–12). (Reprinted from Licklider JCR. Basic correlates of the auditory stimulus. In: Stevens SS, ed. *Handbook of experimental psychology*. New York: John Wiley & Sons; 1951:985–1039; with permission.)

and 140 dB SPL, individuals experience definite sensations of "tickle" or pain. These are considered tactile sensations and may involve nerve endings from the pinna, ear canal, tympanic membrane, and possibly other middle ear structures. Discomfort sensations to loud sound are described as the threshold of discomfort (TD), loudness discomfort level (LDL), and uncomfortable loudness level (UCL) and have an intensity generally about 20 to 30 dB less than the threshold of feeling.

Average Audiometric Thresholds

The curves associated with the studies identified as number 5 on the graph are based on early studies attempting to define the sensitivity of hearing for a group of "normal" hearing listeners from the general population (5), rather than for "laboratory" ears. However, since about 1964 (6), the levels for general population normal sensitivity have been established approximately midway between the MAF and MAP curves and these curves. The implication of this is that 0 dB on the audiometer (expressed as 0 Hearing Threshold Level, or Hearing Level), is represented by varying amounts of sound pressure and that these sound pressures vary with frequency. For example, based on 1969 American National Standards Institute (ANSI) standards for audiometric zero, the following sound pressures exist for 0 dB HTL at the frequencies specified: 250 Hz = 25.5 dB; 500 Hz = 11.5 dB; 1,000 Hz = 7.0 dB; 2,000 Hz = 9.0 dB; 4,000 Hz = 9.5 dB; and 8,000 Hz = 13.0 dB. How these values relate to 0 dB on the audiometer is depicted in Fig. 2-7.

Auditory Dynamic Range (DR)

DR is often described as the area between the absolute threshold and the curve of feeling. However, for hearing aid purposes, the upper tolerance curve that is significant is the threshold of discomfort (TD; LDL or UCL). These thresholds are estimated to be at about 110 dB for normal listeners (Fig. 2-8), with some variation for frequency and degree of hearing impairment (7). It is important to note that the DR is less at the very low frequencies and at the very high frequencies than in the mid-frequency range.

Audible Area of Humans

Figure 2-9 has been developed in part from data in Figs. 2-6 and 2-8 but generalized to show certain critical elements of what is referred to as the audible area of humans. This shows the significant auditory levels and ranges of usable hearing for normal hearing patients. The useful frequency range of hearing is between approximately 20 and 20,000 Hz. Note that the useful DR of hearing (TD minus best hearing threshold) varies as a function of frequency. The frequency range extremes (both low and high) have a much smaller dynamic range than the middle frequencies.

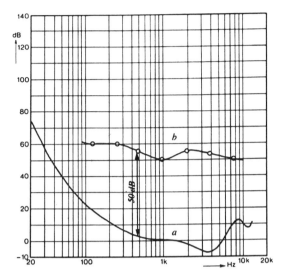

Normal threshold of hearing (a) and an abnormal (poor) hearing threshold (b).

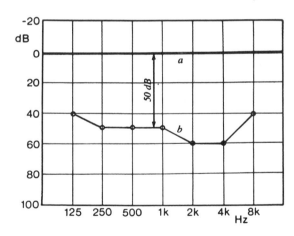

FIG. 2-7. General relationship illustrating the transition of data in SPL (top graph) to HTL (bottom graph) between "normal" thresholds and a moderately severe hearing impairment. (Reprinted from Philips Hearing Instruments, Inc. *Basics of audiology.* Eindhoven, The Netherlands, 1982; with permission.)

For reference purposes, the following examples, all referenced to 20 µbar (SPL), help to understand the levels of sounds:

Sound barely perceptible	0 dB (near 0.0002 dynes/cm², or 20 µbar)
Whisper threshold	20 dB at 5 feet from the speaker
Night noises in a city	40 dB
Normal conversational speech	55–75 dB (65 dB at 1 m)
Pneumatic drill	90 dB at 10 feet
Discomfort	110 dB

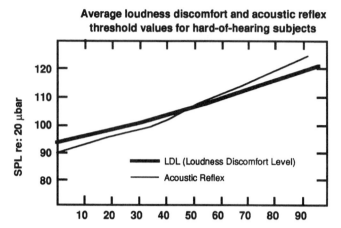

FIG. 2-8. Relationship between LDL and the degree of hearing loss. (Redrawn from McCandless G. Hearing aids and loudness discomfort. Proceedings III: International Otocongress, Copenhagen, 1973:39–44; with permission.)

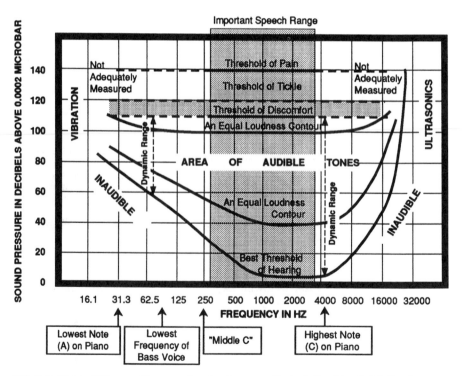

FIG. 2-9. The audible area of humans, showing the generalized relationships that define the range of usable hearing.

The eardrum is exposed to an enormous range of sound pressure variations in sound waves. It has the ability to respond to remarkably small pressure variations (around 0.0002 dynes/cm^2) at 0 dB, which is somewhere around the threshold of hearing, to very loud sounds having pressures of about 2,000 dynes/cm^2 (140 dB SPL).

PHYSIOLOGICAL AND PSYCHOLOGICAL ACOUSTICS

Physical Versus Subjective Properties of Sound

Even though this chapter is devoted to the psychoacoustical aspects of sound, it has been necessary to define three physical properties of sound: the frequency, intensity (or power), and spectrum of sound. These properties can be measured easily and consistently, without the necessity of having a human listener, by physical means using electronic equipment. Regardless, it is also important to understand the subjective correlates of these values: pitch, loudness, and quality. These values are measured only with human listeners.

Frequency and Pitch

Frequency, described as the rate at which air particles vibrate, is measured in cycles per second and recorded in Hertz. Pitch is the subjective correlate of frequency. For most practical purposes, pitch depends on the frequency of the sound source. Generally, as frequency changes—either upward or downward—the subjective sensation of pitch changes in a corresponding manner.

However, factors other than frequency affect judgments of pitch. Intensity, for example, can influence pitch substantially and has more noticeable effects at either very low or very high frequencies. Low-frequency pure tones seem lower as the sound source is brought closer (made louder) to the ear. The pitch of complex waveforms are altered only slightly as intensity changes, which is fortunate for musicians and other individuals who depend on fine pitch differences for their livelihood.

Subjective Pitch Scale: the Mel

Figure 2-10 illustrates the mel scale of pitch, showing how the subjective pitch (recorded in mels) is related to frequency (Hz) for pure tones. The method used to measure pitch consists of presenting to a listener two alternating tones at a fixed loudness level (i.e., 40 phons). With one tone fixed in frequency, the listener is asked to adjust the other tone until its pitch is perceived to be half that of the fixed tone. On a mel scale (mel is the unit of pitch) 1,000 mels is the pitch of a 1,000-Hz

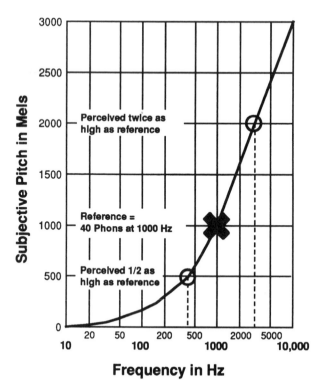

FIG. 2-10. The mel scale of pitch, which shows how subjective pitch (in mels) is related in frequency (Hz) to pure tones.

tone, 500 mels is the pitch that sounds half as high, and 2,000 mels would represent the pitch that sounds twice as high as the 1,000-Hz tone. To assist in understanding the significance of this difference between the physical and subjective scales, using 1,000 mels as a reference, a tone judged to be half as high in pitch is 400 Hz (not 500 Hz). A tone judged to be twice as high in pitch is approximately 4,000 Hz (not 2,000 Hz).

Pitch of Complex Tones

Complex tones (i.e., speech, music, and other sounds) also produce a recognizable pitch. For most, it depends on the frequency of the lowest component, or fundamental frequency of the complex tone. There are some notable exceptions, however. For example, when the complex tone consists of a series of frequencies that are separated by a constant difference (i.e., 200, 400, 600, and 800 Hz), the pitch is judged to be a 200-Hz tone.

Frequency Discrimination

The minimum frequency change a listener can detect for tones is called the difference limen (DL) or just noticeable difference (JND) for frequency. This varies as a function of intensity and frequency (Fig. 2-11). Generally, below 1,000 Hz, and at a moderate intensity level, a 2- to 3-Hz frequency change is detectable by normal listeners. For higher frequencies, the DL tends to be a constant fraction of the frequency, about 1/20 of a semitone (notes on consecutive keys on a piano differ by one semitone) (8).

Pitch Perception and Frequency Resolution

It has long been known that different frequencies are distributed by the cochlea to selected places along the basilar membrane (traveling wave explanation for the mechanical action within the cochlea [9]). This frequency analysis activity forms the basis for the generalized place theory of pitch perception (10). Tuning curves, which show that neurons respond more easily at a particular frequency or narrow band of frequencies, support this concept. However, at higher intensity levels, they are no longer as frequency specific and involve a broader range of nerve activity. Regardless, the information learned from mapping experiments of the higher auditory pathways suggests a tonotopic distribution throughout the entire system; nerve fibers that transmit high frequencies are located in certain locations within each higher auditory center, and those that transmit low frequencies in other locations (11).

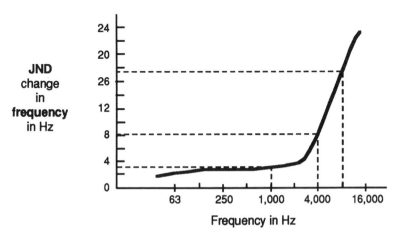

FIG. 2-11. Just noticeable differences for frequency, showing how much the frequency of a tone must change in order to produce a change in pitch.

Because the place theory does not account for all pitch perception phenomena, modifications and alternatives have been suggested. One is the temporal (frequency; rate of neural discharge) theory (12). This theory accepts that the apex and basal ends of the cochlea are maximally stimulated by low and high frequencies, respectively. It also suggests that below 1,000 Hz, nerve fibers at the maximal point of stimulation fire at a rate equal to the frequency (i.e., a 500-Hz tone would cause the nerve fibers to fire at 500 times per second). To compensate for the fact that individual nerve fibers cannot discharge faster than 1,000 times per second, frequencies above 1,000 Hz are considered to discharge (fire) in volleys. The combination of the place (high frequencies) and temporal (low frequencies) theories has come to be identified as the place-volley theory of pitch perception and frequency analysis (13).

Intensity and Loudness Level

Intensity, as described earlier, is the pressure or power of a sound and is measured commonly with different expressions of reference points in dynes/cm^2, Watts/cm^2, or some variation of these. It is expressed in decibels. Loudness is the subjective correlate of intensity. Again, as with frequency and pitch, for most practical purposes, loudness depends on the intensity of the sound source. Generally, as intensity changes—either upward or downward—the subjective sensation of loudness changes in a corresponding manner.

Figure 2-12 illustrates loudness level contours, showing how the loudness level (with the phon as a scale to indicate the increasing magnitude of loudness sensations) is related to intensity (in SPL) for pure tones. The following explanation describes the method by which loudness is related to intensity. Loudness levels are identified by first presenting a tone of, for example, 1,000 Hz to a listener at 40 dB SPL (a reference tone). Tones of different frequencies are then presented, and the listener is asked to match them in loudness to the reference tone. However, just because they are the same in loudness does not mean they are the same intensities. From Fig. 2-12, the numbers associated with each contour are the number of phons (loudness units) representing that contour. At 1,000 Hz, the phon units and the SPL for that sound are identical. For each contour, all points along the contour are represented by the same phon number. And although the SPL associated with the 1,000-Hz tone for the 40-phon contour is 40 dB SPL, it varies with other frequencies (at 30 Hz a loudness level of 40 phons requires about 77 dB SPL; at 100 Hz 63 dB SPL; at 4,000 Hz 37 dB SPL, etc.). Collectively, these loudness contours are called equal loudness contours, meaning that all frequencies along that contour are experienced as being equal in loudness, even though the sound pressure levels associated with them differ. Note also that the 0 phon contour is close to the threshold curve, a curve of equal loudness (just barely heard). Likewise, the 110-phon contour is close to the TD. Collectively, these curves of equal loudness have come to be known also as the Fletcher-Munson curves (14).

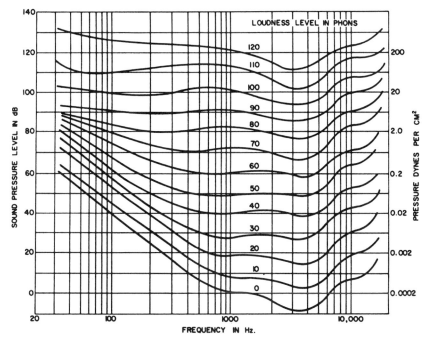

FIG. 2-12. Curves of equal loudness (in phons) and how they relate to sound pressure in decibels and to sound pressure in dynes/cm². Although a number of fairly similar graphs of equal loudness exist, this graph is based on those of Fletcher and Munson and therefore are called Fletcher-Munson curves for equal loudness.

Subjective Loudness Level Scale: the Sone

The subjective scale that expresses loudness levels uses the sone as its unit of loudness. A loudness of 2 sones is judged to be twice as loud as 1 sone; half a sone is half as loud as 1 sone, etc. As a reference, a 40-dB SPL tone at 1,000 Hz has been arbitrarily assigned the value of 1 sone. How does perceived loudness (sones) compare with loudness level (phons) of a tone? The results are shown in Fig. 2-13. To derive a numerical scale of perceived (subjective) loudness, a common method used is to present two tones alternately to a listener and ask that one be adjusted until it is twice as loud (or half as loud) as the other. It is possible to proceed one step further from this graph. By viewing perceived loudness levels on this curve (in sones), it is possible to identify the associated phons, and then, by referring to Fig. 2-12, determine the intensity level in decibels SPL. As an example, the increase in the loudness of a sound from 0.1 sone (about 20 phons) to 10 sones (about 66 phons) is a 100-fold increase in loudness. From Fig. 2-10, this means that a 1,000-Hz tone must be increased by 46 dB, from 20 to 66 dB phon contour (8). This 46-dB sound pressure increase represents a factor of 40,000 as opposed to

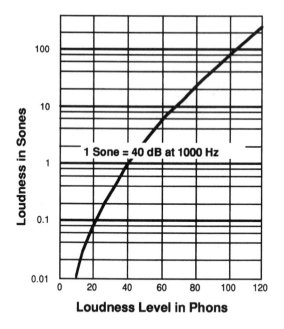

FIG. 2-13. The perceived sensation of loudness (with the sone as its unit of loudness), depends on the loudness level of the stimulus (in phons).

the 100-fold increase in loudness. Therefore, it is obvious that loudness judgments do not change as greatly as do intensity changes.

Intensity Discrimination

The JND or DL for intensity is not a constant and varies with the frequency and intensity of the measured tone. Basically, tones near threshold must be increased substantially in intensity before a loudness change is noticed (i.e., 2–3 dB), whereas tones presented at suprathreshold levels require minimal increases in intensity before a loudness change is noticed (i.e., 0.5–1 dB).

Denes and Pinson (8) reported on the number of pure tones a normal listener can distinguish, based on measured difference limens. With loudness level maintained at 40 phons, there are approximately 1,400 distinguishable pitches. With frequency maintained constant at 1,000 Hz, about 280 perceptually different loudness levels are perceived. The number of difference limens for complex stimuli is substantially greater, but exactly how many is not known.

Loudness Perception

Loudness perception is dependent on the number of nerve fibers activated by the stimulus. The greater the number of nerve fibers activated, the louder the sound.

Spectrum and Quality

The spectrum of a sound refers to the wave shape of complex sounds. Quality is the subjective correlate to spectrum.

Other Characteristics of Sound

A number of other concepts that relate to sound are worthy of discussion because they have significance to hearing aids and hearing aid fittings.

Masking

The fact that it is more difficult to hear sounds in noisy environments should be no surprise. Masking occurs when noise or sound interferes with the audibility of another. Keep in mind that masking effects can be complete, but more likely reduce the ability to hear the primary sound to varying degrees, depending on the efficiency of the masker.

Types of masking include simultaneous and nonsimultaneous masking. Simultaneous masking occurs when two sounds, having different frequency, intensity, and phase, are presented at the same time. Two results of this type of masking are especially of interest here. First, for moderate masker intensities, sounds tend to mask most effectively other similar sounds rather than sounds far removed in frequency. This concept is used often in hearing testing masking. Second, with pure tones and with different types of noises (narrow band, broad band, etc.), it has been shown that low-frequency sources more easily mask higher frequency sounds than vice versa (Fig. 2-14).

That masking tendency is thought to be related to basilar membrane function has been summarized nicely by Preves and Curran (11):

> This masking tendency is thought to be somewhat indirectly related to the behavior of the basilar membrane when it is stimulated at the same time by two tones of different frequencies. Since the traveling wave for low frequency tones is distributed along the entire basilar membrane, it will cause some depression of the membrane in the basal turn of the cochlea where high frequency tones are primarily located. As a result, the wave traveling through the basal area may "use up" some of the capacity of the basilar membrane to initiate a neural response for a high frequency tone.

Upward spread of masking is the term applied to the tendency for low-frequency sounds to mask high frequencies presented simultaneously. And although the physiological mechanism is not entirely clear, the psychological perceptual experience is well documented. It is because of the possible effects of upward spread of masking on critical high-frequency speech sounds that many hearing aid fittings attempt

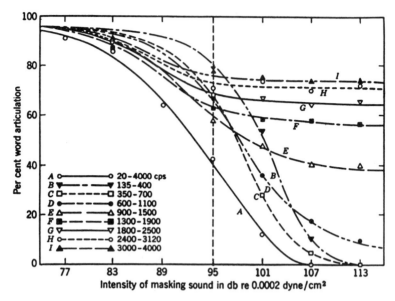

FIG. 2-14. Speech masked by narrow bands of noise at different masking noise intensities. Speech was not filtered and was constant at 95 dB SPL. This shows that wide-band masking (curve A) provides the most effective masking of speech. At low noise levels, the high-frequency bands were more effective. At high noise levels, low-frequency bands were more effective. However, when low-frequency noise is sufficiently intense, it can mask the entire speech range. (Reprinted from Licklider JCR, Miller GA. The perception of speech. In: Stevens SS, ed. *Handbook of experimental psychology*. New York: John Wiley & Sons; 1951:1040–1074; with permission.)

to reduce amplification, especially below about 1,000 Hz, where a disproportionate amount of random background noise exists.

Nonsimultaneous (temporal) masking occurs when sounds follow or precede each other closely in time. When a preceding loud sound masks a following sound that is softer, this is called forward masking. In the word "at," for example, the low-frequency energy of the vowel may have reduced the sensitivity of the broad range of stimulated cells or generated a prolongation of their activity and, especially if overamplified, may cause the softer consonant to be masked. If a loud sound follows a soft sound very closely in time and masks the soft sound, this is referred to as backward masking. Temporal masking can have important implications for hearing aid use in that the sounds of words have almost a 30-dB range, with vowel sounds being louder than consonants. If amplified vowel sounds both precede and follow soft consonants, the possibilities of temporal masking exist, making recognition of the word difficult because of the consonant loss. As with simultaneous masking, temporal masking effects are greatest for low-frequency sounds than for high-frequency sounds.

Phase

Phase is the time relationship between two or more pure tones occurring simultaneously. Figure 2-15 illustrates the combined effect of two sine wave (pure tone) components. Numbers 1 and 2 are of the same frequency but of different phase relationships. The bottom line (R) equals the resultant signal from adding lines 1 and 2. It is seen easily that depending on the phase relationships between 1 and 2 that the resultant signal can be experienced as an increase in amplitude over either sound (Ra), a complete cancellation of sound (Rb), or partial cancellation or reduction in amplitude over either sound (Rc).

Another result of phase differences between sounds, primarily tones, is that of standing waves. Standing waves occur when two wave trains (compression and rarefaction), moving in opposite directions, interfere. Although standing waves can create increases in amplitude, it is also important to understand that amplitude can be reduced as well. This has some significance to sound generated into the auditory canal. To explain, when a pure tone is introduced into a closed pipe having the same length as the wave length of the tone, the wave is reflected back from the closed end 180° out of phase with the original wave. If exactly 180° out of phase, the result is a cancellation of the sound (Fig. 2-15b). With an ear canal of almost 1.5 inches, the wavelength of an 8,000-Hz tone is almost the same. Thus, a possibility exists that an 8,000-Hz tone could be reduced somewhat in amplitude during audiometric testing, depending on the test conditions.

Beats are heard when two tones are presented at the same time but differ from each other by only a few cycles. The listener hears as many beats as there are cycles of difference between the tones. For example, if a 500-Hz and 505-Hz tone were presented simultaneously, the listener would hear five beats. This holds true up to about 16 beats per second. If the two tones are farther apart than this in frequency, a new tone—the

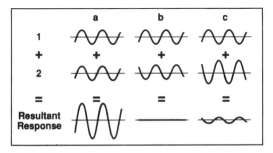

FIG. 2-15. Combined effects of two sine-wave components (1+ 2) having the same frequency, but of different phase and amplitude relationships. **a:** Both in phase with a resultant increase in amplitude. **b:** With opposite phase and equal amplitudes, cancellation results. **c:** With opposite phase but unequal amplitudes, partial amplitude cancellation results.

"difference tone"—will be heard, which represents the difference in frequency between the two original tones. For example, if a 1,500-Hz and 2,000 Hz tone are presented simultaneously, a difference tone of 500 Hz would be heard by the listener.

Resonance

Resonance is the phenomenon in which one body, that has a natural tendency to vibrate at a certain frequency, builds up vibrations with comparatively large amplitudes when it is set in motion by another body that is vibrating at a similar frequency. The closer the frequency of the driving system is to the natural frequency of the resonator, the greater the amplitude. Enclosed volumes of air (such as the ear canal) can resonate as well; acoustical rather than mechanical resonance. Wiener showed the average natural resonance of the ear (including pinna, concha, pinna flange, and canal) to be about 17 dB at 2,700 Hz (Fig. 2-16).

Reflection and Absorption

When sound waves impinge on a surface, they are reflected or absorbed. The amount of reflection depends on the surface composition. That which is not re-

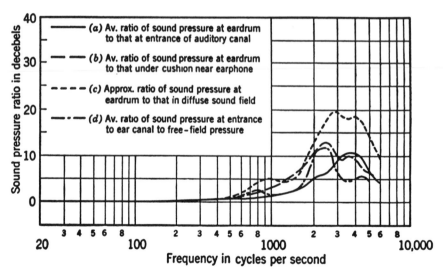

FIG. 2-16. Curves displaying the ratios of sound pressures measured in and around the ear. Curve b is calculated, but recent real ear microphone probe measurements are close. (Reprinted from Wiener FM. On the diffraction of a progressive sound wave by the human head. *J Acoust Soc Am* 1947;19:143–146; with permission.)

flected is absorbed. When reflection is continual or prolonged, it results in rever-beration and echoes (persistence of sound even when the sound source has stopped vibrating). Hard walls and surfaces are highly reflective and result in unintelligible or blurred speech and/or music. Therefore, environments that are highly reflective are not good for hearing aid wearers. Absorptive surfaces (carpets, draperies, acoustical tile, etc.), on the other hand, reduce reflections and echoes and are better for hearing aid wearers.

BINAURAL HEARING EFFECTS

Binaural indicates the use of both ears. Diotic listening involves the use of both ears but presents identical sound waves to each ear. Dichotic listening describes the condition in which different sound waves are presented to each ear and is com-patible with the use of both ears for normal hearing. Normally, sound waves that reach the ears differ primarily in two respects, creating dichotic hearing: (a) there is an intensity difference between the ears, and (b) there is a difference in the time of arrival of corresponding parts of the sound waves.

Sound Localization

This may be the most important binaural effect, and, when functioning, can identify the source of low-frequency tones to within about 10° (8), eliminating far field sounds that are not easily quantified (16). Localization can be performed with reasonable accuracy only by using two ears. Sound localization results from the in-teraural difference in time of arrival of sound waves and from their differences in intensities. Generally, the magnitude of the interaural time difference decreases as the sound source moves from 0° to 90° to 270°. However, a difference in arrival time at the ears can be compensated for by appropriate differences in intensities (when made louder, the sound "moves" toward that ear). Additionally, below ap-proximately 1,500 Hz the interaural time difference could be explained meaning-fully as an interaural phase difference (3). Humes (3) continues by explaining that this could happen because, with sound coming from specified azimuths, interaural time differences cause the signal in the far ear to begin after the signal to the near ear. Thus, even though interaural time differences are the same for all frequencies, the interaural phase differences resulting from these time differences vary with fre-quency. This has led to the duplex theory of sound localization (17), which states that although both cues are used over a wide range of frequencies, interaural time differences predominate at low frequencies and interaural intensity differences predominate at high frequencies.

Head Shadow (Sound Shadows: Far Ear Effect)

When only one ear is being used, whether due to a hearing loss or as a result of monaural amplification, one ear is always on the wrong side of the head. Olsen and Carhart (18) reported that when listening under a monaural-indirect listening condition, the level of a speech stimulus at the far ear was reduced by roughly 6 dB (but as high as 15 dB) because speech loses energy as it crosses from one side of the head to the other. These interaural intensity differences result from a sound shadow being cast by the head (Fig. 2-17). High frequencies tend to travel in a straight line from the source. The result of this is that when an object is encountered in its path, an acoustic shadow is cast, and the area behind the object experiences no sound (19). Therefore, localization is more likely to occur for low-frequency than for high-frequency sounds, because the former are more likely to be heard. Shaw (20) showed that the magnitude of the head shadow created by the head increases with frequency above 500 Hz. For example, for sounds originating from 90° and 270°, the intensity for a 6,000-Hz tone is about 20 dB greater at the near ear versus that measured at the far ear. For a 500-Hz tone, the maximum interaural intensity difference under these same conditions is less than 4 dB. The result is a reported reduction of about 23% in word recognition (21) or the equivalent of about a 6-dB improvement in signal-to-noise (S/N) ratio (19).

Binaural Summation

When a signal arrives at each ear at the same time, the fact that both ears are involved increases the apparent loudness. At threshold this results in an improvement of about 2 to 3 dB, but at suprathreshold levels, it translates to an im-

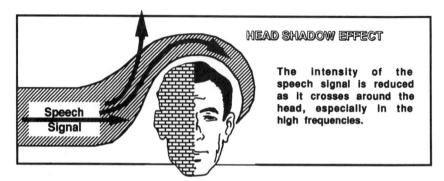

FIG. 2-17. Illustration of a sound shadow being cast by the head when an individual has no hearing on the sound source side and normal hearing on the other. A reduction of all sound intensity occurs as the signal passes around the head, especially in the high frequencies.

provement of about 6 to 10 dB. Additionally, frequency and intensity DLs obtained binaurally are about two thirds the magnitude of those obtained monaurally (22).

Binaural Loudness Squelch Effect

Documented by Carhart (23) with respect to hearing aids, this refers to a release from masking effects or improvement in S/N ratio when two ears are involved rather than one. The S/N improvement is about 3 dB, which in itself may not seem like much. However, under certain circumstances, improvement in word recognition due to the binaural effect can be as high as 20%. This binaural loudness squelch effect is not present if the ears do not have relatively equal sensitivity.

Masking Level Differences

The ability to separate primary sounds from background or unwanted sounds is also attributed to binaural hearing. The masking level difference (MLD) (24) is the dB difference necessary to maintain the listener's performance constant when changes in the interaural listening conditions are introduced (25). The MLD represents the condition under which the removal, reduction, or addition of a masking signal makes the primary signal easier to detect. Mostly, this involves restoring the listening condition to dichotic, making understanding easier. MLDs are greatest at low frequencies from 100 to 500 Hz and increase with the intensity of masking up to an effective masking level of about 40 to 50 dB. It is generally less than 15 dB when the dichotic listening condition is optimal (3).

Binaural Fusion

This concept involves combining similar, but not exactly identical, signals delivered to the two ears into a single sound image. In reality, it might be better defined as binaural resynthesis, rather than fusion (26).

ACOUSTIC CHARACTERISTICS OF SPEECH

Various acoustic characteristics of speech are important to understand because of their implications for hearing aid understanding and use.

Speech Intensity Levels

The acoustic energy of normal speech is low, and when we do speak, that which is available is spread in all directions (Fig. 2-18). Additionally, the range of the

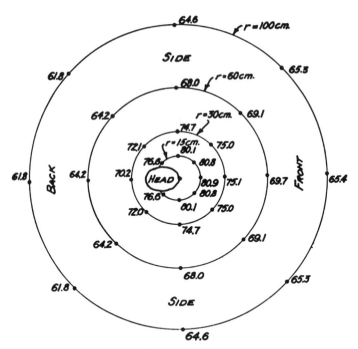

FIG. 2-18. Relative speech intensity levels on the horizontal plane at various azimuths and distances (in centimeters) from the speaker's lips. The shadowing effect of the head on the spoken word is clearly shown. (Reprinted from Fletcher H. *Speech and hearing in communication*. Princeton, NJ: Van Nostrand; 1953; with permission.)

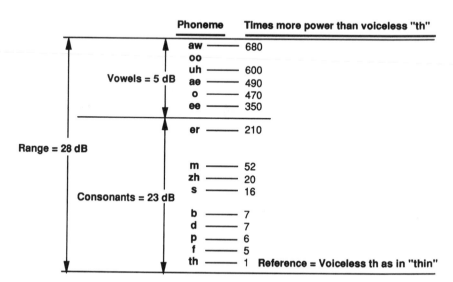

FIG. 2-19. Conversational values of speech power, showing the range of the loudest vowel to the softest consonant, a power difference of 680:1, or 28 dB. (Reprinted from Fletcher H. *Speech and hearing in communication*. Princeton, NJ: Van Nostrand; 1953; with permission.)

strongest vowel sound (the "aw" as in "all," to the weakest consonant (the voiceless "th" as in "thin," is a ratio of 680 to 1. This converts to a 28-dB difference in the range between these speech phoneme extremes for normal conversation (Fig. 2-19). Essentially, this means that for normal conversational speech, a range of almost 30 dB should be expected as a usual condition. Speech intensity levels change also for loud, normal, soft, and whispered speech. These levels are 85 dB, 65 dB, 45 dB, and 25–35 dB, respectively.

Speech Spectrum

As related earlier, the spectrum of a signal identifies its frequencies and intensities. For speech, at least two types of spectra are of interest: the long-term spectrum of speech and spectra of individual phonemes.

Long-Term Average Spectrum of Speech

When speech is analyzed over a long sequence of connected speech, such that all phonemes occur many times, the energy level in each part of the spectrum can be summed to provide an overall spectrum (Fig. 2-20). This long-term average

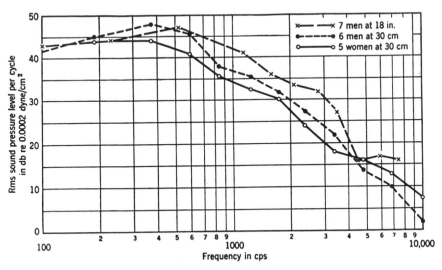

FIG. 2-20. Long-term average spectrum of speech measured 30 cm in front of the talkers. The overall levels, not indicated on the graph, were 18 inches in front of the seven male talkers, 74 dB SPL; 30 cm in front of the six male talkers, 76 dB SPL; and 30 cm in front of the five female talkers, 73 dB SPL. After Dunn and White, 1940, and Rudmose et al., 1944. (Reprinted from Licklider JCR, Miller GA. The perception of speech. In: Stevens SS, ed. *Handbook of experimental psychology.* New York: John Wiley & Sons; 1951:1040–1074; with permission.)

speech spectrum shows that energy is greatest in the low-frequency region with a peak at about 400 to 500 Hz (27). As can be seen, there is little difference between male and female voices. This range includes both the fundamental frequency and the first formant (overtone energy region). At about 4,000 Hz the average energy is lower by about 30 dB, being consistent with the difference between vowel and consonant ratios.

Speech Spectra

The spectra of different speech sounds, primarily vowels, has been widely investigated. Because the vocal tract functions like an air-filled tube, it acts as a resonator. These resonance areas are identified in speech spectra and are called formants, with each configuration of the vocal tract having its own set of characteristic formant frequencies . The lowest formant frequency is called the first formant, the next highest formant frequency the second formant, etc. Formant frequencies are not the same as harmonics (equal multiples of a fundamental frequency). Formant frequencies are determined by the vocal tract, whereas harmonics are determined by the vocal cords, with the understanding that these can move independently of each other. Figure 2-21 illustrates this independent relationship. It shows the wave shapes and corresponding spectra for the vowel "ah" produced with two different vocal cord frequencies (90 and 150 Hz), but showing that the formants and spectral peaks are unchanged because the shape of the vocal tract remained the same (11).

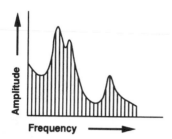

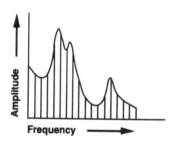

FIG. 2-21. Spectra of the sound "ah" produced from the same speaker with two different vocal fold frequencies: vocal fold frequency at 90 Hz (top), and at 150 Hz (bottom). Even though the frequencies are different, the spectra are the same because the vocal tract that generated them is the same. The vocal tract simply emphasizes the amplitudes of harmonics that are similar to its own natural resonant frequency.

TABLE 2-1. *Average formant frequency values of 10 english pure vowels as pronounced by a number of different speakers*

	ee	I	e	ae	ah	aw	U	oo	^	er
First formant frequency										
Male	270	390	530	660	730	570	440	300	640	490
Female	310	430	610	860	850	590	470	370	760	500
Second formant frequency										
Male	2,290	1,990	1,840	1,720	1,090	840	1,020	870	1,190	1,350
Female	2,790	2,480	2,330	2,050	1,220	920	1,160	950	1,400	1,640
Third formant frequency										
Male	3,010	2,550	2,480	2,410	2,440	2,410	2,240	2,240	2,390	1,690
Female	3,310	3,070	2,990	2,850	2,810	2,710	2,610	2,670	2,780	1,960

Another way to visualize the spectra of speech is by visualization of a sound spectrogram. Figure 2-22 is a sound spectrogram (visible speech) of vowels in isolation and then of a simple sentence. On a sound spectrogram, time is shown along the horizontal axis and frequency along the vertical axis. The darker the images, the greater the energy. Vowels have definite energy regions (formants) corresponding to the resonances of the vocal tract. The first three or four are sufficient for speech recognition, and Table 2-1 identifies the average formant frequency values for 10 English pure vowels. Consonants do not resonate with the vocal tract and therefore have no formant regions. Instead, they show energy, but to a lesser extent, over the entire frequency range. Vertical lines are produced only when the vocal cords vibrate. Blank segments indicate the absence of any sound during a stop-plosive consonant. Nasal consonants tend to show lower intensity segments, and fricative consonants produce fuzzy segments.

SPEECH RECOGNITION

The acoustic features of the speech wave form the bases for speech recognition, but it is also influenced strongly by listener expectations, the speaker, the topic, rules of grammar, etc. Although these are all important considerations, this discussion addresses only the acoustic features that influence speech recognition. These explanations lead us to ask what the important conditions for speech recognition are: what can be eliminated, what can be retained, and what influences speech recognition? Many words can be recognized without any acoustic cues at all. The language, redundancy, grammar, and meaning influence the linguistic information. In many cases the additional information restricts the choices to be made and makes ambiguous acoustic cues even less ambiguous.

Speech recognition tests form the basic building blocks for measurements that allow the previous questions to be investigated. Results of these tests are referred to historically as articulation tests (certainly a misnomer by today's interpretations, especially because they have nothing to do with speech articulation). The stimuli

Spectra of Pure Vowels Spoken in Isolation

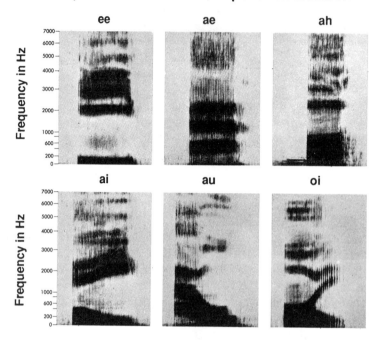

Spectrum of Speech Spoken at Normal Speech
"I can see you"

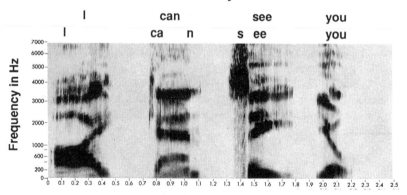

Time in Seconds

FIG. 2-22. Spectra of vowels spoken in isolation (*top six spectrograms*), and the spectrum of normal speech (*bottom spectrogram*). The upper row shows vowels whose quality remains unchanged. The center row shows the changing patterns of diphthongs, and the bottom spectrogram shows how different the patterns can be. (Altered from Denes PB, Pinson EN. *The Speech Chain*. Baltimore: Waverly Press, 1963.)

used for these tests most commonly consists of words, sentences, or nonsense syllables, depending on the task expected. Proper tests should be standardized as to equal stimulus difficulty and representation and quantity of stimuli used, as well as for the speaker. The task is to repeat or write the speech task heard and to record it as a percentage of the number of words correct. Word lists that consist of two-syllable words having equal stress on each syllable (such as "baseball," "cowboy," "inkwell," etc.), are called spondees and are used most often for speech threshold determination. Other lists of words consist of single-syllable words that are selected based on their relative frequency of occurrence in the English language. These are called phonetically balanced (PB) words. A variety of different spondee and PB word lists exist, as do nonsense and sentence lists, to meet varying needs of difficulty, reliability, diagnostic worthiness, age, time involved in use, etc. In terms of speech recognition hierarchy, word differentiation provides information only about how well words in speech can be distinguished. At the other extreme, when listening to speech, one learns about the speaker's identity, the tone of the speech (angry or happy), if asking a question or making a statement, etc.

Vowel Effects on Speech Recognition

It was shown previously in this chapter that vowels are recognized based on their formants. Experiments have shown that the first three formants are more than sufficient to identify vowels. With only the first two formants available, even marginal recognition of the vowel is possible. However, there is evidence that vowels can be identified even if the first two formants are not present. These results are based on synthesized speech from a pattern-playback device built by the Haskins Labs of New York. In other cases vowels that have identical formants can be identified as different sounds, depending on the duration of the formants. The implication of these confusing statements is that speech recognition is possible because of multiple cues and not isolated to a single acoustic component. (That multiple cues should be taken into consideration on all issues related to speech recognition should be evident.) When evaluated on normal and sensorineurally impaired listeners having sloping configurations, the second formant is most important for intelligibility, both for quiet and noise (28).

Consonant Effects on Speech Recognition

Because consonants do not have formants, how are they recognized, and what will be the effect of their modification and/or elimination? Denes and Pinson (8) characterized these consonants as follows. Fricatives are distinguishable by their "hissy" sound. The fricative consonants "s" and "sh" are distinguishable from other fricatives ("f") by their greater intensities, and from each other by spectral differences (the "s" when most of the energy is concentrated above 4,000 Hz, and "sh" when the energy is concentrated in the 2,000- to 3,000-Hz region). Weaker fricatives ("f" and voiceless "th") are influenced markedly by the adjacent vowels' second formant transition. Additionally, the duration of the fricative helps identify it.

Effect of Intensity

Figure 2-23 shows the percentage correct expected from normal listeners at different speech presentation levels (dB SPL) and for different speech stimuli. When comparing the "articulation functions" (curves) of different stimuli, it is noteworthy that the relationship between word and sentence scores depends on a number of circumstances. As a general rule, normal conversation can be achieved under circumstances in which a 50% word-recognition score is recorded. The steepness of the curve reflects the difficulty of the speech task performed; the steeper the curve, the easier the task (material).

Articulation Index (AI)

Because articulation function curves are tedious and expensive to generate, especially in noise, the development of a computational tool was developed to replace or supplement the laborious testing procedures. With articulation functions dependent on the test materials used, the method allowed sentence, word, syllable, and sound articulation scores to be related to a fundamental index that predicted

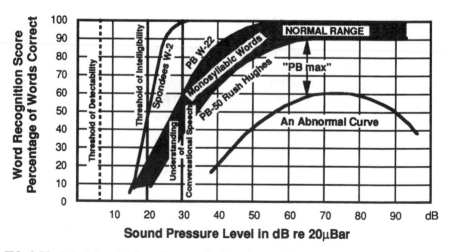

FIG. 2-23. Articulation functions (the growth of word recognition scores with increasing sound pressure levels) for words having different levels of difficulty. The steeper the slope, the easier the word recognition. Other thresholds are indicated as a point of reference.

performance without having to perform the testing (27). The AI as proposed by French and Steinberg (29) is based on the following assumptions: (a) the range of important speech frequencies is from 100 to 6,100 Hz; (b) this range can be divided into 20 frequency bands, each contributing equally to the intelligibility of speech, provided the S/N ratios are equal in each band; (c) a 30-dB change in S/N ratio spans the entire range of word intelligibility scores from 0 to almost 100% [0 assigned when all speech components are poorer than the listener's threshold, and 100 assigned to "normal" sound preference levels (orthotelophonic reference) across the frequency spectrum; and (d) each of the 20 frequency bands contributes 0.05 (5%) to the articulation index, with each decibel of the S/N ratio in the band contributing 1/30 of the 5% articulation index [as described by Newby (30)]. Therefore, to calculate an AI in a given situation, it is necessary to determine the S/N ratio (at the ear of the listener) in each of 20 frequency bands of specified width to arrive at the proportion of the 5% that that band contributes to the total AI. The sum of the contributions of each band then is the AI. The AI is based on having analyzed the intensity and frequency components of both speech and noise and working out their interactions mathematically. If the intensity of the speech in a given band is below the threshold of hearing, the band makes no contribution to intelligibility.

Because determining the S/N ratio for 20 frequency bands is not simple, a speech interference level (SIL) was devised to obtain a computational arithmetic average of the octave-band levels in the bands of 600 to 1,200, 1,200 to 2,400, and 2,400 to 4,800 Hz. Determination had been made that reliable speech communication exists when the overall root-mean-square level of undistorted speech is 12 dB above the SIL at the listener's ear. This is equivalent to an AI of 0.4. Table 2-2 represents the SILs that just permit reliable word recognition at different distances between the speaker and listener, at various speech levels, and assuming that no reflecting surfaces exist. For the speech of women and children, the SILs should be decreased by 5 dB. As if the procedure were not complicated enough, varia-

TABLE 2-2. *Speech interference levels (in dB SPL) that barely permit reliable word intelligibility at the distances and voice levels indicated*

Distance (ft)	Voice level (average male)			
	Normal	Raised	Very loud	Shouting
0.5	71	77	83	89
1	65	71	77	83
2	59	65	71	77
3	55	61	67	73
4	53	59	65	71
5	51	57	63	69
6	49	55	61	67
12	43	49	55	61

tions in the SILs are provided for preferred center frequencies of 500, 1,000, and 2,000 Hz (31) and for using A-weighted and variation sound-level meter readings (32).

Critical Bands

Critical bands are frequency bands making equal (5%) contribution to intelligibility when all bands are at their optimum levels. Table 2-3 shows the critical bands developed by French and Steinberg (31) for 20 bandwidths from 250 to 7,000 Hz, and for a flat signal. In these critical bands, bands below 2,000 Hz contribute a full 50% to intelligibility, and through 3,000 Hz a full 70%. It is suggested that if the bandwidths are not optimum, wider bands would be required for a given critical band. Additionally, cochlear hearing impairment can have dramatic effects on the critical band by making it wider (33).

Although the critical bands of French and Steinberg were obtained using nonsense syllables and form the basis of part of the ANSI S3.5-1969 standard for the calculation of the AI, Studebaker et al. (34) challenged the assumption that the frequency-importance function is the same for all speech material. They found that for a sample of continuous discourse (CD), ". . . lower frequencies were found to be relatively more important for the intelligibility of CD than for identification of nonsense syllables and other types of speech which are available, except for synthetic sentences." Their interpolation of 20 equal contributing 5% bands is presented in Table 2-4. When compared with French and Steinberg's critical bands, they show greater intelligibility contribution at lower cutoff frequencies (70% below 2,000 Hz and 80% below 3,000 Hz). When their data were plotted for one-third-octave-band-importance function (importance/dB), they found the frequency

TABLE 2–3. *Frequency bands making equal (5%) contributions to articulation index when all bands are at their optimum levels: composite data for men's and women's voices*

Band	Frequency limits (Hz)	Band	Frequency limits (Hz)
1	250–375	11	1,930–2,140
2	375–505	12	2,140–2,355
3	505–645	13	2,355–2,600
4	645–795	14	2,600–2,900
5	795–955	15	2,900–3,255
6	955–1,130	16	3,255–3,680
7	1,130–1,315	17	3,680–4,200
8	1,315–1,515	18	4,200–4,860
9	1,515–1,720	19	4,860–5,720
10	1,720–1,930	20	5,720–7,000

Adapted from French NR, Steinberg JC. Factors governing the intelligibility of speech sounds. *J Acoust Soc Am* 1947:19;90–119; with permission.

TABLE 2–4. *Cutoff frequencies of 20 equally contributing (5%) bands*

Band	Band limits (Hz)	Band	Band limits (Hz)
1	150–300	11	1,189–1,407
2	300–355	12	1,407–1,641
3	355–408	13	1,641–1,915
4	408–458	14	1,915–2,234
5	458–515	15	2,234–2,568
6	515–592	16	2,568–2,951
7	592–697	17	2,951–3,390
8	697–824	18	3,390–4,213
9	824–990	19	4,213–5,361
10	990–1189	20	5,361–8,000

Adapted from Studebacker GA, Pavlovic CV, Sherbecoe RL. A frequency importance function for continuous discourse. *J Acoust Soc Am* 1987:81;1130–38; with permission.

region of maximum importance at 400 to 500 Hz, with a suggestion of bimodality with relatively less importance in the 800- to 1,250-Hz region (35).

Effect of Noise

Intelligibility is not affected by noise if the speech intensity is more than 100 times (100:1 S/N ratio, 20 dB) greater than the noise intensity (8). In everyday life and for normal listeners, speech is often intelligible even when its intensity is lower than that of noise. However, for sensorineurally impaired subjects, the effects on word recognition as the S/N ratio becomes less favorable are more pronounced (36).

The relationship between the intensity of the desired signal to that of the undesired signal—generally background or environmental noise—is the S/N ratio. If a signal is 70 dB and the noise level is 50 dB, the S/N ratio is +20 dB. For hearing-impaired listeners, a +14- to +30-dB S/N ratio is required, about 15 dB higher than for normal listening individuals (18,36,37). Figure 2-24 illustrates the significance of distance on the S/N ratio. Because these calculations are made without reflected sound, they may suggest somewhat poorer results than what actually occurs. For hearing aid wearers, broad-band over narrow-band amplification has been demonstrated to provide an 18% (38) to 22% (39) advantage in intelligibility in noise. Binaural amplification has been reported to provide an additional 2- to 3-dB improvement in a diffuse field (40).

Effect of Filtered Speech

Speech can be filtered by passing the lows (low pass), passing the highs (high pass), or passing bands (band pass) between the low- and high-frequency pass bands.

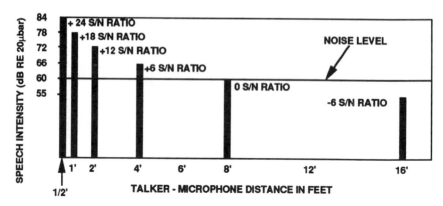

FIG. 2-24. The relationship between S/N ratio and distance. (Adapted from Ross M. Classroom amplification. In: Hodgson WR, ed. *Hearing aid assessment and use in audiologic habilitation.* Baltimore: Williams & Wilkins; 1986:231–265; with permission.)

Figure 2-25 shows the results of low- and high-pass filters on nonsense syllables (29). Effectively, at 1,930 Hz they cross over (recognition score of 67% for nonsense syllables). At this level normal conversation is fully intelligible. What this crossover frequency graph indicates is that at 1,930 Hz, whether only low frequencies below this frequency, or high frequencies only above 1,930 are present, intelligibility will be the same: 67%. When band-pass filtering is used, for example, a narrow band of 1,000 Hz centered around 1,500 Hz can provide 90% intelligibility.

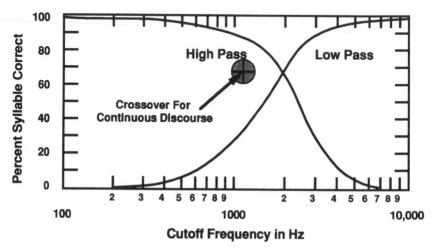

FIG. 2-25. Crossover frequency and syllable recognition for high-pass and low-pass systems operating in quiet and with optimal gain. (Modified from French NR, Steinberg JC. Factors governing the intelligibility of speech sounds. *J Acoust Soc Am* 1947;19:90–119; with permission.)

For continuous discourse, a lower crossover frequency was reported at about 1,189 Hz, with the statement that ". . . although there are exceptions, crossover frequency generally decreases as the redundancy of the test material increases" (34).

Bandwidth and Intelligibility

The effect of bandwidth on intelligibility, depicted by the generalized equal articulation (intelligibility) contours plotted for a bandpass system having a center frequency of 1,500 Hz, is shown in Fig. 2-26. It identifies the condition that as bandwidth is decreased, the intensity must be increased to maintain the word-recognition score constant. For hearing aids, this suggests that the wider the frequency range of a hearing aid, the less gain will be required. If a narrow, high-frequency-emphasis bandwidth is attempted, the gain requirement must be very high, so high that it might cause undue feedback problems (35). This seems to be consistent with Licklider and Miller's (27) statement: "The contribution of a given band of frequencies depends upon the intensity of the speech in the band, as well as upon the width of the band."

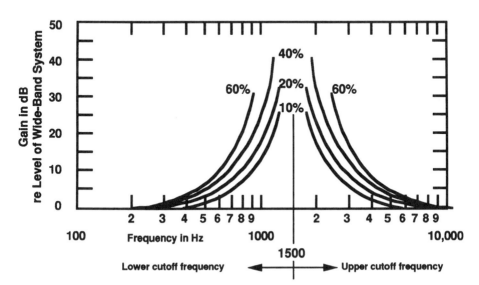

FIG. 2-26. Generalized equal-word-recognition contours plotted for band-pass systems centered at 1,500 Hz. As the bandwidth is narrowed, the intensity must be increased to hold the word recognition score constant. (Modified from Egan JP, Wiener FM. On the intelligibility of bands of speech in noise. *J Acoust Soc Am* 1946;18:435–441; with permission.)

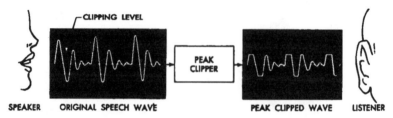

FIG. 2-27. Visualization of the effects of peak clipping on the speech signal. The amplitude of the speech wave can be clipped to varying degrees. (Reprinted from Denes PB, Pinson EN. *The speech chain*. Baltimore: Waverly; 1963; with permission.)

Effect With Distorted Speech

Waveshape distortion of the speech signal also can affect recognition. Although a number of methods could be used to distort the waveform, a common approach has been to use peak clipping to generate square pulses and create harmonic distortion (Fig. 2-27). Surprisingly, even drastic distortion can have little affect on word-recognition scores (remaining as high as 80–90%), even though speech quality suffers dramatically.

Speech Power Versus Intelligibility

Table 2-5, adapted from Fletcher (16), shows the relationship of speech power to intelligibility. This table is used often to justify the use of high-frequency amplification (i.e., because the frequency range from 1,000 to 8,000 Hz represents only 5% of the speech power, but 60% of the intelligibility, high-frequency emphasis should be used). If this line of reasoning were justified, it could as easily be said that the most important frequency range for speech recognition should be 500 to 1,000 Hz, because that single octave contains 35% of the speech power and 35% of the intelligibility.

TABLE 2–5. *Relationship of speech power and intelligibility*

Frequency range (Hz)	% of speech power		% of speech intelligibility	
62.5–125	5 ⎤		1 ⎤	
125–250	13 ⎥ 60		1 ⎥ 5	
250–500	42 ⎦		3 ⎦	
500–1,000	**35**		**35**	
1,000–2,000	3 ⎤		35 ⎤	
2,000–4,000	1 ⎥ 5		13 ⎥ 60	
4,000–8,000	1 ⎦		12 ⎦	

Adapted from Fletcher H. *Speech and Hearing in Communication.* New York: D Van Nostrand; 1929; with permission.

The Effect of Aging

In reviewing the implications relating speech recognition ability in the elderly, the following generalized statements can be made. The prevalence of hearing loss increases with age (Fig. 2-28). Individuals over 57 years of age can expect approximately a 31% prevalence of hearing loss, and it is significantly greater in men (33%) than in women (27%) for the population over 57 years of age (42). The audiometric configurations for the elderly are 29% sharply sloping, 29% flat, 36% gradually sloping, and 6% rising audiograms (43). Most significant changes in hearing thresholds begin between 40 and 50 years of age and continue into the 80s.

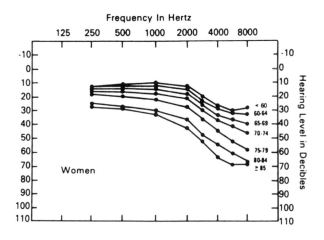

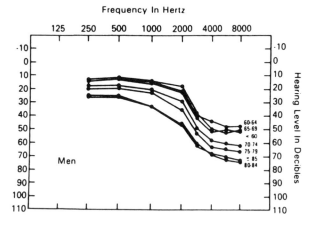

FIG. 2-28. The effects of aging on hearing thresholds for women (top) and for men (bottom). (Reprinted from Moscicki E, Elkins E, Baum H, McNamara P. Hearing loss in the elderly: an epidemiologic study of the Framingham Heart Study Cohort. *Ear Hear* 1985;6:184–190; with permission.)

Additionally, hearing levels in men are slightly poorer than those in women, especially in the high frequencies.

In quiet, a gradual increase in SPL with age is needed to maintain a 60% word recognition score. But when comparing population ages, some investigators (44, 45) found that about a 15- to 16-dB greater SPL was required in older populations than in younger populations.

When listening tasks are made more difficult, speech perception tends to decline with age (46). Therefore, speech materials presented in degraded conditions are more likely to show deficits resulting from the aging process. For example, with longer reverberation times, older patients experienced more difficulty in word recognition than did younger patients (45). Comparing word recognition scores in quiet between younger and older patients, Helfer and Wilber (47) found scores that were about 7% poorer in the elderly population. When the task was made more difficult (+10 S/N, but no reverberation), this difference was 15%; and under a condition of reverberation (T = 1.3 s) but of no noise, the difference was 18%.

When evaluating speech recognition tasks with the elderly, it is important to keep in mind certain issues:

1. Word-recognition testing does not help the patient gain insight into his or her communicative problem.
2. Handicap questionnaire data can complement information and provide useful insights not obtained on other traditional speech recognition tasks.
3. It has been reported that the elderly are more conservative in tasks requiring decision making than are younger adults (48).
4. The materials, presentation level, response format, test paradigm, and conditions under which testing is performed should be designed to show age effects.

Effect of Redundancy

The ease with which a person is able to recognize speech is due in part to the extrinsic redundancy within the speech signal and the intrinsic redundancy within the auditory system (49). When the cues are due to the numerous overlapping cues within speech itself, they are identified as being of extrinsic redundancy. When the cues result from multiple central auditory nervous system pathways and sources of information that are inherent for processing speech, they are identified as being of intrinsic redundancy. Redundant cues result in a message that becomes predictable, and it is this predictability that makes redundancy so powerful (50). When only one of these two types of redundancy has been reduced, an individual performs at or near normal for speech processing tasks (51). However, if both extrinsic and intrinsic redundancy have been reduced, abnormal performance in speech processing tasks is often observed.

Effect of Temporal Characteristics

Normal hearing individuals show about a 10- to 15-dB improvement in threshold as stimulus duration increases from 10 to 500 ms (52). However, with cochlear involvement, such as found in the elderly population, this improvement in threshold with increasing stimulus duration is greatly reduced (53).

REFERENCES

1. Fechner GT. *Element der Psychophysik*. Leipzig: Breithopf & Harterl; 1860.
2. Hirsh IJ. *The measurement of hearing*. New York: McGraw-Hill; 1952.
3. Humes LE. Psychoacoustic considerations in clinical audiology. In: Katz J, ed. *Handbook of clinical audiology*. 4th ed. Baltimore: Williams & Wilkins; 1994;56–72.
4. Licklider JCR. Basic correlates of the auditory stimulus. In: Stevens SS, ed. *Handbook of experimental psychology*. New York: John Wiley & Sons; 1951:985–1039.
5. Beasley WC. *National Health Survey (1935–36), Preliminary Reports, Hearing Study Series, Bulletins 1–7*. Washington, DC: Public Health Service; 1938.
6. Davis H, Kranz FW. The international standard reference zero for pure-tone audiometers and its relation to the evaluation of impairment of hearing. *J Speech Hear Res* 1964;7:7–16.
7. McCandless G. Hearing aids and loudness discomfort. Proceedings III: International Otocongress, Copenhagen, 1973:39–44.
8. Denes PB, Pinson EN. *The speech chain*. Baltimore: Waverly; 1963.
9. Békésy G von. Variation of phase along the basilar membrane with sinusoidal vibrations. *J Acoust Soc Am* 1947;19:452–460.
10. Helmholz HLF. *Die Lehre von den Tonempfindungen als Physiologishe Grundlage für die Theorie der Musik*. 1st ed, 1863. 3rd English ed, 1870. English translation by Ellis AJ. *On the Sensations of Tone*. 2nd English ed. New York: Longmans, Green; 1985.
11. Preves DA, Curran JR. Basic hearing science. In: Sandlin RE, ed. *Hearing instrument science and fitting practices*. Livonia MI: National Institute for Hearing Instruments Studies; 1985.
12. Rutherford W. A new theory of hearing. *J Anat Physiol* 1996;21:166–168.
13. Wever EG. *Theory of hearing*. New York: Wiley; 1949.
14. Fletcher H, Munson WA. Loudness, its definition, measurement and calculation. *J Acoust Soc Am* 1933;5:82–102.
15. Wiener FM. On the diffraction of a progressive sound wave by the human head. *J Acoust Soc Am* 1947;19:143–146.
16. Fletcher H. *Speech and hearing in communication*. New York: Van Nostrand; 1953.
17. Stevens SS, Newman EB. The localization of actual sources of sound. *Am J Psychol* 1936;48:297–306.
18. Olsen WO, Carhart R. Development of test procedures for evaluation of binaural hearing aids. *Bull Prosthet Res* 1967;10:22–49.
19. Staab WJ, Lybarger SF. Characteristics and use of hearing aids. In: Katz J, ed. *Handbook of clinical audiology*. 4th ed. Baltimore: Williams & Wilkins; 1994:657–722.
20. Shaw EAG. The external ear. In: Keidel WD, Neff WD, eds. *Handbook of sensory physiology*. New York: Springer; 1974.
21. Nordlund B, Fritzell B. The influence of azimuths on speech signal. *Acta Otolaryngol (Stockh)* 1963;56:132–642.
22. Jesteadt W, Weir CC. Comparison of monaural and binaural discrimination of intensity and frequency. *J Acoust Soc Am* 1977;61:1599–1603.,
23. Carhart R. Monaural and binaural discrimination against competing sentences. *Int Audiol* 1965; 4:5–10.
24. Hirsh IJJ. The influence of interaural phase on interaural summation and inhibition. *J Acoust Soc Am* 1948;20:536–544.
25. Schoeny ZG, Talbott RE. Nonspeech procedures in central testing. In: Katz J, ed. *Handbook of clinical audiology*. 4th ed. Baltimore: Williams & Wilkins; 1994:212–221.

26. Katz J, Ivey RG. Spondaic procedures in central testing. In: Katz J, ed. *Handbook of clinical audiology.* 4th ed. Baltimore: Williams & Wilkins; 1994:239–255.
27. Licklider JCR, Miller GA. The perception of speech. In: Stevens SS, ed. *Handbook of experimental psychology.* New York: John Wiley & Sons; 1951:1040–1074.
28. Danaher E, Osberger J, Pickett J. Discrimination of formant frequency transitions in synthetic vowels. *J Speech Hear Res* 1973;16:439–451.
29. French NR, Steinberg JC. Factors governing the intelligibility of speech sounds. *J Acoust Soc Am* 1947;19:90–119.
30. Newby HA. *Audiology.* 3rd ed. New York: Appleton-Century-Crofts; 1972.
31. Webster JC. Speech communications as limited by ambient noise. *J Acoust Soc Am* 1965;37: 694.
32. Botsford JA. Predicting speech interference and annoyance from A-weighted sound levels. *J Acoust Soc Am* 1967;42;1151.
33. Hall JW, Tyler RS, Fernandez MA. The factors influencing the masking level difference in cochlear hearing-impaired and normal-hearing listeners. *J Speech Hear Res* 1984;27:145–154.
34. Studebaker GA, Pavlovic CV, Sherbecoe RL. A frequency importance function for continuous discourse. *J Acoust Soc Am* 1987;81:1130–1138.
35. Staab WJ. Significance of mid-frequencies in hearing aid selection. *Hear J* 1988;42:23,25–28, 30–34.
36. Olsen WO, Tillman TW. Hearing aids and sensorineural hearing loss. *Ann Otol* 1968;77:717–727.
37. Carhart R, Tillman TW. Interaction of competing speech signals with hearing losses. *Arch Otolaryngol* 1970;91:273–279.
38. Pascoe DP. Frequency responses of hearing aids and their effects on the speech perception of hearing-impaired subjects. *Ann Otol Rhinol Laryngol* 1975;84(suppl 23).
39. Skinner MW, Karstaedt M, Miller J. Amplification bandwidth and speech intelligibility for two listeners with sensori-neural hearing loss. *Audiology* 1982;21:251–268.
40. Killion MC. The noise problem: there's hope. *Hear Instrum* 1985;36:26,28,30,32.
41. Fletcher H. *Speech and hearing in communication.* New York: Van Nostrand; 1929.
42. Moscicki E, Elkins E, Baum H, McNamara P. Hearing loss in the elderly: an epidemiologic study of the Framingham Heart Study Cohort. *Ear Hear* 1985;6:184–190.
43. Gates G, Cooper J, Kannel W, Miller N. Hearing in the elderly: the Framingham cohort, 1983–85. Part I. Basic audiometric test results. *Ear Hear* 1990;11:247–256.
44. Plomp R, Mimpen AM. Speech-reception threshold for sentences as a function of age and noise level. *J Acoust Soc Am* 1979;66:1333–1342.
45. Nabelek A, Robinson P. Monaural and binaural speech perception in reverberation for listeners of various ages. *J Acoust Soc Am* 1982;71:1242–1248.
46. Dubno J, Dirks D, Morgan D. Effects of age and mild hearing loss on speech recognition in noise. *J Acoust Soc Am* 1984;76:87–96.
47. Helfer K, Wilber L. Hearing with aging and speech perception in reverberation and noise. *J Speech Hear Res* 1990;33:149–155.
48. Botwinick J. Disinclination to venture response versus cautiousness in responding: age differences. *J Genet Psychol* 1969;115:55–62.
49. Bocca E, Calearo C. Central hearing processes. In: Jerger J, ed. *Modern developments in audiology.* New York: Academic; 1963.
50. Miller GA, Heise CA, Lichten D. Intelligibility of speech as a function of the context of the test material. *J Exp Psychol* 1951;41:329–335.
51. Mueller HG, Bright KE. In: Katz J, ed. *Handbook of clinical audiology.* 4th ed. Baltimore: Williams & Wilkins; 1994:222–238.
52. Salvi R, Henderson D, Hamernik RP. Physiological bases of sensorineural hearing loss. In: Tobias JV, Schubert ED, eds. *Hearing research and theory.* Vol. 2. New York: Academic; 1983.
53. Watson CS, Gengel RW. Signal duration and signal frequency in relation to auditory sensitivity. *J Acoust Soc Am* 1969;46:989–997.
54. Philips Hearing Instruments, Inc. *Basics of audiology.* Eindhoven, The Netherlands; 1982.
55. Ross M. Classroom amplification. In: Hodgson WR, ed. *Hearing aid assessment and use in audiologic habilitation.* Baltimore: Williams & Wilkins; 1986:231–265.
56. Egan JP, Wiener FM. On the intelligibility of bands of speech in noise. *J Acoust Soc Am* 1946;18:435–441.

HEARING AIDS: A MANUAL FOR CLINICIANS,
edited by Robert A. Goldenberg
Lippincott–Raven Publishers, Philadelphia © 1996

C H A P T E R ✦*3*✦

Effective Listening

Richard H. Nodar

Department of Otolaryngology and Communication Disorders,
The Cleveland Clinic, Cleveland, Ohio

Key Points _____

Listening strategies for the hearing impaired • methods of aural rehabilitation • techniques of speechreading (lipreading) • identifying freindly
listening environments • approaches to counseling.

This chapter addresses several listening strategies. For the most part, they have applications for the individual who is hearing impaired. However, they also apply to
all listeners; first because we are all exposed to difficult listening situations, and
second, because if we live long enough, we will all have hearing losses as a function of noise exposure and aging (1). Furthermore, this chapter provides the reader
with an overview of concepts and approaches to speechreading and auditory training, with the understanding that the two areas extend far beyond the scope of this
book. In this chapter we differentiate between hearing and listening. Hearing refers
to the broad spectrum of a person's interaction with the world of sound, including
detection, discrimination, adaptation, habituation, auditory fatigue, recruitment,
and processing. This statement underscores the admonition to avoid the phrase
"normal hearing" when looking at a pure-tone audiogram. Listening involves active participation by an individual in attending to a sound or sounds.

Any and all attempts to assist individuals with hearing losses or hearing disorders fall under the broad category of aural rehabilitation/habilitation. Aural rehabilitation has been defined as addressing "the total communication function of
the hearing impaired individual. It may include instrumentation (hearing aids,
cochlear implants (CI), tinnitus maskers, and other assistive devices), training
(speech reading, auditory training, and speech conservation)" (2). Children and infants who have profound hearing losses and who lack an awareness of sound and
its meaning, are candidates for aural habilitation.

The infant with a profound hearing loss does not fall within the pervue of this chapter. They should be referred to an infant stimulation/language program immediately upon discovery of their hearing loss.

Children are dependent on their families and the hearing professionals for support, encouragement, and involvement in the development of their listening strategies. Flexor (3) presents strategies for assessing listening skills in children. Heather Whitestone, Miss America 1995, has a profound hearing loss. In several public addresses, she expressed that her "support team," consisting of her family, friends, and professionals, played a key role in any successes that she has enjoyed.

Adults must be encouraged to admit to and acknowledge their hearing problem. This will provide the backdrop for their behavior, such as requesting preferential seating.

The rest of the chapter presupposes that the persons discussed are wearing hearing aids. Remember, support, encouragement, and appropriate referral are the bywords of this chapter.

SPEECHREADING

The term speechreading was introduced in the United States in 1944 (4). Speechreading is preferred to lipreading because it is more descriptive of the process of understanding spoken language by synthesizing: lip movements, facial expression, context, the environment, time of day, time of year (i.e., season, holiday), body language, gestures, and others. Understanding speech by watching only the lips move is difficult for the following reasons: (a) speech is very fast, (b) many speech movements look alike (homophones), (c) certain sounds are either invisible or nearly invisible on the lips (i.e., h, g, and k), (d) dialects may distort, and, finally, (e) facial hair, pipes and cigarettes, eating food, hand gestures, and head movements may obscure or distort the lips.

Speechreading lessons should be recommended for any person who, even with a hearing aid, cannot understand conversation. It serves to augment the spoken word and helps the listener to focus on the speaker.

AURAL REHABILITATION

The term aural rehabilitation (also called audiologic rehabilitation) broadly encompasses most of this book; that is, hearing aids are at the heart of aural rehabilitation. Therefore, only those aspects of aural rehabilitation not addressed in other chapters are covered here.

Auditory training consists of a seven-step developmental process that begins with the infant and continues through adulthood:

1. An awareness of sound (i.e., sound exists)
2. Sound has meaning

3. Gross discriminations of different sounds
4. Fine discriminations of sounds
5. Gross discriminations of speech sounds (i.e., vowels)
6. Fine discriminations of speech sounds (consonants)
7. Word discrimination/recognition

Steps 1 and 2 are primarily for the child who has a severe to profound hearing loss. The severely handicapped child may never have heard sound and may be frightened by it at first exposure. The concept that sound has meaning involves the complex task of demonstrating meaningful sounds, i.e., door bells, telephones, car horns, smoke alarms, etc. The other five steps are self-evident.

LISTENING ENVIRONMENTS

Most individuals with hearing impairments appreciate the enormous spectrum of listening environments. "Quiet" is rarely silent, and "noisy" may vary from two people speaking to the cacophony of 80,000 voices cheering as a touchdown pass is caught in the end zone. The remainder of this section will be painted with broad strokes, with the understanding that every possible listening situation cannot be addressed.

The Hearing Aid

Regardless of the listening situation, the hearing aid should rarely be removed or taken off. Hearing aids are an adjunct to hearing. One's hearing aid allows hearing sound through walls, around corners from behind, above, and below. However, there are times when the situation mandates prudence. Fireworks displays, power tools, shotguns, discos, etc. require ear protection. In all of these instances, it would be prudent for the hearing aid user to avoid exposure completely. However, when high-impact or high-volume sound cannot be avoided, the hearing aids should be turned off, but not removed. The hearing aid itself may provide some degree of protection.

Unilateral Hearing Loss

Whenever possible, the unilateral hearing loss should be fitted with a hearing aid. If the ear is unable to be fit (deaf ear, canal pathology, etc.), a CROS (contralateral routing of signal) aid should be worn. However, the listening strategy for this individual is to direct the better ear (unaided ear) toward or closer to the sound source.

Programmable Hearing Aids

Programmable hearing aids have two advantages over conventional hearing aids: (a) they allow for modification (fitting) of the hearing aid by the audiologist while the patient is wearing it, and (b) the patient can change programs as he or she moves from one sound field to another.

Preferential Seating

This term implies that the hearing aid user should get the best seats in the house. However, we intend it to reflect the notion that the hearing aid user should select his or her seating based on hearing preference: up front, centered, better ear toward the speaker, away from the air conditioner, away from open doors, leading to noisy corridors or the outside, away from people who talk during the performance, and, if possible, away from "coughers."

The Sound Field

By definition, a sound field is any medium in which sound waves exist, and there is some reverberation within the region containing the sound (5). A free field is one that is free from boundaries or one in which the effects of the boundaries are negligible. Ideally, if the listener can choose the area for communicating, he or she should opt for one in which the reverberation is at a minimum. Below are listed certain "good" and "bad" listening environments for the hearing aid wearer to consider for communication. Granted, there are exceptions; however, these are intended to give the reader a perspective, not an all-inclusive list. The "good" listening environments include a living room, a patio, the library, a den, a private office, a park, and a country road. "Bad" listening environments include anywhere there is an echo (church, an auditorium, long marbled corridors, sporting events, discos), large family gatherings, factories, and shopping malls.

The "bad" listening environments are not listed as places to necessarily avoid. Rather, they are listed to alert the hearing aid wearer to the environments where understanding speech may be difficult.

The six keys to effective listening are as follows:

1. Select the best listening environment.
2. Select a seat close to the speaker of interest.
3. Position your "better ear" toward the speaker(s) of interest.
4. Watch the speaker's face, lips, and gestures.
5. Whenever possible, have prior knowledge of the subject.
6. Do not allow your mind to "drift," but attend to the speaker.

COUNSELING

The approach to counseling varies greatly depending on your personality and the personality of your patients and their families. However, the following general guidelines may assist you. Acknowledging that hearing loss can be an isolating experience will help you convey information with compassion and understanding. Speak slowly. Remember that you and the audiologist compliment each other and that you may be saying the same thing, but with slightly different emphasis. Encourage patients to ask questions. If you do not know the answer, do not guess, but refer to someone who knows, or say "I don't know. I'll find out the answer and get back to you."

The Patient

Many of the suggestions for the patient are also true for the family and *vice versa*. The following suggestions are for the patient. First, remember the six keys to effective listening. Second, do not hesitate to tell someone that you have a hearing problem. It will help them understand your behavior and will raise their consciousness about hearing loss, and they may help you with things you missed. Third, be observant, attend to the speaker, but also be aware of your surroundings (others in the room, and the environment itself). Fourth, if possible, be aware of the topic or subject matter; knowing the context of any discussion will be beneficial to you. Finally, relax. Tension, and trying to hear every word may distract you so that you miss the general point of the sentence or paragraph.

The Family

Advice for the family includes knowledge of the six steps to effective listening as well as the information for the patient. Furthermore, there are three watchwords that will assist the family's interactions with the hearing-impaired individual: assistance, compassion, and tolerance (ACT). Assistance suggests that you try to facilitate communication by (a) facing the listener when you are speaking; (b) speaking to the listener only when you are close enough to touch him or her, or at the very least, when in the same room; (c) keeping your hands from in front of your face while speaking; and (d) speaking slightly slower than you might normally speak. Compassion encompasses the entire spectrum of understanding, or trying to understand, the individual's distress and trying to alleviate it. Individuals with hearing loss may feel left out or may even withdraw from a conversation if they cannot keep up with the conversation. Be aware of this possibility and correct it. Tolerance is essential when interacting with the hearing-impaired person. Remarks such as "I just said that!" or "Turn up your hearing aid" are only humorous to the person with normal hearing. If a person says,"I can't hear you," he are she is asking for help deciphering your message.

Repeat the message, slower and even slightly differently, but do not shout; the hearing aid is supposed to compensate for the hearing loss. Senior citizens may have difficulty understanding single words even with a hearing aid. If that is the case, rephrasing a sentence may help.

CONCLUSION

In conclusion, we have offered a framework for you to build on based on your training, interest, and clinical experience. You may relegate the bulk of counseling to an associate, another physician, an audiologist, a rehabilitation councilor, a nurse, etc. However, it is imperative that you have certain knowledge about this subject so that you can exchange information with your patients, their families, and your colleagues.

REFERENCES

1. Nodar RH. The effects of aging and music on hearing. *Generations* 1987;12:39–40.
2. Nodar RH. Aural rehabilitation. In: Hughes GB, ed. *Textbook of clinical otology.* New York: Thieme-Stratton; 1985:152–162
3. Flexer C. Management of hearing in an educational setting. In: Alpiner JG, McArthy PA, eds. *Rehabilitative audiology in children and adults.* Baltimore: Williams & Wilkins; 1993:176–206.
4. Bunger AM. *Speech reading—Jena method.* Danville, IL: The Interstate; 1944.
5. Hirsh IJ. *The measurement of hearing.* New York: McGraw-Hill; 1952.

HEARING AIDS: A MANUAL FOR CLINICIANS,
edited by Robert A. Goldenberg
Lippincott–Raven Publishers, Philadelphia © 1996

C H A P T E R ✦ *4* ✦

Evaluating the Patient

Linda L. Donaldson

Beltone-Apple Creek Hearing Aids and Audiological, Fairborn, Ohio

Key Points

> Description of audiologic tests • use of the audiologic test battery •
> definition of types of hearing loss • using hearing tests to fit hearing aids •
> science of hearing aid evaluation.

Audiologic tests are building blocks to judge each patient's auditory function. Each evaluation (a series of individual tests), along with the otologic workup, pieces together the patient's rehabilitation course. The entire evaluation is a decision making process. If "X" happens, does the audiologist evaluate for "Z" or for "Y"? The evaluation process helps determine the minimal thresholds for the individual based on normal listeners as well as in comparison with standards (1).

Each audiologic evaluation must be reliable, defensible, valid, and without fault. The total audiologic evaluation must be legally defendable. Test procedures must be consistent in order to provide repeatability. Documentation of standards followed within the scope of practice should be provided. Both the American National Standard Institute (ANSI) and the American Speech Language Hearing Association (ASHA) have auditory assessment standards. Validation must be available for the test procedure. Not only must standards be followed for procedures learned in the university setting, but also for shortcuts used within the scope of practice. No shortcuts may be used until the standards are well understood.

All hearing health-care providers (otologists, otolaryngologists, audiologists, hearing instrument specialists, audiometric technicians, or nursing staff) must be well aware and knowledgeable of required federal and state laws affecting audiologic evaluations and hearing instrument regulations.

Yantis (1) describes variability for auditory sensitivity as either extrinsic or intrinsic. "Extrinsic" implies that equipment must be calibrated to meet ANSI specifications. The methodology and instructions must be valid and consistent. Timeliness is a factor often overlooked by the novice clinician. "Intrinsic" variability refs to the individual's various attributes that may affect either their ability to hear the sound or their response to the sound. Examples of intrinsic variability are listed as follows:

Physiological body activity
Vascular or respiratory abilities
Attention level
Intelligence
Age
Health
Tinnitus
Education level
Motivation
Understanding the task

How motivated is the client to be in the office? Was he or she forced into the office by a family member (1–3)? Variables must be noted because they help determine how well a patient will function with amplification. The process to fit a hearing instrument begins at this initial stage. A properly fitting hearing instrument must not cause physical or perceptual discomfort. All of the patient's needs must be analyzed (4).

Level of hearing is age related and varies from patient to patient. Presbycusis, the term for hearing loss due to increasing age, is a degeneration that causes pathological changes in the cochlear and retrocochlear systems. Figure 4-1 displays the effect of aging on frequencies. The high frequencies are particularly affected with increasing age; the majority of hearing instrument candidates are over 65 years of age (2,3).

The U.S. Food and Drug Administration requires that a patient be referred to a physician if any of the following eight conditions are detected before being fitted with a hearing instrument:

1. Visible congenital or traumatic deformity of the ear.
2. Visible evidence of cerumen accumulation or a foreign body in the ear canal.
3. History of active drainage from the ear within the previous 90 days.
4. Acute or chronic dizziness.
5. Unilateral hearing loss of sudden or recent onset within the previous 90 days.
6. History of sudden or rapidly progressive hearing loss within the previous 90 days.
7. Pain or discomfort in the ear.
8. Audiometric air bone gap equal to or greater than 15 dB at 500, 1,000, and 2,000 Hz.

It is mandatory to note any nonstandard test procedures on a patient's audiogram. The information needed for each audiogram should be easily replicated and understood for future reference. Standards must be followed for validity and not personal testing style.

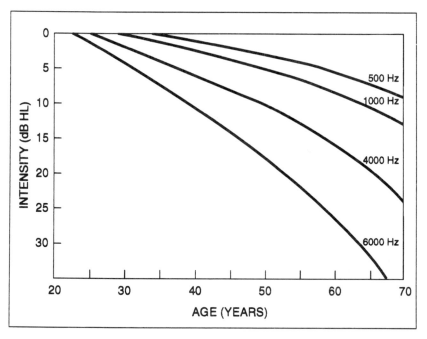

FIG. 4-1. Hearing as a function of age. From Deutsch L, Richards A. Elementary hearing science. Copyright 1979 by Allyn and Bacon. Reprinted by permission.

The American Academy of Otolaryngology and the American Council of Otolaryngology have approved a formula for evaluating hearing handicap. They have also defined the following terms: permanent impairment, permanent handicap, and permanent disability.

A permanent impairment is due to any anatomic or function abnormality leaving hearing thresholds outside of normal limits. A hearing-impaired person unable to perform all activities of daily living has a permanent handicap, whereas a person unable to work full time has a permanent disability. Table 4-1 redefines the formulas to compute percentage of hearing loss (5).

TABLE 4-1. *Percentage of hearing handicap (1979)*

Calculation of average hearing threshold level:
(500 Hz + 1000 Hz + 2000 Hz + 3000 Hz): 4 = average dB HTL
Calculation of monaural impairment:
(Average dB HTL − 25 dB) × 1.5% = monaural percentage of impairment
Calculation of hearing handicap:
monaural % of impairment smaller number (better ear) × 5 = x
monaural % of impairment larger number (poorer ear) × 5 = y

BASIC OTOSCOPIC EXAMINATION

The otoscopic examination is the first step in obtaining a valid assessment of hearing impairment. A clear view of the tympanic membrane should be visible with a notation of any abnormalities or cerumen present in the ear canal. Otologic disorders must be resolved before fitting any hearing instrument. The ear canal must be checked for any sharp bend or narrowing that may be pertinent to fitting the hearing instrument. Note any abnormalities that may affect the fitting of an in-the-canal or completely-in-the-canal hearing instrument. Any protrusion may be flattened during the ear impression procedure and thus may not be present on the actual ear impression. These areas might then create sores or pressure points upon fitting a hearing instrument or earmold.

Collapsed canals are common among very young and very old patients and often result in a mild conductive component. A collapsed canal may occur by mere placement of the earphone on the soft cartilage of the pinna. To work with a collapsed canal, it is best to use some type of specula such as a 1-inch tubing placed in the external auditory meatus or circumaural earphones to keep the canal open, allowing for a valid evaluation. If using tubing, caution must be used when removing it upon completion of the evaluation (3). Sound field testing also may be needed to evaluate a patient with collapsed canals.

RELATIONSHIP OF DECIBELS: HEARING LEVEL TO SOUND PRESSURE LEVEL

Sound intensity is measured in decibels. Stating a specific number of decibels with no accompanying reference is meaningless because sound intensity is measured on a ratio scale (2). Decibels are referenced to decibel sound pressure level (SPL), decibel hearing threshold level (HTL), decibel hearing level (HL), or decibel sensation level (SL). Decibels are referenced to SPL in dynes/cm^2. Zero decibels SPL refers to the minimal audible sound of 0.0002 dynes/cm^2, whereas 140 dB SPL is equated to 2,000 dynes/cm^2. The formula for determining dB SPL is as follows (3,4):

$$dB\ SPL = 20 \times \log \text{pressure measured/pressure reference}$$

Most audiometers are referenced to dB HL, whereas most hearing instruments, master hearing instruments (MHIs), and real-ear measurement (REM) are referenced to dB SPL. A conversion factor exists between the two references. To convert from HL to SPL for speech, 20 dB is added. Therefore, in converting an uncomfortable loudness level (UCL) of 90 dB HL, 20 dB is added to compute a comparable SPL reading of 110 dB.

Normal hearing sensitivity is inappropriately plotted by use of dB SPL measurements due to the decibel variance for each frequency. Decibel variance for SPL identified as normal for specific frequencies may be seen in Table 4-2. It is much simpler to identify each frequency at a zero level scale, hence the dB HL scale. All audiometers are calibrated in dB HL referenced to 0.0002 dynes/cm^2. As an example, a 2,000-Hz tone of 0 dB HL is the same as 9 dB SPL at 2,000 Hz.

TABLE 4-2. *Normal sound pressure levels (reference 0.0002 dynes/cm²)*

Frequency (Hz)	125	250	500	1,000	2,000	4,000	8,000
Intensity (dB SPL)	45.0	24.5	11.5	7.0	9.0	9.5	13.0

Human hearing mechanisms are not equally sensitive to all frequencies across the spectrum. Frequencies below 500 Hz and above 3,000 Hz require more intensity to be audible to the ear than do the mid-range frequencies. Caution must be taken when testing lower frequencies because they are more audible and sometimes project a vibrotactile response due to the longer wavelength of the signal (2).

BASIC AUDIOMETRIC EVALUATION

In air conduction pathways the sound enters the ear canal as acoustic energy that alters to mechanical energy once the sound is received by the middle ear. Upon reaching the fluid-filled inner ear the sound becomes hydraulic energy. Once the hair cells are stimulated, sending the signal through to the eighth nerve, the energy changes to electrochemical.

Testing air conduction pathways requires headphones, which are one of three types: supraural, circumaural, or insert receivers. Each audiometer must be calibrated to a specific headphone. Transferring earphones from one audiometer to another may result in incorrect intensity levels. Supraural headphones rest over the pinna and are generally TDH 39 or TDH 49. Circumaural earphones go around the pinna and are most appropriate for evaluating in noisier environments. Insert receivers (Fig. 4-2) have been evaluated over the past 10 years and are becoming increasingly popular.

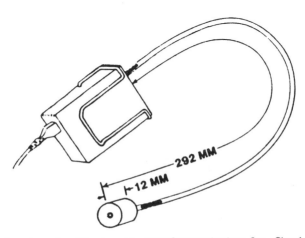

FIG. 4-2. Insert receiver (Courtesy Advanstar Communications, Inc., Cleveland, Ohio).

One of the primary advantages of using insert receivers is that the interaural attenuation (IA) may be as great as 90+ dB, which is 50+ dB higher than that of supraural or cicumaural earphones (Fig. 4-3). IA describes the energy needed for the test signal to cross from the poorer ear via the skull to the better ear. In this situation the better ear will respond for the poorer ear, creating false-positive threshold responses. Appropriate masking procedures must be implemented to ensure that true thresholds are obtained from the poorer ear. The need to use masking procedures lessens with insert receivers (6). Insert receivers also decrease the extraneous noise level when evaluating without a sound booth, as when testing in a home, in a nursing home, or at a hospital bedside. Additionally, using insert receivers decreases difficulties with collapsed canals. However, insert receivers have two prevailing concerns: hygiene and expense (7).

Traditional "sound-proof" rooms are actually sound isolated, sound treated, or sound reducing. These rooms may be commercially built or constructed to fit available space according to calibration requirements. A truly sound-proof room is an anechoic chamber in which there is an absence of reverberation and sound is truly free field.

Sound room systems may be single or double rooms. Most sound room walls are 3 to 4 inches thick, being single or double walled. A single-walled booth 3 or 4 inches thick is generally acceptable. A single-room suite either has the examiner and patient in the same test room or the patient in the sound room and the evaluator

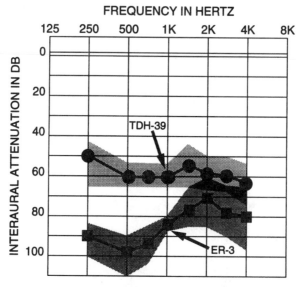

FIG. 4-3. Average and range of interaural attenuation obtained on six subjects with two earphones: TDH-39 and ER-3 with deeply inserted plugs (Courtesy Advanstar Communications, Inc., Cleveland, Ohio).

in a separate room. A double-room suite has the patient in one sound room and the examiner in a second sound room. When the examiner is in a separate space, paneled electrical and acoustical connections or wiring are necessary for the earphones, bone conduction oscillator, talk-over microphone, sound field speakers, and talk-back system. Due to the American Disabilities Act each office is required to provide facilities such as wheelchair accessibility.

During evaluation procedures the patient must not perceive any visual cues from the examiner. A repetitive signal such as a head or hand movement may cue a patient to respond to a particular stimuli (5). Some patients require more positive reinforcement to responses than do others. In some situations visual contact may be necessary for rapport and reinforcement.

TUNING FORK TESTS

Tuning fork testing remains a viable procedure to confirm test results. Weber and Rinne tests remain most common and use a 250- or 500-Hz tuning fork. The Weber Test, developed in 1834, tests lateralization (5). The tuning fork is taped into vibration with the tuning fork stem placed on the frontal bone. One must determine in which ear the patient perceives the sound: right, left, or midline. If the sound presents with greater intensity to the better ear, the ear is suspected to be normal or sensorineural. If the tuning fork lateralizes to the poorer ear, it is suspected of presenting with the greatest conductive component. A midline response represents either normal hearing or a bilaterally equal conductive, sensorineural, or mixed loss (3).

A Rinne test places the tuning fork both on the mastoid process and near (but not touching) the external auditory meatus. The patient is asked to indicate at which location the sound is most intense. If the sound is loudest at the ear canal aperture, then the air conduction pathway is greater than the bone conduction pathway (AC > BC), suggesting a normal or sensorineural ear. If the bone conduction pathway, or sound on the mastoid process, is most intense (BC > AC), then there may be a conductive component (3). The Rinne tuning fork test provides a good measure of the sealing capability of earplugs for children with pressure equalization (PE) tubes as well as earplugs for noise protection.

AUDIOGRAM

Figure 4-4 shows two audiogram forms. One is strictly a graph form, which presents information to the patient simply and straightforwardly, whereas the other audiogram form provides a table, which is more practical and economical for comparing multiple audiograms in the patient's chart. The audiogram form must provide the following pertinent information: name, date of evaluation, date of birth, gender, audiologist name, audiometer used, or any information pertinent to your practice such as REMs, impedance, or master hearing aid results. An audiogram key also must be present on the audiogram (Fig. 4-5).

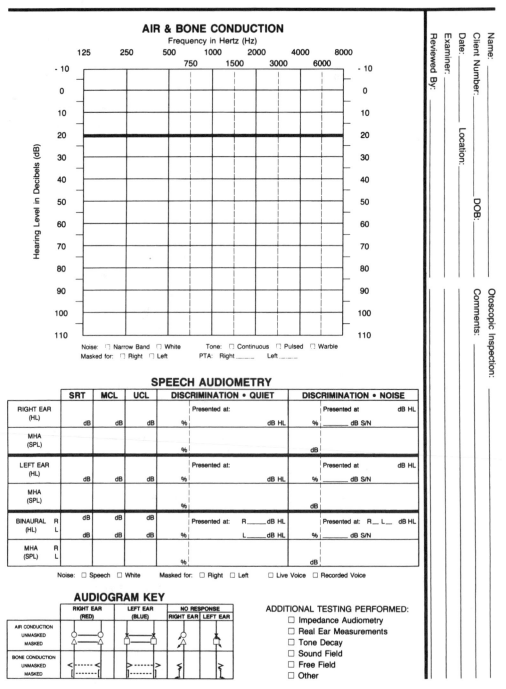

FIG. 4-4. Two audiogram forms.

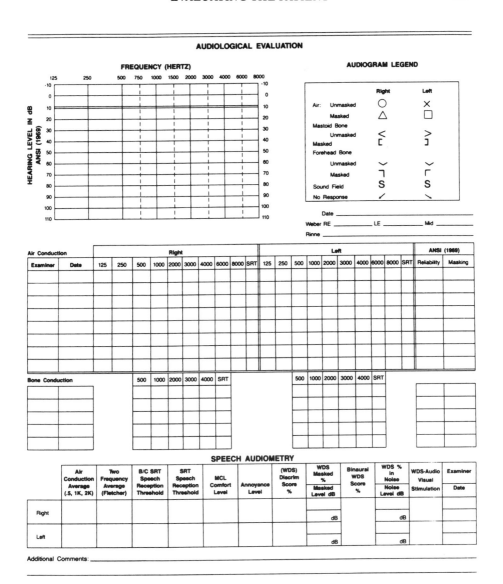

FIG. 4-4. *Continued.*

Whether fitting hearing instruments via a comparative method (using an MHI or programmable hearing instruments) or prescriptive method (applying pure tone responses to a formula), the audiometric values are paramount in determining a hearing instrument's output, gain, and slope. The degree of hearing loss helps determine the amount of power to build into a hearing instrument. Also, slope of loss is needed to properly fit a hearing instrument.

SPEECH AUDIOMETRY

	Air Conduction Average (.5, 1K, 2K)	Two Frequency Average (Fletcher)	B/C Speech Reception Threshold	SRT Speech Reception Threshold	MCL Comfort Level	Annoyance Level	(WDS) Discrim Score %	WDS Masked % Masked Level dB	Binaural WDS Score %	WDS % in Noise Noise Level dB	WDS-Audio Visual Stimulation	Examiner Date
Right								dB		dB		
Left								dB		dB		
Right								dB		dB		
Left								dB		dB		
Right								dB		dB		
Left								dB		dB		
Right								dB		dB		
Left								dB		dB		
Right								dB		dB		
Left								dB		dB		
Right								dB		dB		
Left								dB		dB		

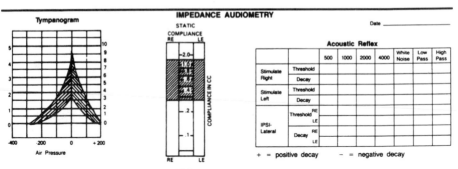

IMPEDANCE AUDIOMETRY

Tympanogram

STATIC COMPLIANCE

Date _____

Acoustic Reflex

		500	1000	2000	4000	White Noise	Low Pass	High Pass
Stimulate Right	Threshold							
	Decay							
Stimulate Left	Threshold							
	Decay							
IPSI-Lateral	Threshold RE LE							
	Decay RE LE							

+ = positive decay   − = negative decay

FIG. 4-4. *Continued*

AUDIOGRAM KEY

	RIGHT EAR (RED)	LEFT EAR (BLUE)	NO RESPONSE RIGHT EAR	LEFT EAR
AIR CONDUCTION UNMASKED MASKED				
BONE CONDUCTION UNMASKED MASKED				

FIG. 4-5. Audiogram key.

Most clinicians evaluate in octaves, so noted on the audiogram. Audiometers test as low as 125 Hz and as high as 8,000 Hz. A few clinical audiometers evaluate as high as 12,000 Hz. Commonly, octaves from 250 Hz to 8,000 Hz are evaluated. Half octaves (750, 1,500, 3,000, or 6,000 Hz) are not routinely tested unless the threshold of the lower octave and next higher octave demonstrates a 20 dB or greater difference. For example, should a 1,000-Hz threshold present at 50 dB HL and a 2,000-Hz threshold present at 85 dB HL, there is a need to determine whether the half octave (1,500 Hz) falls closer to 1,000 Hz or closer to 2,000 Hz.

Evaluating 3,000 Hz and 6,000 Hz is becoming more routine as hearing instrument circuitry becomes more specific in the higher frequencies. This level of testing is especially important to hearing instrument fittings (8). Intensity levels, which will be discussed shortly, have maximum levels of 70 to 110+ dB, each being frequency, decibel standard (dB HL or dB SPL), and equipment specific.

Several testing methods have been suggested regarding the intensity a client should be given, which frequency should be evaluated first, and in which order subsequent frequencies should be given. Although some variability exists within this scope of practice, consistency is the optimum standard. However, standard procedures dictate beginning with the better ear. One standard procedure developed by Hughson-Westlake, the ascending method, presents tones from levels of inaudibility to levels of audibility. A clinical threshold is defined as "the minimal level at which perception is achieved in more than half of the ascents" (8). Deutsch and Richards describe a behavioral threshold as one that is found when a tone is just audible at least 50% of the time (2). The Hughson-Westlake method introduces a new signal to the patient at a level of audibility ascertaining that the patient understands the response task. Beginning at a level of inaudibility, the intensity is increased in 15-dB increments until a response is obtained. Then the intensity is decreased in 10-dB increments until the stimulus is inaudible. Finally, the intensity is increased in 5-dB increments until the stimulus is once again audible. Once this ascent is repeated three times with a response at the same decibel level, a true threshold has been established (8).

It is common practice to begin with 1,000 Hz, which has been established as a frequency with good test/retest reliability. Beyond this point, there is disagreement as to whether the frequencies above or below 1,000 Hz should be presented in subsequent order. Although the clinician can do either, it is important to maintain consistency throughout the evaluation process. Consistency should be maintained within the scope of practice as well as among the clinicians or audiologists on staff. In working with patients of any age, expediency and efficiency are paramount. It is recommended to begin in the first ear at 1,000 Hz and evaluate higher frequencies up to 8,000 Hz (1,000, 2,000, 3,000, 4,000, 6,000, and 8,000 Hz) then to return to 1,000 Hz and evaluate the lower frequencies (1,000, 500, and 250). The frequency procedure should be repeated for the second ear. Each ear should be evaluated separately (9).

The patient should be instructed to respond to pure tone audiometry by raising a hand or finger to indicate a positive response. Some audiologists prefer to use a hand-held response button or switch. The use of the switch sometimes confuses older patients. Older patients often have a longer response time to the pure tone signal. The tone presentation time should range from 500 msec (0.5 sec) to 1,000 msec (1 sec) to lessen the effect of tone duration on the threshold being tested (2). ASHA standards recommend a tone duration of 1 to 2 sec. The time span between the stimuli presentation should be varied but no shorter than the test tone duration (9).

Each clinician must be aware of false-positive and false-negative responses. A response given when no stimulus is presented is a false-positive response. False-positive responses are more likely with a patient who responds to assumed criteria, whereas the person with a more conservative criteria will miss stimuli, resulting in a false-negative response. Both types of responses can result in inaccurate test results. It is often necessary to provide instructions more than once in order to obtain accurate test results (2). The patient should be instructed to respond to the test tone no matter how faint and to cease responding when the test stimuli are no longer present.

Due to IA, a difference between right and left air conduction thresholds of 40 dB or more or a difference between the poorer ear air conduction and the obtained bone conduction threshold of 40 dB or more indicates the need for masking. The better cochlea responds for the poorer ear when the sound crosses through the skull. Narrow band noise is the masking noise of choice for evaluating air and bone conduction audiometry (10).

The headphones must be placed securely over the pinna. Caution must be used when placing the headphones on the patient's ear; a slip of the hand could allow the earphones to hit the ear abruptly, resulting in patient discomfort. Earphones should be sanitized routinely.

BONE CONDUCTION

Bone conduction audiometry determines the cochlear reserve of the patient's auditory system. Bone conduction pathways present with sound directly placed on the mastoid process or the frontal bone to both cochleas. Energy is presented by direct mechanical force to the cochlea, at which point energy is altered to hydraulic energy. The remaining energy pathways occur as they do for previously reported air conduction pathways.

Three modes of bone conduction pathways exist: inertial, compressional, and osseotympanic. Inertial bone conduction is thought to be more effective in the lower frequencies because the skull moves as a whole, with the cochlea and the stapes moving due to suspended ossicles, causing sound to be audible to the cochlea. Compressional bone conduction is considered more effective for the higher frequencies because the skull, especially the forehead, vibrates in an alternately complex fashion. Osseotympanic bone conduction is created by skull vibrations that result in air vibrating in the external auditory canal that in turn stimulates the tympanic membrane. It is felt that bone conduction responses result from a combination of all three bone conduction processes (2).

Frequencies evaluated by bone conduction audiometry differ from air conduction usage because the bone conduction oscillator has limited parameters. The evaluation process may be as low as 125 Hz and as high as 4,000 Hz. Bone conduction oscillators and specific audiometers have lower intensity limits than do air conducting earphones due to harmonic distortion, which occurs mainly in lower frequencies (2). Some systems test only to 60 dB, whereas others may present as high as 70 dB. It is best to review the manufacturer's manuals. Caution must be taken at 250 Hz because it is a less reliable frequency due to calibration limitations; this frequency's longer wavelength may elicit a vibrotactile sensation. These low frequencies are often felt before they are audible, especially with patients who display a more severe or profound hearing loss sensitivity.

Bone conduction audiometry evaluates a smaller range of frequencies than does air conduction audiometry. Again, consistency within one's practice is paramount. Some practices routinely begin at 250 Hz and test to 4,000 Hz, whereas others begin at 500 Hz and test to 4,000 Hz. New practitioners often are taught in basic audiology courses to begin testing for bone conduction at 1,000 Hz, test the higher frequencies, recheck 1,000 Hz, and finally test the lower frequencies. However, field experience proves that beginning at the lower frequencies (250 or 500 Hz) and working to the higher frequencies is efficient and less disconcerting for the patient. Caution must be taken, particularly at high-intensity levels in the lower frequencies, because some patients may perceive an auditory response that is actually a vibrotactile sensation.

ANSI (9) recommends using a continuous tone with a pulsed tone presented only in specific conditions such as with the presence of tinnitus. It is often easier to distinguish between the test tone and tinnitus when the test tone is pulsed. Some audiologists use a descending technique, whereas others use an ascending technique. ASHA recommends beginning at 30 dB HL with an ascending technique. If no response is obtained, the test tone is increased to 50 dB HL. If no response occurs, the decibel level is increased in 10-dB increments until a response occurs. After obtaining a response, the test tone is decreased in 10-dB increments until no response occurs. All final ascending responses are assessed at 5-dB increments. A rule of thumb is "down 10, up five." A threshold is accepted as a true threshold if it is audible 50% of the time. Responses are recorded on the audiogram.

The bone conduction oscillator should be placed on the mastoid process. No earphones should be covering the pinna and ear canals. An exception to this process is made when using masking during bone conduction testing. The procedure for bone conduction masking places the bone conduction oscillator on the mastoid process with the headphones covering the contralateral ear only. The unused earphone rests askew on the head. Early bone conduction literature mentioned placement of the oscillator on either the mastoid or frontal bone (10). Mastoid placement has become the most common for several reasons:

1. The pure tone is more intense at the mastoid when evaluating normal hearing patients (3).
2. The location of the bone conduction oscillator is in the proximity of the ear under test (10).
3. The frontal bone placement requires masking techniques 100% of the time (10).

Due to IA, placing the bone conduction oscillator on the right mastoid process does not indicate that the right cochlea is the only cochlea responding; the response could be obtained from either cochlea because IA for bone conduction occurs at a level as low as 0 dB. This suggests that masking for bone conduction audiometry should be performed 100% of the time, which is quite time consuming. The general rule is to mask for bone conduction audiometry whenever a difference of 15 dB or more occurs between the bone conduction threshold of the better ear and the air conduction threshold of the poorer ear (10).

An occlusion effect (OE), which only occurs in bone conduction testing, happens when placing an earphone on the contralateral ear increases the bone conduction sensitivity below 1,000 Hz. Due to OE, a factor of 5 to 15 is added into the effective masking level (EML) when evaluating bone conduction thresholds (Table 4-3) (10).

Also, based on the bone conduction IA of 0 dB, bone conduction audiometry for a symmetrical sensorineural loss of hearing sensitivity needs to be performed only on one ear. If the test results indicate a 0- to 10-dB difference between the obtained bone conduction threshold and the obtained right or left air conduction threshold, evaluation of both ears for bone conduction audiometry is not necessary. However, if an overly concerned patient questions why both ears were not evaluated, bone conduction for both ears should be evaluated to allay any patient fears regarding the evaluation's validity.

TABLE 4-3. *Occlusion effect*

Study	Frequency (Hz)			
	250	500	1,000	2,000
Huizing (1960)	13.0	15.0	8.0	1.0
Elpern and Naunton (1963)	28.0	20.0	9.0	0.0 (TDH 39 with firm rubber cushion)
Goldstein and Hayes (1965)	19.4	12.6	5.7	1.1
Dirks and Swindeman (1967)	22.9	20.2	8.8	0.5 (MX 41/AR cushion)
Recommended	15	15	10	0

Values are decibel levels.

HEARING IMPAIRMENT TYPES

The degree and type of hearing impairment is based on the relationship between the air and bone thresholds and the level at which they fall on the audiogram. Table 4-4 quantifies degrees of hearing impairment.

As one may discern, there are discrepancies as to the degree of hearing loss, depending on one's reference (3).

Five primary categories of hearing impairment affecting aidable hearing impairments deserve brief description (Fig. 4-6):

Normal: Both air and bone conduction threshold levels fall between 0 and 20 dB with a difference of less than 10 dB between air and bone conduction thresholds.

Conductive: Bone conduction threshold levels fall between 0 and 20 dB with air conduction threshold levels 15+ dB poorer than bone conduction thresholds (e.g., impacted cerumen, otitis media, otosclerosis).

Sensorineural: Both air and bone conduction threshold levels fall below normal limits, with less than a 10 dB difference between them (e.g., presbycusis, noise-induced hearing loss).

Mixed: Both air and bone conduction threshold levels fall below normal limits, with a conductive component displaying a difference of 15 dB or more between the air and bone conduction thresholds (e.g., presbycusis with impacted cerumen or presbycusis with otitis media).

Central auditory processing: This involves not only the degree of loss but the perception of the auditory signal (e.g., auditory discrimination, localization, synthesis, and fusion).

Conductive components indicate a breakdown between the pinna and oval window. Sensorineural components show a breakdown in the cochlea or along the 8th nerve to the brain stem (2).

Patients with low normal hearing impairments may be candidates to be fit for hearing instrument(s), depending on the patient's subjective difficulties. For this type of loss to be aided, word recognition in noise with a +5 signal-to-noise (S/N) ratio and +10 S/N ratio should be evaluated. A +5 S/N ratio presents with the signal

TABLE 4-4. *Degrees of hearing impairment*

Two examples of decibel level of hearing impairment		Hearing impairment
−10–15 dB	0–26 dB	No loss (normal)
16–25 dB		Slight (low-normal)
26–40 dB	27–40 dB	Mild
41–65 dB	41–55 dB	Moderate
	56–70 dB	Moderate severe
66–94 dB	71–90 dB	Severe
96+ dB	91+ dB	Profound

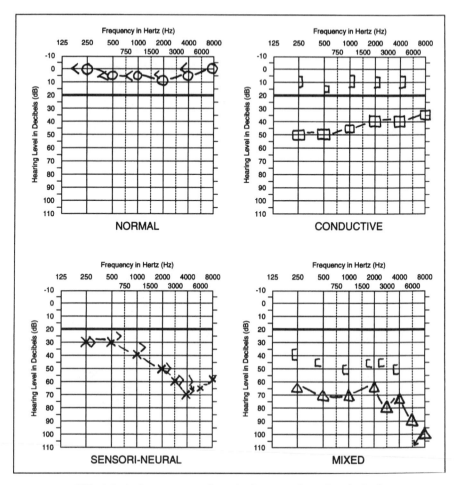

FIG. 4-6. Audiograms: normal, conductive, sensorineural, and mixed.

(speech stimuli) 5 dB louder than the noise. All losses (conductive, mixed, and sonsorineural) are aidable after completion of medical intervention.

Although air and bone conduction threshold levels are good determinants as to the level of hearing impairment, speech audiometry certainly complements the assessment, allowing better determination of patient needs. Speech audiometry uses several types of stimuli, depending on the particular speech test. Specifications call for a flat spectrum during speech audiometry, not a sloped response as used with a MHI or hearing instruments.

Spondee threshold (ST) or speech reception threshold (SRT)	Spondee words

Voice awareness level (VAL)	Continuous discourse
Most comfortable loudness (MCL)	Continuous discourse
Uncomfortable loudness (UCL)	Continuous discourse
Word recognition or speech discrimination	Phonetically balanced words

Speech audiometry may be presented by live voice or recorded voice. Recorded presentation standardized the composition and stimulus material. Intensity levels and speech patterns are more consistent with recorded voice. Caution must be taken with the age or wear of the recorded stimulus. Digitalized stimuli eliminate some of the mechanical difficulties (11). Live voice presentation allows more flexibility in the presentation pace of the stimulus.

The term "word reception threshold" or "Spondee threshold" refers to the material used to obtain the threshold. The SRT is appropriate with Spondee materials. ASHA adopted the terminology "Spondee threshold" to be used in place of SRT, but SRT is commonly used. A starting point for level of presentation of speech audiometry may be established as the pure tone average (PTA) plus 30 dB. Once an SRT is established, another starting point for the MCL level or speech discrimination list is SRT plus 30 dB. A rule of thumb measurement is to begin at 50 dB HL if the patient appears to converse fairly well during the case history or at 70 dB HL if the patient appears to have more difficulty hearing and understanding during the initial interview. These levels are rather conservative, keeping in mind the number of sensorineural losses that may experience tolerance difficulties.

Speech audiometry requires some type of a response from the patient. Response may be verbal, written, or tactile, using picture identification. A verbal or live voice response is much more timely but is subject to error based on the listener's interpretation of the verbal stimuli, the language and articulation level of the patient, and the quality of the equipment used by the clinician. One important positive aspect of the verbal response is the verbal and visual rapport established between the clinician and patient (3).

In speech audiometry, written responses are less likely to be erroneous due to the listener's interpretation. However, scoring is more time consuming than with a verbal response and is affected by the patient's level of written language. Picture identification is more commonly used with children, mentally handicapped people, and stroke patients (3). Speech stimuli should be presented without any visual cues. Each audiometer has a volume unit (VU) meter that monitors the stability of speech signals (12). All speech stimuli should be presented with the VU meter peaking at 0.

The SRT or speech threshold (ST) confirms the validity of the pure tone audiogram (11). ST is the preferred terminology according to the ASHA. The ST and the PTA should be within 10 dB of one another. Depending on the patient's age, auditory ability, and slope of hearing loss, the ST may be poorer than the PTA as in cases of poor discrimination. Conversely, patients with high-frequency hearing impairment may find the PTA poorer than the ST. If poor discrimination may have created elevated STs, a note should be placed on the audiogram. The ST is the lowest level speech stimuli correctly identified 50% of the time.

SRTs or STs are obtained by using Spondee or spondaic words. Spondee words have two syllable with equal emphasis or stress on each syllable, such as "football," "ice cream," or "workshop." Spondee words may be presented with a carrier phrase preceding the stimuli, such as, "Say the word." When using a carrier phrase, the phrase and the Spondee word must peak at 0 on the VU meter. The carrier phrase provides no real advantage (4). The Central Institute for the Deaf in St. Louis, Missouri, compiled a list of these words (Table 4-5) (5).

ASHA standards present an ascending approach to determine a threshold level for speech. This method determines the SRT by beginning at −10 dB (10). A more practical approach would be at a level 10 dB below the obtained PTA. However, current standards have been altered to recommend a simple descending method for use with patients, except for those suspected of pseudohyacusis. Begin by using the measurements of PTA plus 30, 50, or 70 dB HL. Instructions to be given to the patient are provided as follows:

> You will hear a sequence of two-syllable words that are to be repeated verbally to the audiologist. The volume will become softer and softer. However, even at the lower levels if you feel you know what the word is, please take a guess at the word.

ASHA recommends a descending method in 2-dB increments, yet 5-dB increments are acceptable. More audiometers (clinical and portable) can evaluate in 2-dB increments. Chaiklin and Ventry (13) found 5-dB increments to be as valid as previously used 1- or 2-dB increments. An ST is obtained when the Spondee words can be repeated at a level of 50% accuracy.

It is important to remember that the ST is a test to validate the PTA; thus, one need not labor over this evaluation. It is paramount to maintain an expedient evaluation and not to keep the client in a stringent, fatiguing listening situation for long periods of time. The SRT also is the bottom value in determining the range of hearing or dynamic range.

A VAL, speech detection threshold, or speech awareness threshold evaluates a patient's threshold for speech by cold running speech or continuous discourse to

TABLE 4-5. *C.I.D. Auditory Test W-1*

List A		
1. Greyhound	13. Padlock	25. Playground
2. Schoolboy	14. Mushroom	26. Airplane
3. Inkwell	15. Hardware	27. Woodwork
4. Whitewash	16. Workshop	28. Oatmeal
5. Pancake	17. Horseshoe	29. Toothbrush
6. Mousetrap	18. Armchair	30. Farewell
7. Eardrum	19. Baseball	31. Grandson
8. Headlight	20. Stairway	32. Drawbridge
9. Birthday	21. Cowboy	33. Doormat
10. Duckpond	22. Iceberg	34. Hothouse
11. Sidewalk	23. Northwest	35. Daybreak
12. Hotdog	24. Railroad	36. Sunset

Reprinted courtesy of the Central Institute for the Deaf, St. Louis, Missouri.

determine the level of just audible but not necessarily understood speech (4). This section of the speech audiometry evaluation is most often used for clients with profound loss or poor discrimination. Often, a client with poor discrimination may have difficulty with a SRT solely related to discrimination. A VAL determines the threshold by simply stating, "Tell me when you are just able to detect my voice through the headphones."

The MCL gives credence to the belief that a comfortable listening level is related to a hearing instrument's use gain. The MCL uses cold running speech or continuous discourse such as a short speech or declaration. This level may be ascertained using formulas such as the SRT + 30 or PTA + 30. A more interactive way to determine this level is to ask the patient to choose a level of comfort based on two decibel level options. Busy practices often determine a SL, or predetermined MCL. However, using a preset SL does not provide a true MCL for every hearing instrument candidate. Many times a patient, especially one with a sensorineural hearing impairment, displays recruitment, and an actual MCL is extremely important to the hearing instrument fitting; an SL is not always good enough. A low MCL may indicate a hearing instrument candidate with a tolerance to loudness or recruitment.

It is most advantageous to obtain a monaural as well as a binaural MCL. Often the binaural MCL will be approximately 5 dB softer than the monaural MCL. This difference is an important factor in a binaural fitting.

Speech discrimination (also referred to as speech recognition or word recognition) is the speech test most important to the patient. Patients express the most concern about speech discrimination because it effects their ability to communicate effectively. One of the most common case history responses is, "I can hear that the person is speaking to me, but I do not understand the words." Speech discrimination lists, developed in the 1940s, are composed of phonetically balanced words. Phonetically balanced words are single-syllable words that contain phonemic information found in the English language. Each word in the list of 50 is measured in two percentage points. These results provide a score for the amount of speech discrimination or word recognition for each ear as well as a binaural speech discrimination. A binaural speech discrimination may determine binaural fusion capabilities. A score equal to or better than the best ear evaluated suggests binaural amplification. Half lists have proven to be acceptable, with each word providing a 4% score. However, lists using fewer than 25 words have been found to be inconsistent (5). When testing for word recognition, it is important to note which words were obtained in error as a high frequency consonant error, as when a patient responds with "car" for the word "carve." This type of error is common for a high-frequency sensorineural hearing impairment. However, a gross error, as when a patient responds with "rabbit" for the word "down," is of greater concern.

Comprehension is one aspect of understanding speech. A single-syllable word is more difficult to understand than a two-syllable word. Similarly, a four-word sentence is more difficult to understand than a seven-word sentence. The level of understanding is directly related to the amount of information provided.

TABLE 4-6. *C.I.D. Auditory Test W-22*

List 1A

1. An	14. Low	26. You (ewe)	29. None (nun)
2. Yard	15. Owl	27. As	40. Jam
3. Carve	16. It	28. Wet	41. Poor
4. Us	17. She	29. Chew	42. Him
5. Day	18. High	30. See (sea)	43. Skin
6. Toe	19. There (their)	31. Deaf	44. East
7. Felt	20. Earn (urn)	32. Them	45. Thing
8. Stove	21. Twins	33. Give	46. Dad
9. Hunt	22. Could	34. True	47. Up
10. Ran	23. What	35. Isle (aisle)	48. Bells
11. Knees	24. Bathe	36. Or (oar)	49. Wire
12. Not (knot)	25. Ace	37. Law	50. Ache
13. Mew		38. Me	

Reprinted courtesy of the Central Institute for the Deaf, St. Louis, Missouri.

Word recognition is affected by binaural fusion, binaural summation, and degradation. Binaural summation, the comfort level for binaural word-recognition presentation, is 3 to 6 dB better than the monaural level. A degradation effect results when a binaural word recognition score is poorer than the monaural results. Binaurality is affected by localization and word recognition in noise (2). A patient with poor discrimination or word recognition should not be considered unaidable. The clinician should monitor which sounds were missed in the word. For example, a patient with a high-frequency hearing impairment will miss high-frequency consonants, especially when using flat verbal input or the audiometer. It is best to document in writing the errors made by the patient in order to analyze this area of error.

Speech discrimination lists are available from the Central Institute of the Deaf's Auditory Test W-22 (Table 4-6). Word lists also are available that are suitable for a high-frequency hearing loss. The high-frequency lists generally use a vowel that contains sounds with higher frequency emphasis.

MASKING FOR SPEECH AUDIOMETRY

Masking is necessary whenever a conductive component or an asymmetrical loss is present. The procedure is needed for SRT, MCL, and speech discrimination. Masking is generally not used when determining the UCL. As a rule of thumb, masking is used for speech audiometry whenever a difference of 40 dB or more occurs between the SRT or PTA of the better ear and the presentation level (PL) of the poorer ear. The EML is defined by the amount of masking noise necessary to "cover" or mask the better ear from responding for the poorer ear. The EML for speech audiometry is determined by using the following formula:

$$EML = PL - 20 \text{ dB}$$

However, should the patient experience recruitment or a low UCL, the formula may be altered as follows (10):

$$EML = PL - 30 \text{ dB, low TD}$$

UCL has been called many things: threshold of discomfort (TD), tolerance level, or loudness discomfort level (LDL). This level is not merely where sound is "too loud," but where it is "almost certain that dimensions other than the loudness of perceptually abusive sound might elicit the unfavorable response [including] annoyance, harshness, or noisiness, among others" (14). UCL is the ceiling figure in determining the range of hearing or dynamic range (DR):

$$UCL - SRT = DR$$

It is also important to determine the patient's practical dynamic range (UCL 2 MCL). How close is comfortable to uncomfortable? Determining this range is as important to properly fitting a hearing instrument as is determining the DR. The DR for people with no hearing loss is much greater than that for people with sensorineural loss. Setting the maximum power level on a hearing instrument is an essential aspect of fitting a hearing instrument. Establishing a UCL for tones is recommended. However, this process is quite time consuming. Mueller and Bentler recommend an abridged procedure in which testing the UCL at 500 Hz and/or 2,000 or 3,000 Hz using either narrow band noise or warble tones. A method discussed by Hawkins and Schum (4) follows three basic considerations:

1. The patient must be able to make loudness judgements.
2. Clear instructions with categories of loudness must be given to the patient.
3. LDLs or UCLs must be expressed in useful values (insert earphones are ideal).

UCLs expressed in 2-cc values is helpful in selecting the approved saturation sound-pressure level 90 (SSPL90) curve for a hearing instrument. Hawkins stated that "people are happier with a hearing aid that makes speech audible and limits the output below a level of uncomfortable loudness." Because correct output limiting is important for optimal acceptance of the hearing instrument, it deserves more testing time than is routinely given. This evaluation process often is not performed, is overlooked, or is given only fleeting attention. Output trimmers may be placed on the hearing instrument for more versatility and postfitting monitoring of the maximum power output (4).

The TD should be routinely evaluated both unaided and aided because this level may change after the patient has used a hearing instrument (14). Watch for facial expressions when evaluating for TD because the patient often will react with a wince long before a verbal or hand response occurs.

IMPEDANCE AUDIOMETRY

Impedance audiometry is a set of objective measurements based on the transfer of energy from pressure exerted on the tympanic membrane that stimulates the inner ear's hearing mechanism. This procedure shows the amount of space in the middle ear cavity, the presence of fluid in the middle ear, and any disarticulation of the ossicles. It can be used to predict the degree of hearing impairment. This test procedure (in addition to basic audiometry) assists in determining the middle ear function. Being an objective measurement, it is especially helpful in evaluating children and the mentally handicapped.

Tympanometry creates an airtight seal of the ear canal with the probe tip, resulting in a pressure change on the tympanic membrane. More restriction in the middle ear cavity signals less reflection of the acoustic wave. A normal, or type A, tympanogram demonstrates a peak pressure between -100 and $+40$ daPA. Zero daPA is optimal for mobility of the tympanic membrane and hearing mechanism. A type

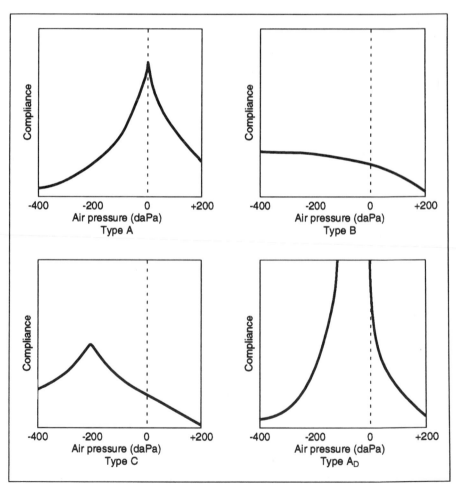

FIG. 4-7. Tympanograms.

B tympanogram has no peak present and appears flat. Middle ear disorders such as fluid in the middle ear cavity present with a type C tympanogram. Tympanograms with a peak pressure lower than -100 daPa display a type C tympanogram. The height of the curve also determines the mobility within the middle ear mechanisms. A stiff system displays a shallow curve, whereas a mobile system creates a taller type A response curve (Fig. 4-7).

Static acoustic immittance measures the acoustic energy in the middle ear cavity. Normal static acoustic immittance occurs from 0.25 cm³ to 2.0 cm³. Levels below normal are considered low acoustic immittance, or very little mobility. Conversely, above normal acoustic immittance results in hypermobile responses.

The stapedius muscle contracts bilaterally with acoustic stimulation of higher intensities. Both ipsilateral and contralateral contractions may be measured. This measurable contraction is based on acoustic immittance changes in the middle ear system and elements associated with the stapedius reflex arc.

The acoustic reflex result measurements are objective and give important information for the hearing instrument fitting. Acoustic reflexes may not be present in sensorineural losses of greater than 60 dB. The greater the hearing impairment, the less chance of obtaining an acoustic reflex. If no conductive component is present, the hearing instrument's gain (power), frequency response, and output (ceiling) may be set either at or lower than the obtained acoustic reflex threshold. This level should be below the point at which sustained muscle contraction occurs, whereas periodic reflexes may occur due to short bursts of energy (15). Although this information assists in hearing instrument fitting, the data should not stand alone in determining the hearing instrument's output.

DISCUSSION OF REHABILITATION PATHS

Although a patient's decision cannot be forced, it certainly may be guided. Well-presented, easy to understand, comprehensive advice affects positively the quality of a patient's rehabilitation. Presenting information and providing recommendations differ greatly from patient to patient. A bedridden 90-year-old in a health-care facility very likely will want only basic information, whereas a 65-year-old retired engineer may want significantly more detail and may have many more questions before ultimately choosing a hearing instrument. However, the clinician should be careful not to plan a patient's rehabilitation course based on a predetermined judgment. As an example, one might assume that one hearing instrument might suffice for the 90-year-old patient even though two would be more appropriate. However, although this patient is bedridden, he or she may receive a large number of visitors and want to communicate with them effectively.

Very often patients misinterpret the statement "there is nothing medically that can be done for your hearing" as "nothing can be done for your hearing." The patient and other interested parties must be made to understand that even after the limits of medical intervention have been reached, hearing instruments may still provide an effective solution to their problem. Binaural amplification should be recommended to all patients with bilateral hearing impairment unless degradation effects or poor binaural fusion exist. The benefits of binaural amplification include better localization skills, better discrimination abilities, better distance hearing (such as in churches and theaters), and optimal functioning in both ears. Whether a patient can or cannot afford two hearing instruments must be the consumer's decision. The audiologist, hearing instrument specialist, and physician must always recommend the optimum course of action for the patient and then allow the patient to decide on the fitting.

VARIABLES

Picture boards and nontraditional responses may be needed when working with children, patients who have sustained a stroke, patients with Alzheimer's disease, or other less responsive patients. As always, the clinician should document any evaluation process that deviates from normal.

As the non–English-speaking population in the United States increases, practices must adjust their evaluation processes to accommodate these people. Too often speech audiometry is not performed due to language limitation. Digital audiometry and available language test batteries assist with this dilemma. It is unfair to require non–English-speaking patients to repeat English words because the evaluator may misinterpret a response given as patients attempt to mimic sounds alien to them.

ARTICULATION INDEX

The AI establishes a patient's speech energy. Mueller and Killion have simplified the complicated ANSI standards for computing AI (16). Mueller and Killion's AI (Fig. 4-8) places 100 dots between 250 and 6,000 Hz. The patient's audiogram is then superimposed on the AI audiogram. The dots above the patient's threshold should be counted and multiplied by 0.01. This AI method places less importance on extreme frequencies, which are not important for speech recognition. This method also examines hearing instrument candidacy by using either a three- (500, 1,000, and 2,000 Hz) or four- (500, 1,000, 2,000, and 4,000 Hz) frequency measurement. Fifty-five dots fall between 500 and 2,000 Hz in a three-frequency measurement, whereas 84 dots fall between 500 and 4,000 Hz in a four-frequency measurement. In either calculation the dots above the obtained threshold should be counted and divided by either 55 or 84, which will provide an AI calculation. If the patient has an unaided AI of 0.80 when using the three-frequency test or 0.70 when using the four-frequency test, the patient is a candidate for being fitted with a hearing instrument. A low unaided word discrimination result does not rule out the necessity for a hearing instrument. A high AI score also does not rule out a hearing instrument fitting. No single test should be relied upon to determine hearing instrument candidacy.

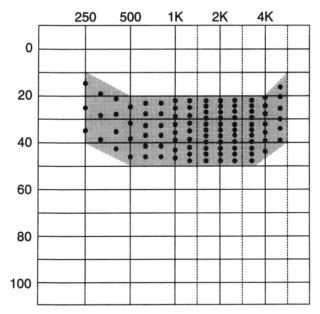

FIG. 4-8. Articulation index. (Reprinted from Mueller G, Bentler R. Measurements of TD: how loud is allowed? *Hear J* 1991;44:19–21.)

Although many variations for measuring AI exist, one must only use methods as described above that are both expedient and valid. AI methods are also used in REM, thereby presenting the patient with a tangible measurement of hearing ability.

No single form or statute for determining hearing instrument candidacy can stand alone. All of the following variables must be established:

Motivation of a client
Degree of hearing impairment
Work environment of the patient
Type of hearing impairment
State of the ear canal
Speech audiometry results
DR
AI

HEARING AID EVALUATION

The term "hearing aid evaluation" (HAE) is not standard. It encompasses different evaluation processes to different audiologists. For some clinicians, HAE describes the entire testing battery (audiologic evaluation, real ear, impedance audiometry, sound field evaluation, and taking the earmold impression), whereas for others it is only the evaluation process after a standard audiologic evaluation, which may include REM, MHI, sound field audiometry, or LDL workups. For now assume that HAE represents the evaluation process after the basic audiologic workup. The components of the step-by-step process are listed as follows:

1. Otoscopic evaluation
2. Otologic workup
3. Audiologic evaluation: (a) pure tone air and bone conduction (bone may be performed after speech audiometry); (b) STs or SRTs; (c) word recognition or speech discrimination; (d) MCL; and (e) UCL
4. Audiologic assessment (review results with patient and significant parties)
5. Master hearing aid or pressure measuring instrument (provide recommendations of treatment and hearing instrument options: monaural vs binaural and hearing instrument style

MASTER HEARING INSTRUMENT

An MHI, or pressure-measuring instrument, is a fitting tool that measures SPL. An MHI allows for a quick and effective demonstration of the benefits of hearing instruments to a patient. Too often the MHA has been promoted as a sales tool because it is the only piece of equipment available to simulate hearing instruments. Unlike 20 or 30 years ago, a hearing instrument can no longer be taken off the shelf and put on a patient. Now that hearing instruments are custom fit, the MHA is necessary to enable patients to experience improved hearing before making a final decision regarding their fitting. The MHA demonstrates increased perception, alters the slope of the speech stimuli more in line with the persons loss (simulating microphone slopes), and demonstrates monaural versus binaural amplification. Although many audiologists have discarded this equipment, it has been found to be a viable tool for demonstrating increased hearing to a patient.

REAL-EAR MEASUREMENT

Probe microphones and REM are used to determine the correct matrix for the hearing instrument, to verify the hearing instrument fitting, to resolve patient complaints, and to troubleshoot the hearing instrument after the actual fitting. All REMs are calculated in dB SPL (17). REM makes the art of fitting hearing instruments more scientific. It offers validity, objective accuracy to hearing instrument fitting, and reliability or repeatability of the evaluation process.

Real-ear equipment is composed of a computer, video screen, sound isolated box for 2-cc coupler measurements, external speaker, and printer. REMs require placement of a probe microphone in the patient's ear canal 8 mm from the tympanic membrane, which measures the hearing instrument's function. The ear canal, concha, and head-resonating characteristics as well as the ear's impedance all affect hearing instrument performance. A measurement was obtained previously using a 2-cc coupler made of hard steel. A 2-cc coupler, being larger than the average ear canal, may increase the dB SPL reaching the tympanic membrane. The 2-cc measurement was determined in the 1940s to approximate an adult ear canal. The average adult ear canal measures 1.2-cc, whereas a child's ear canal measures approximately 0.66 cc with skin and soft cartilage. The 2-cc coupler underestimates low frequencies and accentuates high frequencies (17).

Patients like REM because it is tangible and objective and is a measurement that they can visualize. Probe microphone measurements provide data regarding resonating characteristics that occur in an ear canal. The patient's audiogram is plugged into the equipment from which a target-fitting response is calculated. Even minor changes to the hearing instrument can be visualized by both audiologist and patient (17).

The real-ear unoccluded response (REUR) is found by inserting the probe microphone, held in place with silicone tubing, into the ear canal 8 mm from the tympanic membrane. The real-ear unoccluded response measures the resonating characteristics (diameter, length, and impedance) of the ear canal, tympanic membrane, and concha in dB SPL without any hearing instrument in the ear canal. A primary response peak should be seen at 2,700 Hz with 17 dB of sound. It is this primary peak that becomes altered with a hearing instrument in place. A secondary response peak occurs between 4,000 and 5,000 Hz with an increase of 12 to 14 dB (17).

A second measurement should be given, which is called the real-ear occluded response (REOR). The hearing instrument should be placed in the ear canal in the "off" position. The amount of decibels lost may be determined by inserting the hearing instrument.

The real-ear aided response (REAR) measures the hearing instrument with gain flowing through the hearing instrument. This measurement is expressed in absolute dB SPL with a 70- or 90-dB 1,000-Hz stimulus determining comfort levels. Identical hearing instruments on different patients respond differently.

The real-ear saturation response (RESR) measures the hearing instrument using a high input signal and evaluates the maximum output level in dB SPL. This SSPL90 reading should be below the patient's UCL and must allow for an adequate dynamic range. Also, normal speech should not saturate the hearing instrument (17). This measurement is extremely important because if the patient leaves the office with this level too high, an unhappy patient will return.

The real-ear insertion response (REIR) calculates the difference in decibels between the real-ear unoccluded response (REUR) and the REAR for the entire frequency response. The real-ear insertion gain is the closest to traditional functional gain response, showing aided versus unaided response in sound field. This response is compared with the target fitting.

The real-ear results are ultimately tested by the patient: Does the patient like how the hearing instrument is sounding even with the ultimate match to a target response for that individual? REMs verify the hearing instrument fitting at all frequencies across the hearing instrument's spectrum and are less time consuming than traditional sound field-aided versus -unaided information. A determination may be made as to whether the complaint is due to the patient's hearing system or hearing instrument.

SOUND FIELD AUDIOMETRY

Sound field audiometry places signals in a room environment with the use of speakers rather than earphones. Most audiometers need to be coupled with an amplifier to be appropriately calibrated for sound field. This environment must be calibrated appropriately just as the evaluation equipment does.

The sound field evaluation process varies among practitioners as well as the terminology for the test procedures. Basic audiometric procedures may be performed in sound field, especially when working with children or adults with earphone intolerance. The ASHA tutorial on sound field measurement as reported by Rochlin (18) makes the following recommendations:

1. Warbled pure tones or narrow bands of noise are the stimuli to be used.
2. Warble tone characteristics should include sinusoidal or triangular waveforms, small frequency deviations, and large modulation rates.
3. Patient placement should be a consistent distance from the loudspeaker to assure test signal consistency at the pinna. The azimuth must be consistent at 0, 45, or 90 degrees.
4. Warble tone calibration should be routine through electroacoustic measurements with published normative value data.

Sound field aided testing should be performed with frequencies from 250 to 6,000 Hz to evaluate functional gain. Functional gain is the difference between aided and unaided thresholds or speech audiometry in the sound field. Sound field testing is a subjective, behavioral response.

Sound field testing encompassed the HAE of 92% of those surveyed and included word recognition in noise, measurements of functional gain, and a check of thresholds with collapsed canals. Rochlin reported that most audiologists use a 90 degree azimuth for speaker placement and indicated that the speaker placement was dependent on the procedure under test (18). Pure tones used in sound field may create standing waves. Sound field testing uses a variety of stimuli, lacks standardization, and requires consistent calibration methods.

The term "hearing aid evaluation" has been used for the antiquated procedure of trying three to four different hearing instruments on a patient in the sound field. Each instrument is evaluated with pure tones and speech audiometry to determine which hearing instrument is most appropriate. In today's marketplace, this is not only impractical but costly (both in money and in time).

Manufacturers cannot afford to make several custom-made products for a particular client, knowing that only one instrument will be retained. Hearing instruments are currently fit by prescription matrices or target gains based on formula methods. Based on the particular prescriptive method, a target is prescribed that may be checked as previously mentioned by REM. In sound field, speech audiometry, and pure tones (caution must be given to standing waves), warble tones or narrow band noise may be used to determine the parameters of a particular hearing instrument. The evaluation process may be presented in the aided condition at the patient's functional gain and compared with unaided parameters. The process may include thresholds for narrow band noise or warble tones as well as speech audiometry in quiet or noise:

1. Aided sound field thresholds should use narrow band noise or warble tone at 500 to 6,000 Hz; 250 Hz may be evaluated, but if the hearing instrument has little gain at 250 Hz, then no improvement would be suspected.
2. Aided sound field speech audiometry should include (a) SRT, (b) word recognition in quiet and noise, (c) uncomfortable loudness (if the limits of the sound field system will allow), and (d) MCL
3. Steps 1 and 2 should be repeated in an unaided state.

The patient should not turn the volume control of the hearing instrument(s) too low or too high. A level must be achieved between these two variables at functional gain. Most conversation occurs at −5 to +5 dB S/N ratio. Older patients often require a better S/N ratio than normal listeners.

Binaural amplification should always be recommended for bilateral losses unless a medical difficulty or central deafness causes a binaural degradation effect. The output of the hearing instrument must be kept below the UCL. Sound quality for good listening is found within a hearing instrument when low-frequency sound levels are perceptually balanced with high-frequency sound levels.

Some practitioners feel that the HAE is an ongoing process of determining need(s) as well as each individual's reaction to real-life situations, whereas others feel that sound field-aided versus -unaided responses in addition to REM indicates the acceptable or unacceptable deviations (4).

REFERENCES

1. Yantis P. Puretone air conduction threshold testing. In: Katz J, ed. *Handbook of audiology.* 4th ed. Baltimore: Williams & Wilkins; 1994;97–108.
2. Deutch L, Richards A. *Elementary hearing science.* Newton, MA: Allyn & Bacon; 1979.
3. Martin F. *Introduction to audiology.* 3rd ed. Englewood Cliffs, NJ: Prentice Hall; 1986.
4. Hawkins D, Schum D. LDL measures: an efficient use of clinic time? *Am J Clin Pract* 1991;1:8–10.
5. American Academy of Otolaryngology Committee on Hearing and Equilibrium and the American Council of Otolaryngology Committee on the Medical Aspects of Noise. *JAMA* 1979;241:2055–2059.
6. Killion M, Wilber L, Gudmundsen G. Insert earphones for more interaural attenuation. *Hear instrum* 1985;36:34–36.

7. Killion M. New insert earphones for audiometry. *Hear Instrum* 1984;35:28–46.
8. Carhart R, Jerger J. Preferred method for clinical determination of pure-tone thresholds. *J Speech Hear Disord* 1959;24:330–345.
9. American Speech and Hearing Association, Committee on Audiometric Evaluation. Guidelines for Manual Pure Tone Threshold Audiometry. *ASHA* 1978;20:297–301.
10. Larson Donaldson L. Masking: practical applications of masking principles and procedures. Michigan: National Institute for Hearing Instrument Studies; 1988.
11. American Speech and Hearing Association. Guideline for determining threshold level for speech. *ASHA* 1988;30:85–89.
12. Wilbur, L. Calibration, Puretone, speech and noise signals. In: Katz J, ed. *Handbook of audiology.* 4th ed. Baltimore: Williams & Wilkins; 1994:73–94.
13. Chaiklin J, Ventry I. Spondee threshold measurement: a comparison of 2 and 5 dB methods. *J Speech Hear Disord* 1964;29:47–59.
14. Mueller G, Bentler R. Measurements of TD: how loud is allowed? *Hear J* 1994;47:10–44.
15. Northern J, Gabbard S. The acoustic reflex. In: Katz J, ed. *Handbook of audiology.* 4th ed. Baltimore: Williams & Wilkins; 1994:300–316.
16. Berger K. Some objective guidelines for determining hearing aid candidacy. *Hear J* 1991;44:19–21.
17. Northern J. Real ear measurement. Acapulco, Mexico: Beltone Video Library; 1994. Hearing as a function of age.
18. Rochlin G. Status of sound field audiometry among audiologists in the United States. *J Am Acad Audiol* 1993;4:59–68.

HEARING AIDS: A MANUAL FOR CLINICIANS,
edited by Robert A. Goldenberg
Lippincott–Raven Publishers, Philadelphia © 1996

C H A P T E R   ✦ 5 ✦

How Hearing Aids Work

Joel M. Mynders

West Chester, Pennsylvania

Key Points

Hearing aid anatomy • use of different circuits for special needs • description of batteries and their use • how earmolds and case shells work • how hearing aid function is measured.

Hearing aids work by collecting and electronically boosting sound (speech, music, or any other sounds) from the environment. This chapter addresses the fundamental aspects of an amplifier, physical style differences in hearing aids, circuit option differences, hearing aid batteries, the role of earmolds and case shells in the function of hearing aids, and the ways to measure a hearing aid electroacoustically to determine if it is working.

The most basic hearing aid amplifier works in response to an input signal, which is sound of any type, that hits the microphone. The microphone then transduces that sound to electrical current. This current passes into the amplifier circuit, which increases the incoming sound. This increased sound, in turn, passes onto the receiver (speaker), which transduces the electrically increased sound into sound waves again (1). Figure 5-1 shows the flow.

The range of components involved in hearing aids includes some or all of the following: input transducers, which are microphones, tele-coils and audio input sockets; output transducers, which are the hearing aid's receiver or speaker; the power supply, which is batteries; amplifiers, which may include preamplifiers, circuit limiters, signal-processing circuits, monitoring circuits, filtering circuits, programming circuits, memory circuits, etc.; variable resistors, which are present as trimpots for audiologic adjustment; and patient controls, which are volume controls, tone switches, directional microphone switches, telephone switches, off/on controls, and remote controls. The location of these components is shown in Fig. 5-2.

Among the available controls are the telephone coil and the remote control. The telephone coil allows the patient to switch from collecting sound through the hear-

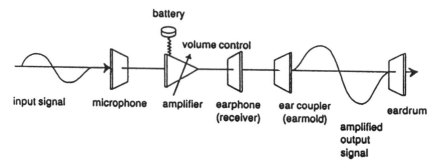

FIG. 5-1. Flow diagram of a hearing aid. (Reprinted from Sandlin RE, ed. *Hearing instrument science and fitting practice*. Livonia, MI: National Institute of Hearing Instruments, 1985; with permission.)

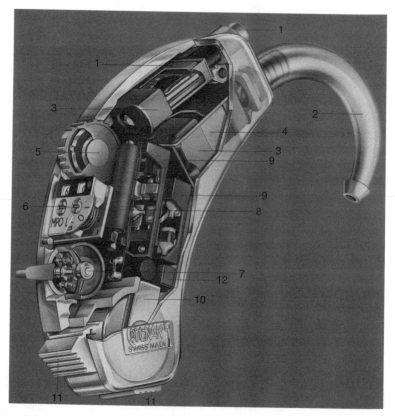

FIG. 5-2. Hearing aid cross-section (courtesy Phonak, Inc., Naperville, IL).1, microphone; 2, tone hook; 3, transducer suspension system; 4, high-performance receiver; 5, volume control wheel; 6, audio programmer; 7, 3-mode switch (M, microphone only; MT, microphone and telecoil; T, telecoil only.); 8, telecoil; 9, amplifier coils; 10, batter contacts; 11, on-off switch; 12, audio-input.

ing aid's microphone to using an induction coil. The induction coil, a small rod wrapped with fine copper wire, responds to magnetic rather than acoustic signals. These magnetic signals are transduced to the amplifier, where they are increased in strength and then sent to the receiver as a louder telephone signal. The telephone coil helps eliminate feedback and the unwanted background sounds while listening on the phone.

Remote control devices, a fairly new patient control in hearing aids, send operational signals to digital programmable hearing aids that increase or decrease loudness, change frequency response, change signal-processing function, turn the aids on or off, and activate or deactivate the telecoil. Figure 5-3 illustrates three different hearing aid remote controls. Because each remote control device is specific to a particular hearing aid design, they are not interchangeable. Remote controls are usually found in more sophisticated and expensive hearing aids.

Hearing aids differ in physical appearance as a result of both style and operation (2). It is important to note that today all hearing aids do not look alike or work alike. The names of the wearing styles are self-descriptive: in-the-ear (ITE), accounting for at least 60% of hearing aids now worn; behind-the-ear (BTE), accounting for 12% to 14% of hearing aids now worn; in-the-canal (ITC), accounting for 10% of hearing aids now worn; completely-in-the-canal (CIC), currently accounting for 8% to 9% of hearing aids now worn, but representing the fastest growing type of hearing aid style; eyeglass hearing aids, accounting for only 0.5% of hearing aids now worn; and body aids, which are worn on the chest and account for only 0.2%. Figure 5-4 shows samples of body, ITE, BTE, ITC. and CIC styles of hearing instruments.

In addition to these wearing style differences, clinicians may encounter two other physical differences: the presence or absence of a volume control or the presence of a remote control. Most hearing aids will have a patient-operated volume control. However, in some hearing aids the the circuitry adjusts up and down electronically. Figures 5-5 and 5-6 show ITE hearing aids in and out of the ear. The volume control is clearly visible in Fig 5-5. In Fig. 5-6 it is absent. The second physical difference of some hearing aids is the presence of a remote control. Some hearing aids that use remote controls do not work without them (Fig. 5-3). The clinician and the patient work together to determine the hearing aid's style and patient controls.

The subject of circuit choice now available to audiologic hearing aid clinicians is complex. A recent tally of hearing aid models available showed more than 600 listed. The *1994 Annual Directory of the Hearing Journal* reported 62 companies and brand names engaged in hearing aid manufacture. Furthermore, there are multiple hearing aid technologies. The demographics underscore the need for a simplified hearing aid circuit categorization for clinicians. Although no professional organization is developing an agreement on these categories, the following five circuit categories are offered as a simple generic list: linear circuits, traditional compression circuits, adaptive compression circuits, automatic signal processor (ASP)

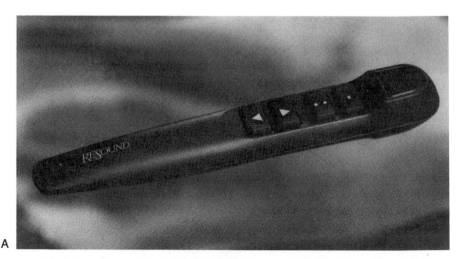

FIG. 5-3. Remote control devices used with hearing aids (courtesy Maico Hearing Instruments, Minneapolis, MN; ReSound Corp., Redwood City, CA; and Widex Hearing Aid Co., Long Island City, NY).

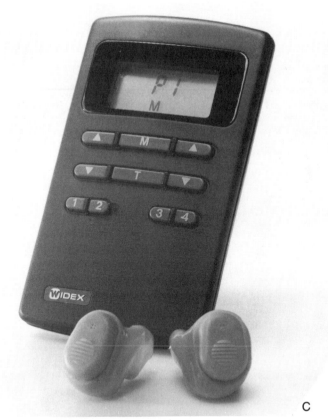

FIG. 5-3. *Continued.*

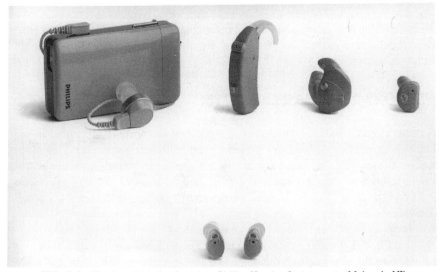

FIG. 5-4. Hearing aid styles (courtesy Philips Hearing Instruments, Mahwah, NJ).

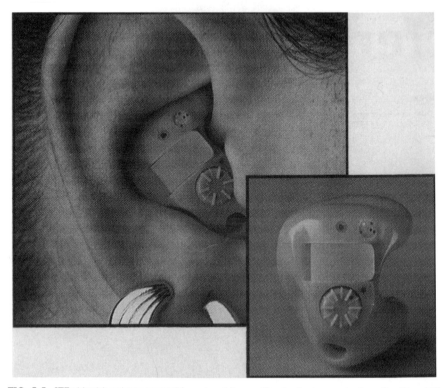

FIG. 5-5. ITE aid with volume control (courtesy Marcon Hearing Instruments, Inc., Hopkins, MI).

K-Amp and filtering circuits, and digital programmable circuits. For those seeking greater detail on the electronics of specific circuit designs, the individual laboratories should be contacted.

CATEGORY 1. LINEAR CIRCUITS

A linear circuit amplifies what enters the microphone without changing the signal beyond increasing its loudness (Fig. 5-7) (3). All linear circuits have an output limit above which the increased signal will not go. At the output limit, the hearing aid is in saturation and the amplified sound distorts. In 1993, 75% of all hearing aids fitted had linear circuits. Linear circuits amplify both speech and background sounds at the same level.

A schema or flow chart provides an easy method for comparing circuit differences. See Fig. 5-8 for a linear circuit schema. Not all linear circuits are basic. Figure 5-9 shows the schema for a three-channel linear hearing aid design that allows

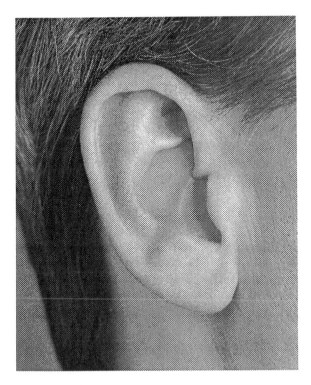

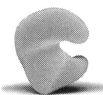

FIG. 5-6. ITE aid without volume control (courtesy Rexton Hering Instruments, Plymouth, MN).

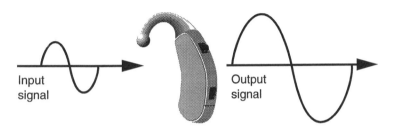

FIG. 5-7. A perfect amplifier. (Reprinted from Sandlin RE, ed. *Hearing instrument science and fitting practice.* Livonia, MI: National Institute of Hearing Instruments, 1985; with permission.)

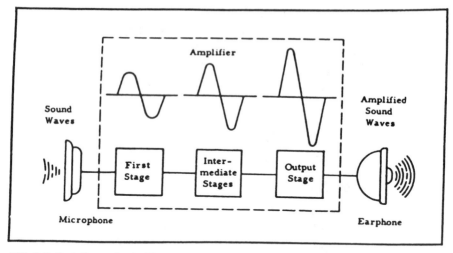

FIG. 5-8. Basic linear circuit. (Reprinted from Staab WJ. *Hearing aid handbook*. Blue Ridge Summit, PA: Tab Books; 1978; with permission.)

for significantly greater adjustment by the hearing aid clinician for the individual patient. Most linear circuits have one or more trimmers for adjustment.

CATEGORY 2. TRADITIONAL COMPRESSION CIRCUITS

A traditional compression circuit softens some of the incoming sounds. Generally these circuits work like a linear circuit in that they make incoming sounds louder. However, compression circuits also contain monitoring circuits that reduce the gain and/or output when a certain loudness level is reached. The compression function is automatic and occurs in milliseconds. The three types of traditional

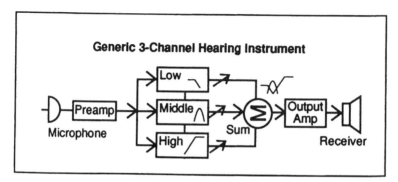

FIG. 5-9. An adjustable linear circuit (courtesy Argosy Electronics, Inc., Eden Prairie, MN).

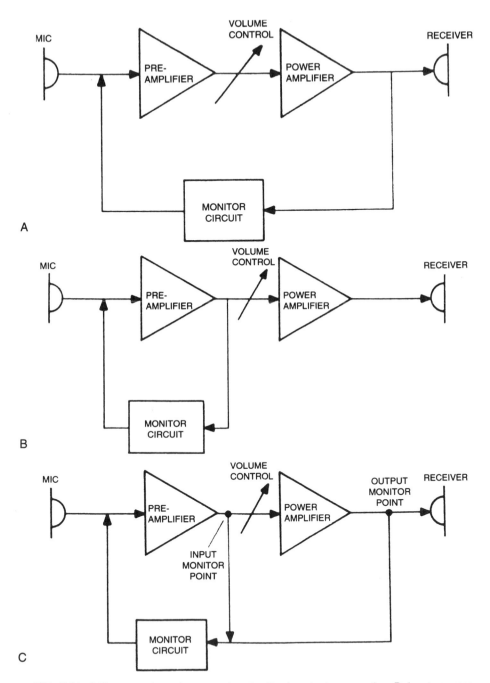

FIG. 5-10. Different traditional compression circuits. **A:** output compression; **B:** input compression; and **C:** input and output compression. (Reprinted from Pollack MC. *Amplification for the hearing impaired.* 3rd ed. New York: Grune & Stratton; 1988.)

compression circuitry are: (a) output compression, which reduces the sound at the output stage of amplification; (b) input compression, which allows the patient to set the level at which compression occurs by setting the volume control; and (c) a combination input/output compression circuit (4). Figure 5-10 illustrates the differences in these circuit designs.

Many patients who use these circuits report hearing a pumping sound when compression occurs. Other patients report that they do not hear as well when sound is compressed. Because compression circuitry is not standardized from laboratory to laboratory, it is difficult to compare and analyze circuit differences. Also, literature on clinical effectiveness of compression hearing aids is sparse.

CATEGORY 3. ADAPTIVE COMPRESSION CIRCUITS

Adaptive compression circuits were developed after engineers and speech scientists recognized that there are temporal differences in loud unwanted sound. Some loud sounds are of short duration and high impact level and others are of longer duration and lower sound pressure. The adaptive compression circuits differentiate between the incoming loud sounds and then compress those sounds differently. This differentiation task occurs in the circuit's monitoring part. This circuitry analyzes incoming sounds and makes electronic choices about how amplification is modified, making it an advanced signal processor (4). Figure 5-11 is a schematic representation of an adaptive compression circuit.

CATEGORY 4. ASP K-AMP AND FILTERING CIRCUITS

This category includes all the nondigital, programmable hearing aids that perform more advanced signal processing than the preceding three categories. The clearest description of the variable circuit designs is the block diagram shown in Fig. 5-12 (5).

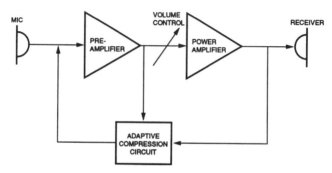

FIG. 5-11. Schematic diagram of an adaptive compression aid. (Reprinted from Pollack MC. *Amplification for the hearing impaired.* 3rd ed. New York: Grune & Stratton; 1988.)

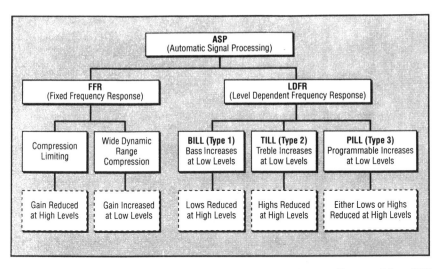

FIG. 5-12. Outline of recommended classification system for ASP type. (Reprinted from Killion MC, Staab WJ, Preeves DA. Classifying automatic signal processors. *Hear Instrum* 1990;4, with permission.)

An ASP hearing aid circuit monitors the incoming sounds and then electrically changes or alters those sounds in frequency, intensity, or time. These circuits were designed to create more noise suppression than previous circuits. Before the invention of ASP circuits, users often complained that the amplified noise overpowered the speech signals that they wanted to hear.

The classic ASP circuit functions to make soft sounds louder, to make loud sounds softer by compression, and, finally, to reduce the low-frequency amplifica-

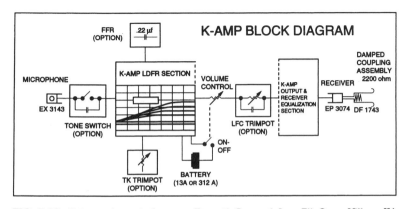

FIG. 5-13. K-Amp schematic (courtesy Etymotic Research Inc., Elk Grove Village, IL).

tion in the presence of different levels of noise. The classic ASP circuit design changes gain, output, and frequency response in changing acoustic environments automatically. Other ASP circuits are often fitted without volume controls because the circuitry performs an automatic volume control function (6).

The K-Amp differs from the classic ASP and other circuit designs in that it has a built in sensor that detects and amplifies only quiet sounds and is acoustically transparent for loud sounds. Gain for loud sounds is available but generally not necessary. Recent versions of the K-Amp design incorporate adaptive compression as well. This circuit design includes a low-battery warning circuit that generates a low "motor-boating" sound that increases in loudness and beeping rate as the voltage drops. Figure 5-13 shows a K-Amp schema.

CATEGORY 5. DIGITAL PROGRAMMABLE CIRCUITS

Digital programmable circuits function to program and not to perform signal processing. The signal-processing advances of these circuits are accomplished through analog circuitry. Pure digital hearing aids will be available in the near future.

Digital programmable hearing aids look like other hearing aids but differ greatly in their use of computer hardware and software programming. Figure 5-14 shows a

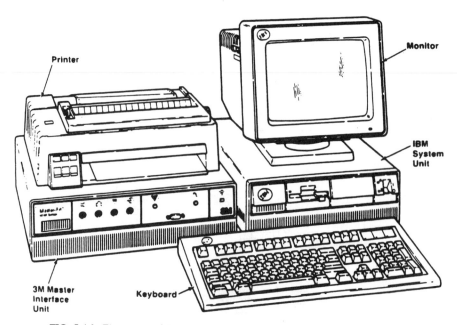

FIG. 5-14. The original 3-M system (courtesy 3-M Hearing Health, Eagan, MN).

personal computer and interface system used with one of the digital programmable instruments.

The improved precision of adjustability enhances patient benefit from these circuit designs. Note that there is not a single uniform circuit with digital programmable instruments. The circuit designs and signal processing goals all differ. Figure 5-15 provides a schema of the 3-M digital programmable hearing aids, demonstrating the increasing complexity of circuit designs. All 3-M programmable hearing instruments are a two-channel design. As indicated in the block diagram, the BTE uses microphone, telecoil, or direct audio input, whereas the ITE uses microphone input only. The input stage contains a programmable microphone-limiting adjustment that functions as a transient remover and also provides overload protection. After this variable-gain input stage, the signal is divided into a low-pass and a high-pass channel. The programmable crossover frequency defines the dividing point between the low-pass and high-pass channels. Each channel contains an independent compression circuit with variable AGC threshold and AGC release time.

The maximum power output and gain in each channel are also programmable. These various parameters can be independently adjusted in each of the eight programs of 3-M instruments. This programming flexibility affords the opportunity to provide a variety of hearing aid responses, differing in frequency shaping and compression characteristics within the same instrument for use in various listening environments.

Figure 5-16 shows the block diagram for the ReSound digital programmable hearing aids. Note the differences from the 3-M design. The arrows in the bottom half of the figure indicate the programmable parameters. Selecting circuitry is the

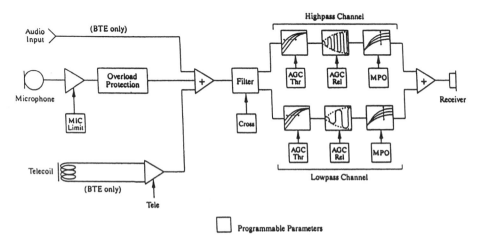

FIG. 5-15. 3-M block diagram (courtesy 3-M Hearing Health, Eagan, MN).

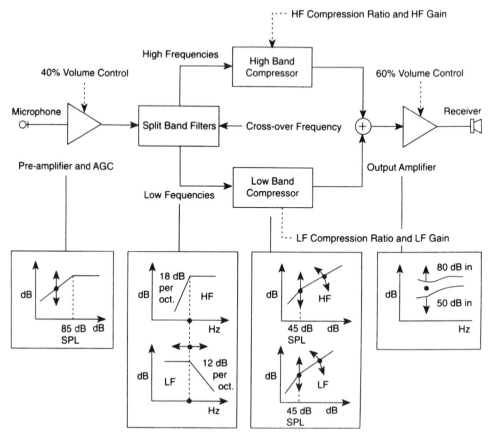

FIG. 5-16. Block diagram of ReSound's sound processing (courtesy ReSound Corp., Redwood City, CA).

most complex task for hearing aid clinicians. The newer technologies are more interactive and flexible than the older hearing aid technologies.

HEARING AID BATTERIES

To non–hearing aid personnel who have contact with hearing aid patients, batteries are a focal point. Hearing aids use batteries that have to be changed regularly. At present, there are three physical battery types: button cells, cylindrical cells, and nickel-cadmium cells. Figures 5-17 and 5-18 show button cells. Figure 5-19 shows a cylindrical cell.

The button cells are the most prevalent type of battery currently used. Different hearing aids use different battery types. These different types are described by a

MS76B

Specifications

System:	Silver Oxide
Voltage:	1.5
Diameter/Width:	.455"
Height:	.210"
Capacity:	180mAh
Primary Usage:	Photo, Electronics

FIG. 5-17. Button cell (courtesy Duracell, USA, Bethel, CT).

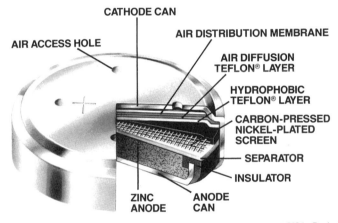

FIG. 5-18. Cross-section of a zinc-air button cell (courtesy Duracell, USA, Bethel, CT).

MN1500

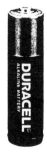

FIG. 5-19. A cylindrical cell (courtesy Duracell, USA, Bethel, CT).

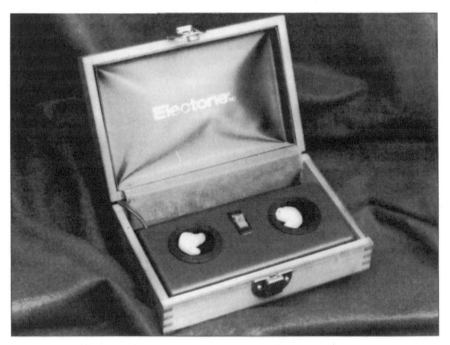

FIG. 5-20. Attractive, easy-to-use charging system (courtesy Electone, Inc., Longwood, FL).

size number and chemical make-up usually represented by letters before or after the size number. The most common sizes are #675, #13, #312, #230 and #10A. The chemical names are mercury, zinc-air, silver oxide, alkaline, lithium, and nickel-cadmium. Each of these chemical compounds may cause voltage differences that result in hearing aid performance differences. The battery size number alone is not enough to assure effective amplification for a given hearing aid.

The question of battery life in different hearing aids requires specific information. Generalizations about hours of battery life do not work. The range of battery life is 45 to 2,000 hours, depending on the circuitry, battery size, and amount of input sound processed by the hearing aids.

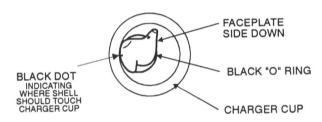

FIG. 5-21. The charger position for recharging (courtesy Electone, Inc., Longwood, FL).

Nickel-cadmium batteries are most commonly used with a recharger. A charge of 8 to 10 hours will give 16 to 20 hours of usage. Figures 5-20 and 5-21 show a hearing aid recharger.

EARMOLDS AND CASE SHELLS

Apart from the physical and electrical aspects of how hearing aids work, one must also examine the various acoustical aspects. The major element in hearing aid fittings acoustically is the earmold or the caseshell.

An earmold is the individually fabricated ear insert that sits in the pinna and canal to channel amplified sound down to the eardrum (7). A case shell is the individually fabricated hearing aid case molded to the contours of the patient's ear. The electronic components are then implanted into this case shell.

The earmold provides an acoustic seal, couples the hearing aid to the ear, secures behind the ear aids on the outer ear, acoustically modifies the response of the aids for fine tuning, helps to provide comfortable fit for hours of use, and allows for an aesthetically acceptable fit to the patient. The functions of the case shell are almost the same except for the retention of the aid on the ear because all shells are in the ear at one level or another.

Earmolds are used with BTE, eyeglass, and body-type hearing aids. They are not used with ITE, ITC, and CIC instruments. These last three types all use the case shell. The mold and the case shell of hearing aids perform the role of an acoustic coupler.

Although the majority of hearing aids now fitted do not use earmolds, knowledge of earmolds and their role in hearing aid fittings is still essential. The hearing aid literature is rich with articles on earmold effect differences. The two goals the hearing aid clinician has in fitting earmolds are physical comfort and acoustic modification of the patient's fit. There are many ways in which the clinician can accomplish these goals. For a complete description of options, the reader is referred elsewhere (7).

Figure 5-22 illustrates some of the options available when considering patient comfort. Although there are many different mold styles for specific applications, this drawing shows three general styles of earmolds the clinician will encounter. Because many of today's BTE instrument fittings are power units, earmold choices to prevent and reduce feedback are indicated and available.

The second goal of fitting earmolds is acoustic modification (Fig. 5-23). Earmold research showed that it is possible to acoustically adjust a hearing aid's response by the three methods shown in Fig. 5-24. The earmold selection process has four parts. First, the clinician must help choose the physical shape or design of the earmold. This choice is dictated by (a) the shape of the concha bowl and canal, (b) the patient's manual dexterity, and (c) the power of the hearing aid circuit. Second, the clinician must select acoustical modification; earmold acoustics allow significant modification of the signals sent to the ear. Third, the clinician must select the

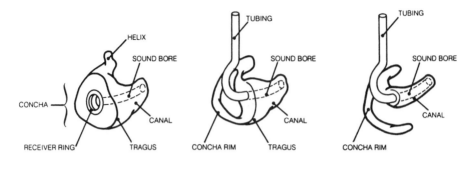

TYPICAL STANDARD MOLD   **TYPICAL SKELETON MOLD**   **TYPICAL NON-OCCLUDING MOLD**

FIG. 5-22. Basic earmold types. (Reprinted from Mynders JM, ed. *Custom earmold manual.* 5th ed, revised. Ambridge, PA: Microsonic; 1994; with permission.)

actual material from which the earmolds will be fabricated. The choices of materials are based on the firmness of the patient's ear, the existence of allergic conditions, and the possible presence of whistling or feedback. The fourth and final step in earmold selection is the tubing choice. There are multiple choices here. Horn theory and reverse horn theory are controlled by the tubing selection (Fig. 5-25).

In musical acoustics it has long been known that the "belling" of a tube will enhance a high-frequency signal passing through that tube. The reverse is also true in that the narrowing of the end of a tube will reduce the high-frequency components (3).

With many of today's hearing instruments reproducing high-frequency signals up to 7,000 to 9,000 Hz, it is particularly important that the tube and earmold not restrict the resonance in the sound channel and cut off high frequencies. With these instruments, incorporating a horn of some type is critical to achieving a successful fitting. In some cases, audiograms show a slope upward in the higher frequencies

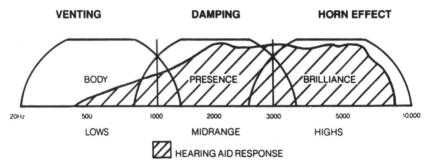

FIG. 5-23. Control areas of earmold acoustics. (Reprinted from Mynders JM, ed. *Custom earmold manual.* 5th ed, revised. Ambridge, PA: Microsonic; 1994; with permission.)

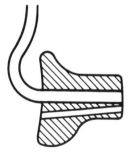 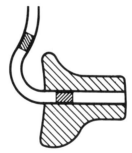 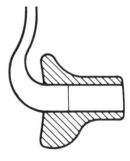

VENTING
- Non-Occluded
  Physical Options
- Parallel Vent
- Diagonal Vent
- External Canal Vent
- P.V.V.
- S.A.V.

DAMPERS
- Lamb's Wool
- Knowles Acoustic
  Dampers
- Sintered Steel
  Inserts
- Damped Earhooks

HORN EFFECTS
- Acoustic Modifier
- Belled Bore
- Horn Bore
- Libby Horns
- C.F.A. Molds
- Wide Range Mold

FIG. 5-24. Acoustic options in earmolds venting-damping-horn effects. (Reprinted from Mynders JM, ed. *Custom earmold manual.* 5th ed, revised. Ambridge, PA: Microsonic; 1994; with permission.)

and need to be reduced instead of enhanced. In these cases the reverse horn must be used.

In discussions of the role of earmolds and case shells in how hearing aids work, the area of impression taking is crucial. Impression taking now falls into two categories: standard impressions used for most earmolds and ITE aids and the deep-canal impressions needed for CIC and peritympanic-type instruments. The process of impression taking is illustrated in Fig. 5-26. The effectiveness of all hearing aid fittings hinges on the clinician's impression technique.

The second category of impression process is the deep canal technique. In Holland, Philips developed a new technique, materials, and some hardware to take a whole impression of the auditory canal up to the tympanic membrane. This technique requires special training. The CIC hearing aids do not go to the same canal depth as the Philips X-P instruments. To observe the difference, see Fig. 5-27.

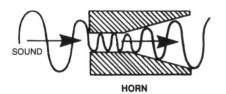 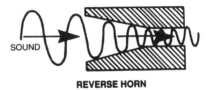

HORN   **REVERSE HORN**

FIG. 5-25. Horn and reverse horn effect. (Reprinted from Mynders JM, ed. *Custom earmold manual.* 5th ed, revised. Ambridge, PA: Microsonic; 1994; with permission.)

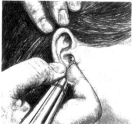

STEP 1
A cotton or foam block is an ABSOLUTE NECESSITY when using the syringe. Set a tight block just past the second bend. Foam blocks MUST be compressed to insure proper results. Be sure to use the correct size foam block even though it may appear to be larger in diameter than the ear canal.

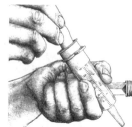

STEP 2
Mix the impression material according to instructions and place in the barrel of the syringe. The quicker you can use the material the better the impression.

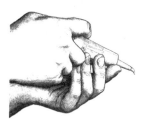

STEP 3
Insert the plunger and gently push the material into the nozzle to remove air pockets.

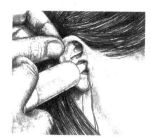

STEP 4
Place the nozzle into the canal and fill the canal.

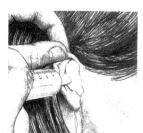

STEP 5
As the material fills the canal, slowly withdraw the syringe and fill the helix and concha areas completely. Then cover the tragus.

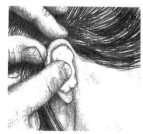

STEP 6
When the external ear has been filled completely, press your finger GENTLY in the concha and helix areas. BE CAREFUL NOT TO PRESS HARD AS IMPRESSION WILL DISTORT.

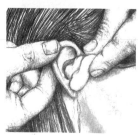

STEP 7
Allow a FULL 10 MINUTES of curing time before removing. The impression can be distorted if removed too soon. To remove, gently press ear away from the impression. Remove helix curl slightly. Bring impression straight out while holding thread. Take your time. Don't strain the impression with a long steady pull.

HELPFUL TIPS FOR BETTER IMPRESSIONS
- If the client wears glasses or dentures, make sure these are in place while taking the impression.
- NEVER flatten or smooth out the finished impression with the palm of your hand while impression material is in the client's ear.
- Ask your client to talk and chew after the impression material is in place. This is to help assure a comfortable fitting custom earmold which will not unseat when the jaw muscles constrict the ear canal.
- Children are sometimes fearful and can be hard to work with. Let the child watch you take an impression of mother's ear to alleviate his fears. Let him play with a piece of the "dough". NOTE: It is difficult to use a block with SOME children. The impression may be better formed without it in these cases.

FIG. 5-26. The standard impression process. (Reprinted from Mynders JM, ed. *Custom earmold manual.* 5th ed, revised. Ambridge, PA: Microsonic; 1994; with permission.)

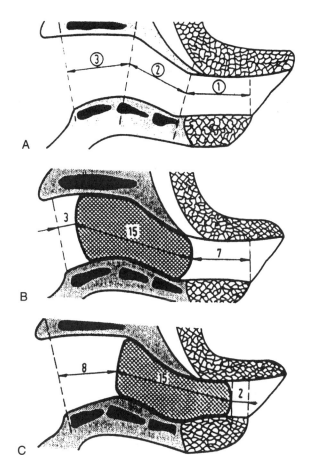

FIG. 5-27. A: Depth zones of the ear canal. B: Depth of CIC instrument. C: Depth of a peritympanic instrument. (All courtesy Philips Hearing Instruments, Mahwah, NJ.)

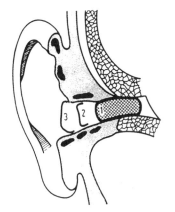

FIG. 5-28. Ear canal position for ITC (no. 3), CIC (no. 2), and peritympanic Instruments (all courtesy Philips Hearing Instruments, Mahwah, NJ).

The general rule for CIC aids is that the impressions for these aids must extend beyond the second bend of the canal. The silicone impression materials for these CIC hearing aids is a different consistency in order that it will flow deeper into the canal. Figure 5-28 shows the positions of ITC, CIC, and Peritympanic (X-P) instruments. The whole thrust of these types of hearing aids is that there are acoustic benefits due to microphone and receiver placement.

ELECTROACOUSTICAL MEASUREMENTS

The next area of how hearing aids work acoustically is electroacoustic measurement. The measurement standards for hearing aids are provided by the American National Standards Institute (ANSI). The actual standards are referred to as ANSI S3.22-1987. This standard measures the following performance characteristics: maximum SSPL 90, high-frequency (HF) average SSPL 90, HF average full-on gain, reference test gain, frequency range, total harmonic distortion, equivalent input noise level, battery current, attack time, and release time. The results of these measurements allow for some comparison of different hearing aids. In the beginning, these measurements were made by hearing aid manufacturer laboratories to

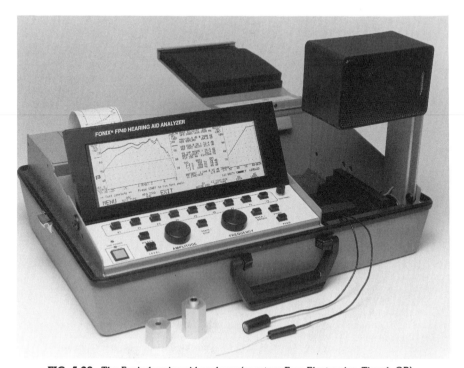

FIG. 5-29. The Fonix hearing aid analyzer (courtesy Frye Electronics, Tigard, OR).

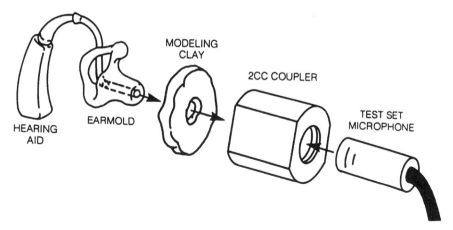

FIG. 5-30. Set-up for checking a hearing aid. (Reprinted from Mynders JM, ed. *Custom earmold manual.* 5th ed, revised. Ambridge, PA: Microsonic; 1994; with permission.)

aid in quality control. Today electroacoustic measurements are made clinically as well. Figure 5-29 shows a hearing aid analyzer used by hearing aid clinicians.

Finally, how well a hearing aid works is related to the individual hearing aid's performance. Clinicians measure hearing aid responses for the fitting process and for maintenance after the fitting. In the fitting process, the electroacoustic measurements are made to target gain. In the maintenance process, measurements are made to determine if the fitted hearing aid is working according to the specifications of the original fitting (8).

How, for example, does a clinician evaluate a BTE hearing aid? The hearing aid analyzer is made up of electronic modules and a test chamber. Inside the test chamber is placed a microphone. The microphone is attached to a standard coupler. The earmold and aid can be attached to the coupler. This is all placed inside the test chamber. Figure 5-30 shows the set-up.

The electronic modules then present a series of signals that pass through the aid and earmold. The output is then sent to another part of the electronic module, and a printout is generated. With current analyzer systems, it is possible to evaluate a hearing aid in a minute or two.

REFERENCES

1. Staab WJ. *Hearing aid handbook.* Blue Ridge Summit, PA: Tab Books; 1978.
2. Pollack MC. *Amplification for the hearing impaired.* 3rd ed. New York: Grune & Stratton; 1988.
3. Sandlin RE, ed. *Hearing instrument science and fitting practice.* Livonia, MI: National Institute of Hearing Instruments Studies, 1985.
4. Pollack MC. Special applications of amplification. In: Pollack M, ed. *Amplification for the hearing impaired.* New York: Grune & Stratton; 1975.
5. Killion MC, Staab WJ, Preeves DA. Classifying automatic signal processors. *Hear Instrum* 1990; 4.

6. Mynders JM. Fitting automatic signal-processor hearing aids—field report. *Hear J* October, 1985.
7. Mynders JM, ed. *Custom earmold manual.* 5th ed, revised. Ambridge, PA: Microsonic; 1994.
8. McCollom H, Mynders JM. *Hearing aid dispensing practice.* Danville, IL: Interstate; 1984.
9. Beilin J, Jensen GR. *Recent developments in hearing instrument technology.* 15th Danavox Symposium 1993. Copenhagen, Denmark: Stougard Jensen, 1993.
10. Grob B. *Basic electronics.* New York: McGraw-Hill; 1971.

HEARING AIDS: A MANUAL FOR CLINICIANS,
edited by Robert A. Goldenberg
Lippincott–Raven Publishers, Philadelphia © 1996

C H A P T E R ✦ *6* ✦

Selecting a Hearing Aid

Ed W. Johnson

Sherman Oaks, California

Key Points

History of hearing aids • evolution of hearing aid electronics • evolution of earmold and case shell design • description of "specific need" hearing aids • speech recognition problems and solutions • emphasis on binaural amplification.

HISTORICAL PERSPECTIVE

Attempts to enhance hearing dates back to at least the ancient Greeks. Cupping the hand behind the ear or placing the small end of an animal horn in the ear were among the early efforts to improve hearing. In the later part of the 19th century musical instrument manufacturers began to make mechanical hearing aids. These instruments were in the form of metal ear trumpets, speaking tubes, horns, or ear scopes (Figs. 6-1 to 6-3). In some cases, these devices were made from shells rather than metal. With the invention of plastic, this material was used more often than metal. The first true binaural hearing aids consisted of metal ear scopes attached to a headband with one scope inserted into each ear.

Carbon Hearing Aids

The first electrical hearing aid is attributed to the invention of the telephone by Alexander Graham Bell. Bell intended to build an electrical hearing aid that used a carbon granule with a magnetic receiver. This work led to the telephone but it also resulted in the first carbon type hearing aid.

Small granules of carbon responded to the pressure of a diaphragm by producing variations in resistance to an electric current. The intensity and frequency of the sound waves resulted in electrical pulsations from the carbon transmitter to the magnetic earphone and was then converted back to sound waves.

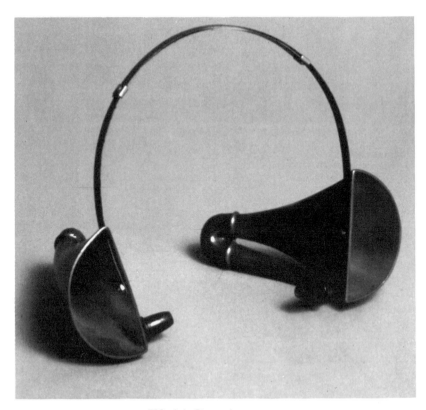

FIG. 6-1. Binaural ear scoops.

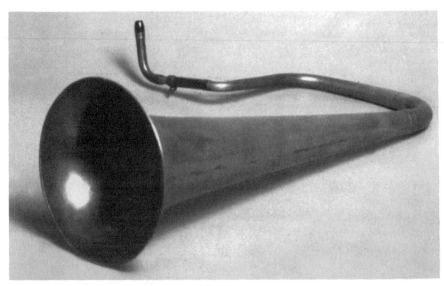

FIG. 6-2. Ear trumpet.

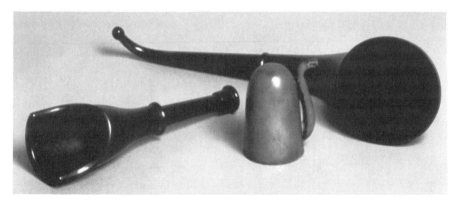

FIG. 6-3. Ear horns.

The carbon hearing aids (Fig. 6-4) were a distinct improvement over mechanical aids but presented many difficulties in wearing. The frequency range was limited, distortion was a major problem, and sudden surges in power output were disturbing.

Vacuum Tube Hearing Aids

The next significant step in the development of hearing aids occurred with invention of the vacuum tube. The standard size vacuum tubes used in radios were adapted to hearing aids early in the 1920s. This resulted in large, expensive, and nonportable devices. The initial instruments used the 110-volt electric current, but later models used large radio batteries.

English manufacturers are credited with the development of vacuum tubes small enough to be used in wearable hearing aids. Before long, however, U.S. companies adapted the English invention to their own purposes and produced even smaller vacuum tubes for smaller, more compact wearable hearing aids. The Aurex Company was the first in the United States to extensively market these wearable aids.

The other important development at this time to allow for small wearable units was the design and manufacturing of tiny, light-weight crystal microphones and receivers. At this stage it was necessary for the patient to wear two separate packs. One pack contained the amplifying device and the second pack contained the A and B batteries. Continued development centered on smaller tubes and reduction of battery drain so that smaller batteries could be used.

These improvements led to the first all-in-one hearing aid. This was a significant step forward in terms of comfort and ease of wearing and encouraged greater acceptance of hearing aids with the elimination of the separate battery pack.

By the early 1940s, it was recognized that individuals varied greatly in maximum tolerance for amplification and that it would be necessary to adjust maximum

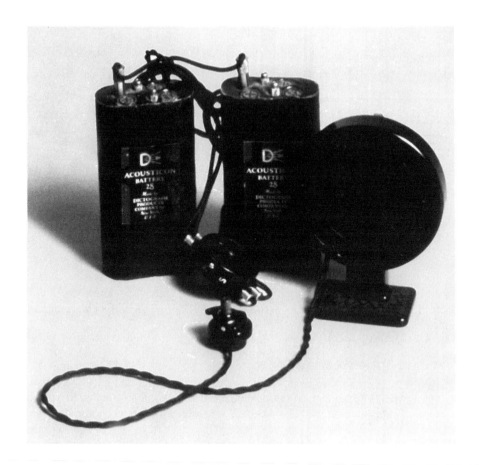

FIG. 6–4. Carbon hearing aid with two battery packs.

output of the hearing aids to avoid discomfort in wearing. The most widespread use of output limiting at this time was peak clipping.

Transistor Hearing Aids

Bell Telephone Laboratories pioneered the development of transistors (Fig. 6-5) and then granted free license for its use to the hearing aid industry. The transistor was a major step forward in hearing amplification. Transistors permit the flow of electrons through a crystalline material (semiconductor) rather than the electron flow through a vacuum or gas in the electron tubes. The advantages of transistors over vacuum tubes is that they are much more efficient. They are much smaller in size than vacuum tubes, they are activated almost immediately as compared with

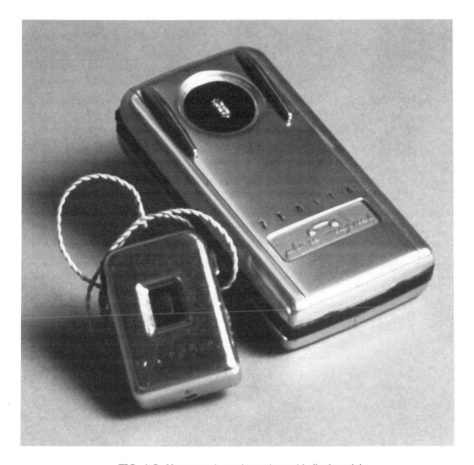

FIG. 6-5. Vacuum tube and transistor aids (body style).

the warmup type required by vacuum tubes, and they are more stable and have a longer life expectancy. Another advantage of transistor aids is that only one battery is required rather than the necessary A and B batteries in vacuum tube instruments. This results in a significant reduction in operating costs for the hearing-impaired patient.

The first transistor aids on the market appeared in the early 1950s and were part vacuum tube and part transistor. These instruments consisted of one transistor and two vacuum tubes and therefore required little circuit change. Within 2 or 3 years, however, all hearing aids produced in the United States were fully transistorized.

The first transistor aids used a germanium base, which was replaced by silicon transistors by about 1957. The advantage of silicon transistors was increased amplification, lower operating currents, and fewer required components. The development of the transistor required a change in the microphone of the aid from a crystal microphone to a magnetic microphone so that the impedance of the microphone could be matched to the low impedance of the transistor.

An additional advantage of the transistor aids was that for the first time a magnetic coil could be placed in the aid to provide for much greater effectiveness in the use of the telephone.

The transistor hearing aid resulted in a major change in the manner in which hearing aids were worn. Initially all transistor aids were body style instruments with a wire running to a receiver snapped onto a custom-made earmold. This system was modified by substituting a plastic tube for the wire, which was considered a cosmetic improvement. An additional cosmetic change involved placing the receiver internally in the body aid to eliminate the need for wearing an external button at the ear.

Before long, manufacturers began to experiment with aids that could be worn at the ear rather than on the body. The first efforts were clumsy, large instruments, but they did provide microphone, circuit, receiver, and battery in a single package worn on the head. Thus the first postauricular [behind-the-ear (BTE)] and eyeglass aids (Fig. 6-6) were introduced. Bone conduction aids also were offered in the eyeglass format but never received widespread use. In 1960 about a quarter of all aids sold were body aids, approximately 45% were eyeglass aids, and roughly 30%

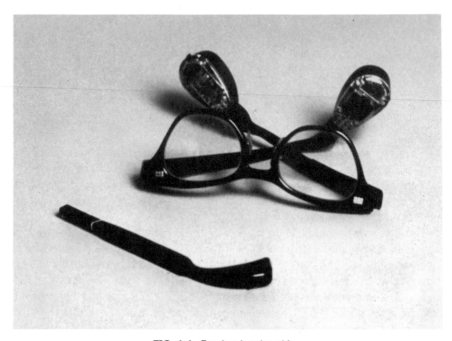

FIG. 6-6. Eyeglass hearing aids.

were postauricular aids. In fewer than 10 years these percentages were drastically changed. BTE aids accounted for more than half of all sales, eyeglass aids about a quarter of all sales, and body aids and the first crude at-the-ear aids making up the remainder of aids sold. The first at-the-ear aids looked like an enlarged receiver and were designed to snap directly into a custom made earmold.

This bit of history brings us up to the modern or current hearing aids now available to the hard-of-hearing public.

Current Hearing Aids

There are three different types of hearing aids presently on the market for hard-of-hearing patients. By far the largest number of instruments have analog components. However, an increasing number of aids have part analog and part digital components. Totally digital aids comprise the smallest group. The all-digital aid is limited by power sources currently available. The completely digital instrument requires much more power to operate than the analog or analog–digital system. Full development and use of the all-digital aid awaits the introduction of a high-power source that can be contained in a small package.

The continued miniaturization of transistor aids led to the invention of the integrated circuit. This significant development resulted in smaller postauricular aids as well as eventually all in-the-ear (ITE), in-the-canal (ITC), and deep canal aids.

METHODS OF WEARING HEARING AIDS

Body-Worn Aids

The first wearable type of aid, the body aid, now accounts for a small part of current hearing aid sales. This method of wearing a hearing aid is used only if a head-worn instrument cannot be used. Patients with a profound or severe loss may require so much power output and gain that it is impossible to eliminate feedback in instruments worn on the head.

In some infants and young children it may be necessary to use a body aid. Adult patients with constantly draining ears that cannot be medically or surgically corrected may need to use bone conduction body aids. Children with atresia of the ear canals (Figs. 6-7 and 6-8) also may need body-worn bone conduction aids until surgery can be performed. Generally speaking, the use of body aids is a last resort, used only if head-worn instrumentation cannot be used.

Postauricular Hearing Aids

BTE aids (Figs. 6-9 to 6-11) still are used by a large number of hard-of-hearing patients. Some of these instruments are very small and are considered by many to

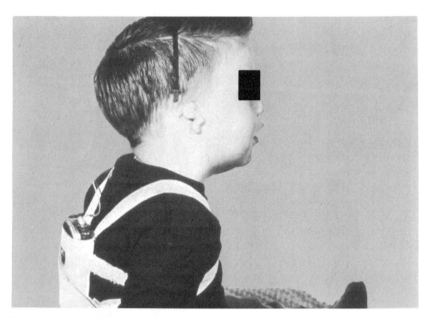

FIG. 6-7. Child with congenital atresia using body aid with bone conduction oscillator.

be less conspicuous than ITE aids. In some cases more gain may be used without feedback problems with this type of amplification. It is also possible to provide more adjustability with a BTE than with an ITE by using an adjustable analog instrument. Programmable analog–digital components are also widely used in BTE aids. Many patients that could use ITE aids simply prefer to wear postauricular aids.

Eyeglass Aids

Eyeglass aids, either air conduction or bone conduction, are seldom used today. The BTE or ITE aids are simply easier and more effective methods of amplification. Occasionally an eyeglass bone conduction aid may be tried, but many individuals have difficulty placing the bone oscillator and still getting a good fit with the glasses.

ITE Aids

The three methods of placing aids in the ear are the full ear system, the ITC aid, or, the most recent innovation, the deep canal aid. All of these methods have been developed due to further miniaturization of the integrated chip circuit and other components. This section discusses the full ear instrument.

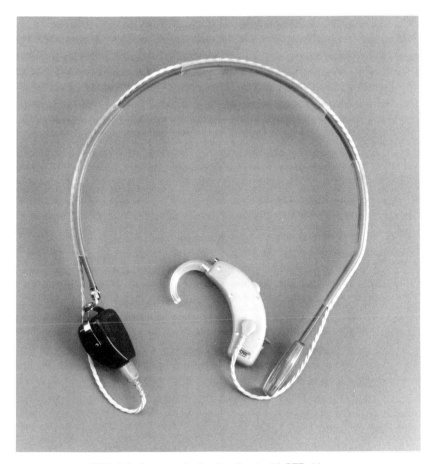

FIG. 6-8. Bone conduction headband with BTE aid.

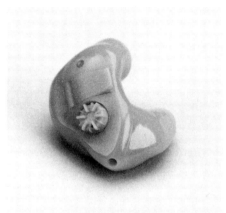

FIG. 6-9. ITE aid.

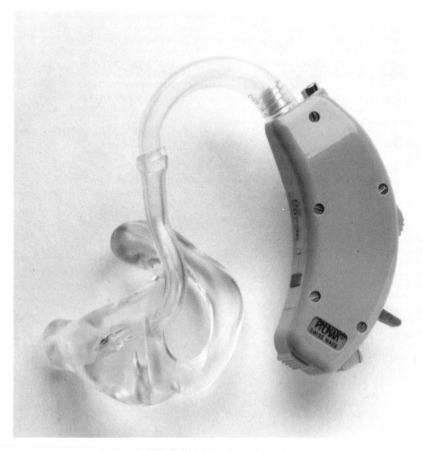

FIG. 6-10. BTE aid with earmold.

Most of the full concha type aids are built within a custom earmold. This requires excellent impressions of the ears to be sent to the manufacturer. Some modifications of the aids may be made by the dispenser, but good initial impressions help to assure comfort in wearing and reduce feedback problems.

As a general rule, more adjustments may be made with a full shell or even a half shell aid than with an ITC type aid. Adjustments may include shaping the frequency response or activating a volume-limiting system such as automatic volume control or peak clipping.

Some patients will reject the full ITE aid strictly on the basis of cosmetics. If the individual insists on an ITE aid but will not accept the full concha type instrument, then the ITC or deep canal type aid may be tried.

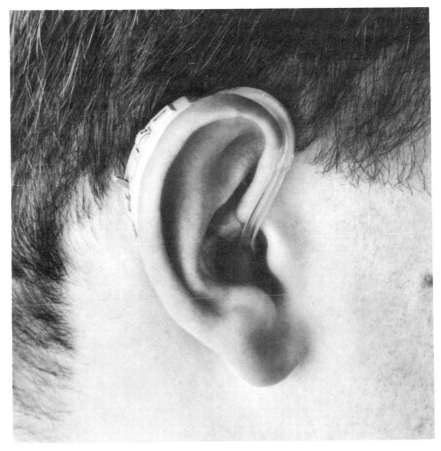

FIG. 6-11. BTE aid on wearer.

ITC Aids

The introduction of tiny custom-made hearing aids that could be contained in the ear canal (Figs. 6-12 and 6-13) spurred many hearing impaired individuals to try hearing aids. The basic appeal of this aid was cosmetic. Many patients with marginal hearing loss who were able to get by in many situations unaided but still experienced hearing difficulties were motivated to try to improve their communication abilities. Otolaryngologists, audiologists, and hearing aid specialists were suddenly confronted with a significant increase in demands for evaluation. Hearing aid manufacturers likewise experienced a marked increase in the number of hearing aids produced.

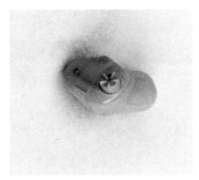

FIG. 6-12. ITC aid.

In 1983 and 1984 there was an important shift in the types of hearing aids manufactured and dispensed. This trend accentuated the reduction in body aids and eyeglass aids and greatly increased the all-in-the-ear aids, including the intracanal instruments.

The demand for ITC aids also introduced new problems for dispensers and manufacturers. Individuals with hearing loss too great for this type of aid insisted on trying canal aids. Many aids were ordered on a trial basis and then returned to the manufacturers because they could not meet the needs of the patient. A certain num-

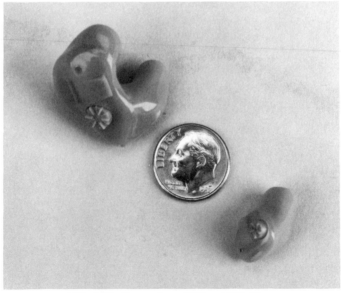

FIG. 6-13. Comparison of ITE and ITC aids.

ber of people simply did not have the manual dexterity to insert and remove the small aids from the ear canal. Many patients could not tolerate the occlusion effect in the ear. In some instances the ear canals were too small to provide space for even a tiny vent. In other instances patients with excellent low-frequency hearing but high-frequency loss could not live with the occlusion effect of the canal aid. This type of instrument is contraindicated for patients with tempromandibular joint problems. With these people, chewing, smiling, or swallowing often resulted in pushing the instrument up from the canal, resulting in feedback.

This is still an excellent method of fitting hearing aids provided the patient is carefully selected to be sure the canal size is adequate, that he has the manual dexterity to handle the aid, and that the hearing loss is appropriate for this type of fitting.

The importance of fitting binaurally cannot be over emphasized. Many of the failures in this method occurred when the patient insisted on a monaural fitting. In most instances, because many of the cosmetic objections are overcome, the individual accepts the use of two ears.

In some instances monaural fittings are appropriate. Patients with one unaidable ear may use a monaural canal aid. This may also be true for the individual with normal hearing on one ear and a moderate loss on the contralateral side.

Many of the fittings for canal aids were for first-time users. Some of these individuals could not successfully use this type of aid but would then go on for a full shell or postauricular fitting. The introduction of the canal aid has resulted in the fitting of many individuals who had previously rejected hearing aid help because of cosmetic objections.

Deep Canal Aids

The latest innovation in hearing aid style is the transcanal, or deep canal aid (Fig. 6-14). Many hearing-impaired individuals who could benefit from amplification rejected even the ITC aid because it could be seen in the ear. The development and marketing of the deep canal aid was in response to the public's continual demand for a hearing aid that could not be detected when placed deep in the ear canal.

The deep canal aid is placed as close to the tympanum as possible so that the end of the mold is in the bony rather than in the cartilaginous portion of the ear canal. A clear plastic line is attached to the end of the aid to facilitate removal from the canal. A small or torturous configurated canal would be contraindicative to fitting this aid.

The deep canal placement of this aid has resulted in a number of apparent benefits to the users. Many patients are unaware of the occlusion effects that are so troublesome to ITE and ITC aid wearers. Manufacturers and dispensers claim that lower gain settings may be used by the patients because of the placement of the end of the instrument so close to the tympanum. One other significant advantage of

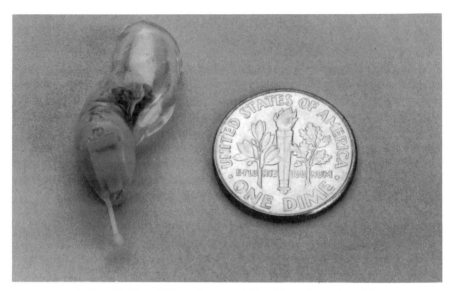

FIG. 6-14. Completely-in-the-canal aid (with hypoallergenic mold).

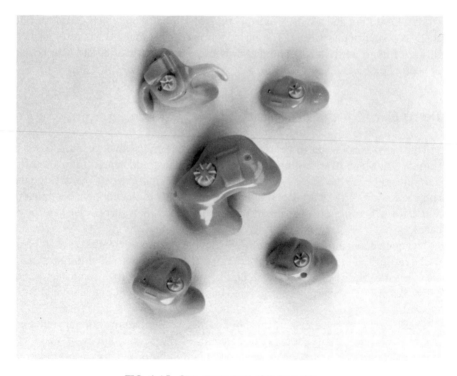

FIG. 6-15. Size comparison of various aids.

the deep canal instrument is in the use of the telephone. ITE and ITC aid users may experience feedback when the telephone receiver is placed against the ear. Deep canal aid wearers may place the telephone receiver in the normal position against the ear and not worry about feedback problems.

This is an interesting and significant development in hearing aids (Fig. 6-15), and time will tell as to the effectiveness and public acceptance of this type of instrumentation.

SPECIAL HEARING AIDS FOR SPECIAL PROBLEMS

CROS Type Hearing Aids

Patients with unilateral hearing loss may function well in quiet environments but have communication problems in the presence of noise. If the impaired ear is aidable, then a conventional hearing aid may be tried in that ear. If the ear has a total loss of hearing or is essentially unaidable, a CROS type instrument may be tried.

CROS stands for contralateral routing of signals and was first suggested in 1960. The first application of CROS was accomplished by using either an eyeglass or a postauricular type of hearing aid. If an eyeglass aid was used, the microphone was placed in the temple of the glasses on the impaired side of the head with the amplifier, receiver, and sound conduction tube on the contralateral side. A wire running from the microphone to the amplifier was embedded in the temples and front piece of the eyeglasses. The sound tube from the receiver was bent to fit into the ear, or a ring mold was made to hold the tubing in place.

If a postauricular fitting was used, the microphone was placed in the hearing aid case on the impaired side and connected to the second aid case by means of a wire that was usually run across the back of the head. The method of sound induction into the ear was the same as in the eyeglass aids. The wire behind the head was cosmetically objectionable to many patients. In response to this negative aspect of CROS, one hearing aid manufacturer introduced a small radio transmitter that could send the signal from the impaired ear to the better hearing ear without the necessity of a wire connection. The system of CROS just described was labeled classic CROS but a number of modifications to this basic method was devised.

One modification was called focal CROS. This system was an attempt to make use of the shielding effect of the pinna by placing the microphone opening into the external meatus rather then at the top of the ear. It was believed that this would lessen the impact of background noise and would therefore be more acceptable to patients with excellent hearing in the better ear.

The mini CROS aid was a further development in the effort to minimize the effect of noise for the CROS aid user. This system simply angled the receiver nozzle of the aid downward toward the ear opening without the plastic tube extension from the receiver nozzle to the opening of the ear canal.

Another modification of classic CROS was the introduction of power CROS (Fig. 6-16). The rationale for power CROS was to allow a patient with severe to profound hearing loss to use an eyeglass or postauricular aid rather than a body instrument. Individuals with severe hearing loss were often denied the use of head-worn instruments because they could not use adequate gain without feedback problems or because of inadequate threshold shifts. The power CROS made use of the head shadow to provide higher gain hearing aids with fewer fitting problems. In this system the sound insertion into the ear required an occluded earmold rather than open tubing to prevent feedback problems.

High CROS was another variation from classic CROS. This aid was designed to help the patient with severe high-frequency impairment. These individuals needed

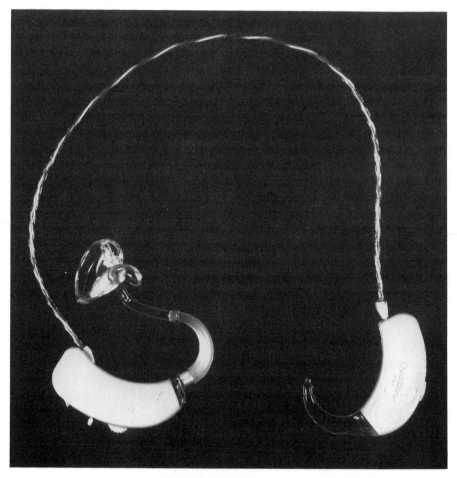

FIG. 6-16. CROS hearing aid.

significant high-frequency gain but experienced feedback unless occluded molds were used. Occluded earmolds were generally intolerable to wear because the low frequencies normally heard were attenuated and the amplified background noise was unacceptable. The high CROS was an effort to enable these people to receive amplification without feedback. This type of fitting is rarely used today because advances in technology have permitted amplifying even severe high-frequency loss with head-worn instruments.

IROS (ipsilateral routing of signals) was still another modification of the original CROS aid. This was devised to help patients with excellent low-frequency hearing but with a moderate dropping loss in the mid- to high-frequency range. High-frequency amplification was used with an open tube in the ear but fitted ipsilaterally rather than across the head. Usually bilateral IROS fittings were used to provide binaural amplification.

Bi-CROS and open bi-CROS were both natural developments of the CROS aid. The bi-CROS system was devised for patients who had an unaidable ear on one side with impaired hearing that needed amplification on the other. The principle was to use two microphones, one on the unaidable side and the other on the aidable ear. Sound from the nonfunctional ear was then routed to the aidable side, and together with the amplified signal on that side was conducted to the ear by means of an occluded (or vented) earmold.

The open bi-CROS was simply a modification of the basic bi-CROS aid. The principle is the same as the bi-CROS except that sound insertion was through an open tube rather than an occluded earmold.

One other modification of the bi-CROS aid was the multi-CROS instrument. This aid was used if the patient had one unaidable ear and one ear that needed amplification. This was essentially a bi-CROS aid with the addition of a three-way switch. The wearer was able to use the aid as a monaural input from the unaidable side, as a monaural instrument from the better ear, or as a true bi-CROS hearing aid. This device provided maximum flexibility in determining input of sound signals but could be used only by discerning patients who knew when to direct hearing reception in the most advantageous way.

There are potential problems and pitfalls in fitting CROS hearing aids. The first step is to determine the cause of the unilateral loss. Patients with an occluding plug of cerumen have been fitted with a CROS aid. Medical evaluation must be the first step because many monaural hearing losses can be successfully treated.

The major inhibitor of fitting CROS is the reluctance of many patients on cosmetic grounds. Placing a wire across the back of the head does not present an attractive fitting solution. The attempt to use a radio transmitter to eliminate the use of a wire resulted in such large postauricular instruments that they were still rejected on cosmetic grounds.

The other major problem with CROS is the noise problem. The motivating factor in fitting CROS is to provide improvement of communication in daily living situations. Unfortunately, background noise of varying intensity is present in almost all normal conversational situations.

The patient with a unilateral loss, even with normal hearing on the contralateral side, is hearing handicapped in the presence of noise. Some highly motivated individuals have learned to accept CROS and have experienced help in communication. An alternate to CROS tried by some clinicians is a hearing aid in an ear with a profound loss or even an ear with no response. In some instances the patient has reported benefit from sound input in the generally considered unaidable ear and this has been attributed to the binaural effect.

CROS is of great value in patients with chronically draining ears who cannot tolerate earmolds. These individuals have not responded to medical or surgical treatment but must have amplification to meet daily living needs.

Children with congenital stenosis of the ear canals must have sound stimulation, and that need may be met with CROS instruments or bone conduction aids.

Bone Conduction Aids

Generally speaking, air conduction amplification is preferred to bone conduction hearing aids. Bone conduction aids are more difficult to wear, and the hearing response is more limited than with air conduction. Bone conduction aids were used initially by means of a body hearing aid with a wire connected to a bone oscillator placed on the mastoid bone. This method is still used in many cases in which bone conduction is the only way to amplify. One alternate system places a bone conduction instrument on a headband on one side of the head and the bone oscillator on the other end of the headband on the opposite ear.

Bone conduction must be used in patients with uncorrectable chronic draining ears, in children with stenosis of the ear canals, and in some long-time users of bone conduction who prefer to continue with this method even though they might be able to use air conduction. Some individuals are able to use eyeglasses with the bone oscillators built into the temple of the glasses. In many cases, this method presents problems in fitting, in placing the oscillator in the most sensitive position, and in getting pressure sufficient for a good hearing response, but not so tight that it is intolerable.

Bone conduction fitting is usually considered the method of last resort. It is a significant help if air conduction cannot be used, but if possible, air conduction is the better solution.

APPLICATION OF HEARING AIDS TO THE PATIENT

Types of Earmolds

In air conduction hearing aids, there must be some method of inducting the amplified sound from the receiver of the hearing aid into the ear canal. This is accomplished by means of custom-made earmolds or through open plastic tubes, except for the all-in-the-ear aids. All other instruments, whether worn on the body or on the ear as eyeglass or postauricular aids, need custom-fitted earmolds.

The early custom-made molds were composed of a rubberized material called vulcanite and came in only one color and one style. Today earmolds come in many different colors and styles. When earmolds were first introduced, all hearing aids, whether body style or eyeglass or BTE instruments, came with an external receiver. The finished earmold therefore had an indentation in the outer surface so that the receiver could be snapped into the mold. Today all postauricular or eyeglass aids have internal receivers so that all that is necessary is to attach the plastic tubing from the earmold to the nubbin of the receiver.

Taking a good impression of the ear is crucial to obtaining a comfortable fit for the patient and to effectively seal off feedback. Impressions were taken with plaster of paris for many years. Fortunately, today impression taking is much easier with current impression materials. Manufacturers provide two vials for impression purposes: one vial contains the powder and the other the fluid to be mixed with the powder. Silicone impression material is also widely used.

There are many different styles of earmolds. If high-gain hearing aids are needed, the earmolds will be the standard (or conventional) molds that essentially fill the concha. It is necessary to occlude the ear, or feedback occurs when the gain of the aid is turned up. If more moderate gain is required, then a smaller mold such as a half shell or a phantom mold may be used. If very little gain is needed, an open mold may be the style of choice. The open mold may use a plastic ring to hold the tube in place and to securely hold the mold in the canal. Another option is to extend the plastic tubing from the receiver nubbin directly down the ear canal.

Venting may be used in most earmolds (except for high-gain aids, where feedback may be a problem). Venting is particularly important if the patient has good hearing in the low frequencies. Venting usually relieves the occlusion effect and relieves the patients "down in the barrel" sensation. Many clinicians feel that venting should always be used if feedback is not a problem. Vent sizes vary from pinhole size to extremely wide openings. It must be recognized that vent size and placement probably change the frequency response of the instrument.

All-in-the-ear aids, whether full shell, half shell, canal, or deep canal all require careful and excellent ear impressions. All of these instruments are built into molds that fit comfortably into the ear of the patient.

Adjustable Hearing Aids

Adjustments in the basic response pattern of hearing aids have been available for many years. This is true for both postauricular and ITE aids. These adjustments (Fig. 6-17) may be made either with a mechanical switch or with a small screwdriver. One switch that the patient can manipulate results in a substantial reduction of low-frequency gain. Another switch permits the user to select microphone input or telephone coil or to turn off the aid. The introduction of fitting controls that

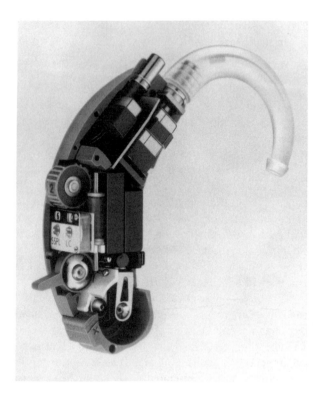

FIG. 6-17. BTE aid cutaway demonstrating components.

could be changed with the turn of a screwdriver introduced much more flexibility in changing response to meet the needs of the patient.

The initial use of a screwdriver control was for a single control that would change an aid with a relatively broad band response to a pattern that dropped the lower frequencies and accentuated the higher frequencies. A further refinement added a second control that could adjust volume limiting by means of peak clipping, usually in two steps, from 0 to 6 to 12 dB. Another development involving three fitting controls permitted changes in a continuously variable input compression control, a continuously variable frequency control, and a separate peak clipping control that could change the peak clipping ceiling by as much as 15 dB.

Probably the ultimate in screwdriver adjustment (Fig. 6-18) was the introduction of an aid with automatic noise suppression (ASP) with four interrelated adjustment controls. This instrument provided the patient with a two-channel aid for maximum performance in either a quiet environment or in the presence of background noise. One channel was a high-frequency channel allowing the low end to be shifted from 800 to 1,600 Hz. The second low-frequency channel was input com-

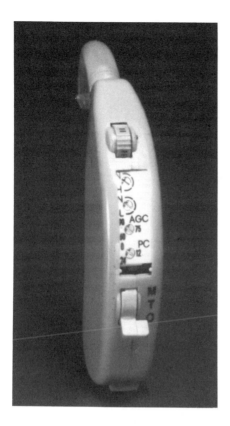

FIG. 6-18. BTE aid with screw-driver-adjustable controls.

pression and permitted as much as 20 dB variability. Activation of ASP in the presence of noise provided a fast attack time (0.3 msec) and a slow recovery time (700 msec), permitting smooth adjustment back to the linear channel. The separate output peak clipping control was a safeguard against the maximum tolerance threshold of the patient.

Programmable Hearing Aids

There has been confusion in definition of adjustable versus programmable hearing aids. Programmable hearing aids (Fig. 6-19) for this discussion refers to all instruments that are electronically controlled, whether they have fully digital or digitally controlled analog circuitry. A number of manufacturers market fairly low-cost single-channel programmable aids. As many as four electronic acoustic options may be used in some of these instruments. This may be adequate to fill the needs of many patients.

Multichannel, multiple-memory aids provide for the largest number of programmable acoustic parameters that have ever been devised for the hearing im-

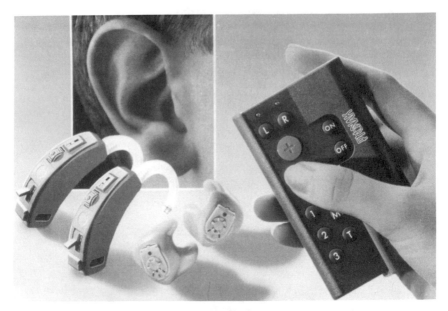

FIG. 6-19. Programmable BTE and ITE aids with remote control.

paired. This explosion of technological options for fitting also introduce a number of problems. Patients that need and may benefit from this type of fitting must be carefully selected and evaluated. The procedure requires a thorough understanding on the part of the dispenser as well as more time in fitting and in return appointments for subsequent fitting changes. Because there is no universal programmer, the dispenser has to purchase each manufacturer's programmer and/or the manufacturer's computer software system. The cost to the patient is significantly more than that incurred with conventional or even single-channel programmable aids.

Having considered the problems in fitting the multi-channel, multi-memory hearing aids, what are the benefits to the patient? The benefits are many (Fig. 6-20). A number of different frequency response patterns may be stored in the aid and permit the patient to select the appropriate configuration, depending on his listening situation. The dispenser has the option of programming a number of different volume-limiting systems. One company offers four different limiting systems (two types of compression and two types of peak clipping) in the same hearing aid.

Once the audiogram is entered into the programmer, there are a variety of fitting formulas that may be selected. Or the clinician may use his own formula. Whatever formula is chosen will be shown on the monitor as target insertion gain. Many systems calculate the Kemar open ear canal resonance and preselect venting size and tubing type for postauricular or receiver types of ITE or ITC aids.

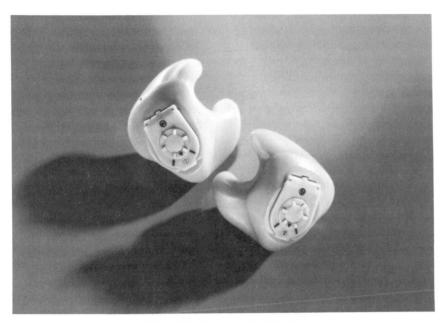

FIG. 6-20. Programmable ITE aids.

Fine tuning of these instruments provides a number of distinct advantages. Gain curves can be changed and optimized and compared with initial settings with the aid in the patient's ear. Output can be modified and/or output-limiting systems may be changed. Some manufacturers provide for a precise loudness balancing system when binaural fitting is used, and this can be a significant benefit to the patient.

Most programmable instruments provide for a number of different program options than can be stored in the aid and selected by the patient when appropriate. The basic audiologic program may be supplemented by programs designed to enhance listening in noise, in group conversations, music listening, telephone use, and so forth.

In most systems, the patients may select the various options by means of a remote control device. Some instruments provide both a remote control and manual controls.

Programmable instruments provide for the best fitting possible for difficult-to-fit patients. Many individuals who are currently using conventional or adjustable aids may significantly benefit from binaural fitting of programmable hearing aids.

GROUP HEARING AIDS

The first group hearing aids can be traced back to the carbon type aids when installations were made in churches and auditoriums. A number of microphones were mounted at the pulpit or lectern and they were wired to earphones at certain designated seats for the hearing impaired. Vacuum tube aids and transistor instruments were used in a similar manner. Further development involved installations in school classrooms. FM instrumentation provided additional impetus, but the invention of infrared technology launched the modern era of group amplification.

Infrared listening systems use infrared light rather than auditory sound. The great advantage of this system is the elimination of disturbing background noise. The listener is given the advantage of a wireless, high-fidelity, broad-frequency sound, with almost no harmonic distortion.

This system may be used in classrooms, churches, theaters, large auditoriums, and conference halls, or as a personal listening device.

Equipment required to run an infrared system includes a transmitter, receiver, and power source. A single transmitter is generally adequate for a personal system in a living room or office area. A classroom or small meeting hall (up to 900 square feet) requires an additional transmitter booster unit. Additional booster units are required to cover large areas such as theaters or auditoriums. The power source for infrared is a 110-volt alternating current power supply.

There are three basic receiver systems. The most widely used is a binaural headset receiver fitted with either foam rubber or silicone cushions. The receiver band

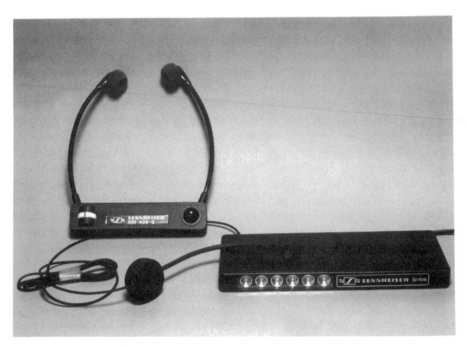

FIG. 6-21. Infrared transmitter and binaural receiver.

has a volume control so that the listener can adjust loudness to his comfort level. There is also a receiver that may be used with a hearing aid by means of inductive coupling or direct coupling. With inductive coupling the hearing aid is simply switched to the "T" position. Direct coupling requires an aid equipped with an audio input so that the cord may be plugged directly into this input.

There are limitations in the infrared systems. This method cannot be used outdoors because bright sunlight inhibits infrared transmission. In addition, light conditions in the room must be evaluated to determine the number of booster transmitters needed. Incandescent light includes a great deal of infrared light, whereas fluorescent light includes only a small amount of infrared light. A room illuminated with incandescent light requires additional infrared transmitters.

Infrared listening systems (Fig. 6-21) provide excellent high-fidelity binaural listening with freedom from annoying and interfering background acoustical signals. Whether this is used as a group hearing aid or as a portable, personal device, it is a superior amplifying system.

BINAURAL AMPLIFICATION

The selection of hearing aids must include evaluation of the patient for binaural amplification. The literature on hearing aids for nearly 40 years has advocated the use of binaural aids in hearing aid fitting. The reality is that far fewer than half of the aids sold in this country are for binaural instruments.

Otolaryngologists traditionally recognize the advantages of binaural hearing. If the physician is able to restore hearing either medically or surgically in one ear, he will inevitably make an attempt to restore hearing in the other ear to provide the patient with true binaural hearing. The physician's rationale for surgery or treatment to restore hearing in both ears is to provide maximum hearing and communicative ability for the patient. It is logical and natural to approach hearing instruments, the third treatment option, using the same rationale.

Assumptions frequently are made that patients with minimum or mild hearing loss need just a little hearing help, so one aid should be adequate. This attitude is also often expressed by the patient. Experience has shown that monaural aids for these patients are seldom satisfactory. In some instances, the monaural instrument simply exacerbates the problem, and amplification will be rejected. The application of two aids provides true binaural effect and with proper counseling usually is accepted by the patient.

Another type of hearing loss that requires binaural input is good to excellent low-frequency hearing but with marked high-frequency roll-off. The use of two instruments, particularly in the presence of background noise, is imperative.

Some clinicians have contended that binaural aids should never be used unless the binaural loss is symmetrical. This myth has been disproved by thousands of successful fittings of individuals with substantial asymmetrical losses. This is true not only of asymmetrical pure tone patterns but of grossly variant speech discrimination scores as well. There are even extreme cases of fitting patients binaurally when there is no functional hearing in one ear. These individuals attest to the benefit of sound input in the greatly impaired ear because they are receiving true binaural effect.

Unless there are specific contraindications for fitting both ears, every candidate for hearing aids should be considered a candidate for binaural amplification. If eyeglasses are needed, we do not resort to a monocle. It should be considered a disservice to hearing-impaired patients with two usable ears to make only a monaural recommendation.

HEARING AIDS: A MANUAL FOR CLINICIANS,
edited by Robert A. Goldenberg
Lippincott–Raven Publishers, Philadelphia © 1996

CHAPTER ✦ 7 ✦

Fitting the Hearing Aid

C. Marke Hambley and Richard E. Cole

Island Acoustic Hearing Services, Victoria, British Columbia, Canada

Key Points

Art and science of hearing aid fitting • use of audiologic tests • establishing a prescriptive target • subjective and objective measurement of fitting parameters • concept of a hearing health team

Selecting and fitting hearing instruments involves a fine balance between art and science. Today's hearing instrument dispenser requires a solid background in many areas: the anatomy and physiology of the ear, hearing disorders, the physics of sound, audiometric testing protocols, electronics, the psychology of the hearing impaired, the art of counseling, and the science and theory of selecting and fitting hearing instruments. The past few years have brought tremendous advances in hearing instrument technology. New products and fitting protocols seem to be introduced almost monthly, with each promising to be better than the last. With so many new products and protocols to choose from, it is becoming increasingly difficult for today's dispensers to determine what is the best fit for a particular patient. To complicate things further, a wisely chosen hearing instrument does not ensure a successful fitting. When you fit a hearing instrument, you are fitting an individual, not just an ear. A successful hearing instrument fitting requires good communication and cooperation between patient and dispenser. A patient's hearing loss, attitude, age, life-style, and motivation all play a big part in the success of a hearing instrument fitting.

It would be wonderful if there were one, single fitting protocol that would guarantee a perfect fit for everyone, every time. Unfortunately, such a universal fitting methodology does not yet exist. Until one does, different dispensers will follow different fitting strategies based on what they find works best.

To discuss all the current strategies for fitting hearing aids and evaluating these fittings would take more than a single chapter; indeed it would take an entire book. For this reason, only a basic introduction to the most common principles and methods for fitting hearing instruments will be provided here. We hope that the information presented in this chapter will help health-care professionals make informed recommendations to their patients regarding the fitting of hearing instruments.

HEARING INSTRUMENT QUALITY CONTROL

In-Office Examination

When the hearing instrument is received in the office, the first thing to do is to check that the make and model are correct and that all requested options have been provided by the manufacturer. Options could include switches or trimmers, which are designed to electronically alter frequency response, gain, output, compression, or other special functions of the hearing instrument. In conventional, nonprogrammable hearing instruments, trimmers are adjusted using a small screwdriver. In programmable hearing instruments, these trimmers are adjusted electronically by computer. In addition to these electronic options, many nonelectronic options also can be ordered (Table 7-1).

Once it has been confirmed that the correct hearing instrument has been received, the hearing instrument must be checked to ensure that it is performing up

TABLE 7-1. *Nonelectric hearing aid options and their purposes*

Finger nail grooves	Grooves etched into the shell to help facilitate removal of the hearing instrument from the patient's ear
Microphone cover	A screen or cover placed over the microphone to help reduce noise caused by wind blowing over microphone
Elevated volume control	To allow for easier adjustment of volume control for people with dexterity problems
Extended receiver tube	To help direct the sound farther down into the ear canal and facilitate wax removal from the instrument
Hypo allergenic shell	A special type of shell material, or a coating placed over regular shell material that is intended to reduce the likelihood of an allergic reaction between the ear and the shell material of the hearing instrument
Flex canal	A soft coating applied to a shell or a shell that is actually made soft with the intention of increasing comfort and/or reducing feedback by providing a more secure fit
Wax guard	Some type of system is placed over the receiver tube opening or placed down inside the receiver tube that is designed to keep wax from getting into and damaging the receiver of the hearing instrument
Removal handle	A handle affixed or built into the battery door or faceplate of a hearing instrument used to help facilitate removal of the hearing instrument from the patient's ear

Typical nonelectric hearing instrument options available with many of today's custom in-the-ear products. Different manufacturers may have different names for these products, but their purposes are the same.

to the manufacturer's stated specifications. This is accomplished by conducting both a biological listening test and an electroacoustical test.

Listening Test

Despite the sophisticated equipment available to test and analyze hearing instruments, there is nothing quite as quick, inexpensive, and valuable as a carefully performed listening check. The main purpose of a listening check is to determine if there is something wrong with the hearing instrument. By listening to the instrument you can determine if it is not working at all, if its output is weak, intermittent, or distorted, or if it has internal feedback. With a little practice a competent dispenser can actually determine the gain, output, frequency response, distortion, and signal-to-noise level of a hearing instrument. An experienced ear can even tell if a hearing instrument has a linear amplifier or an input or output compression circuit. For more detailed information on how to conduct listening tests please refer to Duhamel and Yoshioka (1).

Electroacoustical Measurement

Once the hearing instrument has passed the listening test, electroacoustical measurements should be made. These tests confirm that the instrument functions according to the manufacturer's American National Standards Institute (ANSI) specifications for that particular instrument. The ANSI standard for hearing instruments was first established in the 1960s and has evolved as hearing aid technology and measurement techniques have progressed. The ANSI standard S3.22-1987 (specification of hearing instrument characteristics) is the one in use today (2).

The ANSI standard states that all hearing instrument measurements must be made in a 2-cm^3 metal coupler with a standard connector joining the hearing instrument to the coupler. Although the 2-cm^3 coupler is viewed by many as being representative of the typical human ear, its main purpose is to serve as a standard for quality control. This allows direct comparisons between different manufacturers' products.

Hearing aid manufacturers must supply the following ANSI test measurements for their hearing instruments:

1. Saturation sound-pressure level 90 (SSPL90) curve
2. Peak or maximum saturation SSPL90 (at Hz)
3. High-frequency average SSPL90 (HFA SSPL90)
4. Full-on gain curve (FOG)
5. Peak or maximum gain
6. High-frequency average full-on gain (HFA-FOG)
7. Reference test gain curve

8. Frequency response curve
9. Equivalent input noise
10. Total harmonic distortion
11. Battery current drain
12. Input/output curve [for Automatic Gain Control (aids only)]
13. Attack time (for AGC aids only)
14. Release time (for AGC aids only)

For definitions of these tests and detailed instructions on how they are determined, please refer to ANSI S3.22-1987 in *American National Standard: Specification of Hearing Aid Characteristics* (2).

If the ANSI measurements performed on a hearing instrument agree with those specified by the manufacturer, you can proceed with the fitting of the hearing instrument. If they do not agree, the hearing instrument should be returned to the manufacturer for modification or replacement.

FITTING THE HEARING INSTRUMENT

Currently, the fitting of most hearing instruments is based on a prescriptive method. Prescriptive methods state that for a given hearing loss at a given frequency, a given amount of gain is required to achieve maximum understanding. Some of these prescriptive methods are based on pure-tone thresholds, others on most comfortable loudness levels (MCLs), and still others on uncomfortable loudness levels (UCLs). No matter which prescriptive method is chosen, nearly all make the general assumption that the maximum intelligibility of speech is achieved when average conversational speech is amplified to the listener's MCLs (3). In addition, for a prescriptive procedure to be practical and effective in a clinical setting it must be (a) easy to calculate, (b) simple to administer, (c) logically sound and verifiable, and (d) based on easily acquired audiological information.

The hearing instrument also should (a) provide good sound quality at a comfortable volume, (b) improve clarity of speech presented at average conversational levels, (c) never be uncomfortably loud, and (d) not be so loud as to cause further damage to the patient's hearing.

Many popular prescriptive methods determine amplification gain and frequency characteristics based on pure-tone threshold data from the audiogram. Audiometric pure-tone thresholds are generally accurate, repeatable, and easy to obtain. These prescriptive methods make the assumption that MCLs can be predicted using pure-tone threshold data. In other words, patients with the same pure-tone thresholds should have the same MCLs. Accurate MCLs are often difficult to measure, but one study has shown that MCLs varied by about ±8 dB between subjects. Based on this information, if a hearing instrument has 15 dB of reserve gain, individual differences between users' most comfortable listening levels should theoretically be compensated for by adjustments to the volume control (4).

Other prescriptive procedures are based on suprathreshold MCL or UCL measurements. Several comparisons between threshold and suprathreshold MCL-based procedures have resulted in similar patient satisfaction (5,6,7). However, MCL and UCL measurements generally take longer to complete and tend to have poorer test–retest reliability. They are also more difficult to obtain from some patients, particularly very young children and special populations. For these reasons, threshold-based prescriptive procedures have gained favor over suprathreshold measures and are the method described here.

Threshold-Based Prescriptive Method

More than two dozen threshold-based prescriptive formulas exist. To illustrate the similarities and differences between these formulas, a comparison of four threshold-based prescriptive methods [Berger; Libby ⅓ gain; National Acoustics Laboratory, revised (NAL-R); and prescription of gain and output (POGO)] is presented here. All of the threshold-based prescriptive formulas listed are for use with linear hearing instruments. It has been estimated that 80% of all hearing instruments sold as recently as 1991 were linear instruments (8). By definition, a linear hearing instrument provides a specific amount of amplification at each frequency for all sounds up to the limit of the instrument's amplifier. Thus, if a linear hearing instrument has 25 dB of gain, it will amplify a sound of 40 dB to 65 dB or a sound of 50 dB to 75 dB. The trick in fitting linear instruments is to set the gain high enough to allow the patient to hear important sounds, but not so high that the instrument becomes excessively loud. Put another way, sounds should be amplified so they fall within the user's MCL range. An individual's preferred listening level for amplified sound depends on many factors. On average, preferred listening levels amount to about one-half of the average hearing threshold (9). Lybarger formalized this half-gain rule into a prescriptive fitting formula over 50 years ago. It still forms the basis of many of today's fitting formulas. Figure 7-1 illustrates the rationale behind the half-gain rule. This graph clearly shows that increasing the gain on a 55-dB hearing level (HL) input to half the threshold matches the MCLs for hearing losses up to 60 dB HL. For hearing losses of greater than 60 dB HL, more than half gain is required to reach MCL.

Berger Method

The Berger method (10) is based on the assumption that amplification should raise sounds toward average conversational speech levels. Amplification of low frequencies should be reduced slightly because of their potentially detrimental masking effect on the recognition of speech. This masking of high-frequency sounds by more powerful low-frequency sounds is referred to as upward spread of masking. The Berger method also advocates more amplification at frequencies having greater

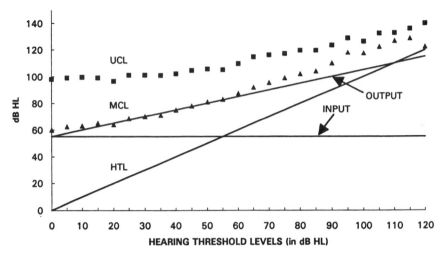

FIG. 7-1. Mean MCL and UCL levels obtained for a range of different hearing losses. Applying the half-gain rule increases a 55-dB hearing level speech signal close to the average MCL for mild to moderate losses. [Modified with permission (28).]

hearing loss. Desired prescriptive gain is calculated for 500, 1,000, 2,000, 3,000, 4,000, and 6,000 Hz, with 10 dB of reserve gain added at all frequencies.

Libby ⅓-Gain Method

The ⅓-gain rule proposed by Libby (11) is based on the rationale that people with mild hearing loss use little gain in real-life situations. Libby maintains that only ⅓-gain, not half gain, is required for people with mild hearing loss. The ⅓-gain method makes no attempt to restore average conversational speech to the average MCL level at discrete frequencies. The Libby ⅓-gain formula specifies ⅓ times the hearing threshold level (HTL) less 5 dB at 250 Hz, ⅓ the HTL less 3 dB at 500 Hz, and ⅓ the HTL at all other frequencies between 1,000 and 6,000 Hz.

Libby also proposes a ⅔-gain rule, stating that individuals with greater hearing impairment require more than half gain. Figure 7-1 supports this hypothesis, although the amount of gain to reach MCL for individuals with hearing losses greater than 60 dB HL is not exactly two thirds. Also, Libby does not clearly specify at what thresholds the ⅔-gain rule should be applied.

NAL-R Method

The NAL-R (12) approach uses a half-gain rule combined with a ⅓ slope rate. It uses less gain in the low frequencies to avoid potential upward spread of masking effects. By applying gain constraints based on the steepness of the slope, the NAL-R formula attempts to control excessive gain for patients with steeply sloping hearing loss. Gain calculations for the NAL-R are more complicated than the other methods shown. However, with the use of computers these calculations can be easily determined. Gain specifications are made at frequencies from 250 to 6,000 Hz. The HTL for each frequency is multiplied by 0.31, and added to this is a value of 0.05 × (HTL at 500 Hz + HTL at 1,000 Hz + HTL at 2,000 Hz). Frequency-specific constants are then subtracted from these results.

POGO Method

POGO (13) is similar to the half-gain rule with 10 dB of gain subtracted at 250 Hz, 5 dB of gain subtracted at 500 Hz, and half gain applied to frequencies of 1,000 to 6,000 Hz. An additional 10 dB of reserve gain is added to all frequencies. The formulation for the POGO method was in part based on the results of real-ear gain data obtained from successful hearing aid users with a variety of hearing losses.

Figure 7-2 shows a typical mild to moderately sloping, sensorineural hearing loss. Figure 7-3 shows the required or insertion gain (often called the target gain) for each of the prescriptive methods discussed. These responses show considerable variation. However, when one considers that the person with the hearing instrument is able to adjust the volume control, the range of variability is not as extreme. Figure 7-4 shows the four prescriptive target curves normalized at 1,000 Hz. Although normalized curves provide less variability, there is still a significant difference between the curves.

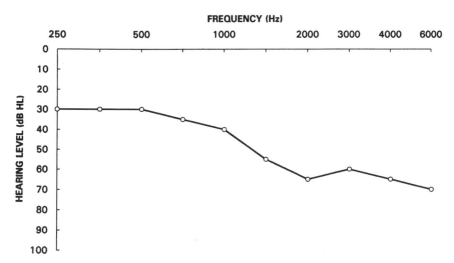

FIG. 7-2. Pure-tone audiogram illustrating a mild-to-moderately sloping hearing loss.

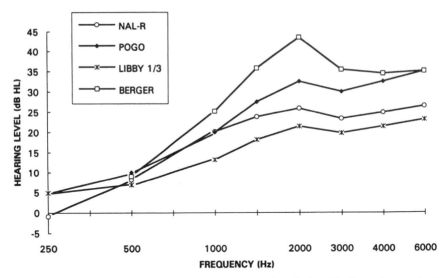

FIG. 7-3. Insertion gain targets for four prescriptive formulas calculated for the audiogram shown in Fig. 7-2.

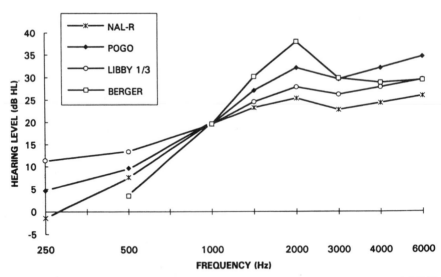

FIG. 7-4. Insertion gain targets for four prescriptive formulas used in Fig. 7-3 normalized at 1,000 Hz.

Deciding which particular prescriptive method is best for a given patient is often difficult. In any case, the prescriptive formula chosen serves only as a starting place for fitting a hearing instrument. The dispenser needs to work closely with the patient to fine-tune the instrument to meet the patient's particular needs. Other hearing instrument factors, such as distortion, bandwidth, damping characteristics, trimmer settings, venting, and amplifier noise, affect the patient's subjective impression of the fitting. All these issues must be addressed to achieve a successful hearing instrument fitting.

Functional Gain

Once a prescriptive formula has been chosen, a method must be used to determine if the hearing instrument is delivering the amount of gain specified by the prescriptive target. The two most common methods of measuring hearing instrument gain in the ear are referred to as functional gain and insertion gain measurements.

Functional gain is a psychoacoustic measure of the difference between unaided thresholds (patient not wearing a hearing instrument) and aided thresholds (patient wearing a hearing instrument) as measured in a sound field. A sound field is the area in which a signal from a loudspeaker radiates in a sound-treated room. Functional-gain threshold measurements are determined in much the same way that audiometric pure-tone thresholds are determined. The two main differences between these two types of tests are the type of signal used and the source of the signal. Functional-gain measurements typically use warble tones or narrow-band masking noise, as opposed to pure tones. The signal is presented through a loudspeaker rather than through headphones. Warble tones or narrow-band masking noise is used instead of pure tones to reduce measurement errors due to the possible presence of standing waves.

Functional-gain threshold measurements are first determined with the patient not wearing a hearing instrument. Threshold measurements are then determined again, this time with the patient wearing a hearing instrument adjusted to a comfortable or preferred listening level. The difference between the unaided threshold measurement and the aided threshold measurement at a given frequency is the functional gain provided by the hearing instrument. In Fig. 7-5, at 2,000 Hz the unaided threshold is 65 dB, whereas the aided threshold is 40 dB. This results in a functional gain measurement of 25 dB (65 dB minus 40 dB) at 2,000 Hz. In other words, the patient's threshold for warble tones improves by 25 dB when listening with the hearing instrument.

Functional-gain measurements are based on behavioral responses. As such, factors that affect the participation level of a patient can greatly affect the accuracy of the test results. Measurements on a patient who is unmotivated, ill, tired, or medicated may not clearly reflect the actual gain being provided by the hearing instrument. Other factors also can affect functional-gain measurements:

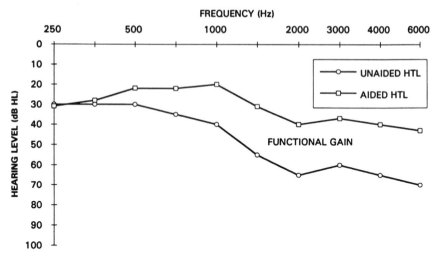

FIG. 7-5. Comparison of aided and unaided hearing thresholds. The difference between these two lines is a measure of the improvement in hearing provided by the hearing instrument and is referred to as functional gain.

1. Masking from the internal circuit noise of the hearing instrument, shifting true hearing thresholds
2. Masking from environmental noise in the sound field, shifting true hearing thresholds
3. Subject head and body movement between aided and unaided conditions
4. Less precise measurements of threshold because of the use of 5-dB attenuator steps
5. Unmeasurable hearing thresholds at some frequencies beyond the range of sound-field audiometric equipment when measuring profound hearing losses.

Functional Gain Under Headphones

With the arrival of completely-in-the-canal (CIC) hearing instruments, many of the inherent problems of conducting sound-field–based functional gain measurements can now be alleviated. For conventional hearing instruments, circumaural headphones cannot be used for measuring functional gain because of the feedback produced when the headphones are placed over the hearing instruments. Today's CIC instruments typically have low-gain requirements and little if any venting. Also, their microphones are placed inside the opening of the ear canal. For these reasons, circumaural headphones can now be used to conduct aided and unaided threshold measurements without producing feedback.

Insertion Gain

Insertion gain is an electroacoustic measurement of the difference in decibels between sound-pressure levels (SPLs) measured in the ear canal with and without a hearing instrument in the ear. Insertion gain is measured using computerized probe–microphone equipment. Like functional gain, insertion-gain measurements are made with the volume control adjusted to a comfortable or preferred listening level.

Unlike functional-gain measures, insertion-gain measurements are based on quantifiable physical measures obtained in the ear canal, not behavioral responses.

For some individuals there can be large differences between functional gain and insertion gain, but on average they are approximately equal (14–16). Functional-gain and insertion-gain measurements are conducted on real ears, not in 2-cm^3 couplers. For this reason they are referred to as real-ear measurements.

Both insertion-gain and functional-gain measurements attempt to determine how much gain a hearing instrument provides across a range of frequencies for a given patient. Real-ear insertion-gain measurements are the measurement of choice for verifying most hearing instrument fittings. However, functional-gain measurements have an advantage over insertion-gain measurements for patients with severe hearing loss and for those fitted with CIC instruments. For these patients, insertion-gain testing can be unsatisfactory. Inaccurate measurements may result because the tightly fitted earmold required by those with severe hearing loss may flatten the probe-tube during testing. Also, feedback may occur because the thickness of the tube being placed alongside the earmold can break the seal with the ear canal. Another problem with insertion-gain measurements is that they require the tip of the probe-tube to be at least 5 mm past the end of the shell or earmold (17). This length is difficult to achieve with a CIC instrument, when its tip is less than 5 mm from the tympanic membrane.

Real-Ear Probe-Tube Measurements

To understand real-ear probe-tube measurements, it is important to understand some basic definitions.

Real-Ear Unaided Response

Real-ear unaided response (REUR) is measured by placing a probe-tube microphone into the ear canal and measuring the SPL, as a function of frequency, when a sound of known intensity is presented. The REUR is primarily a measure of the resonance characteristics of the ear canal and the concha. When a sound is presented to the ear, its natural resonance characteristics amplify certain frequencies.

For the average adult ear, the REUR shows a peak around 2,700 Hz of about 17 dB (Fig. 7-6). The REUR is an important measure for the fitting of hearing instruments because it often serves as a reference value for other insertion-gain measurements.

Real-Ear Aided Response

Real-ear aided response (REAR) refers to the SPLs measured across a range of frequencies with a probe-tube microphone placed in the aided ear canal (Fig. 7-7).

Real-Ear Insertion Gain

Real-ear insertion gain (REIG) is the difference between SPLs measured at a given frequency with a probe-tube microphone placed in the ear canal with and then without a hearing instrument in place (Fig. 7-7). These are the values calculated by the different prescription formulas discussed earlier.

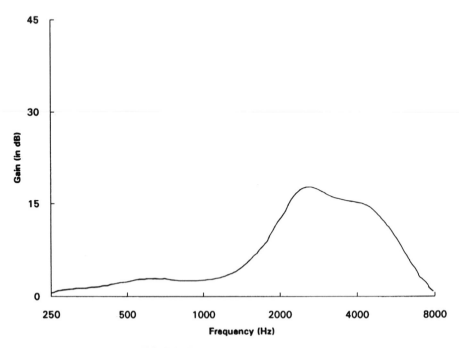

FIG. 7-6. Example of an average REUR.

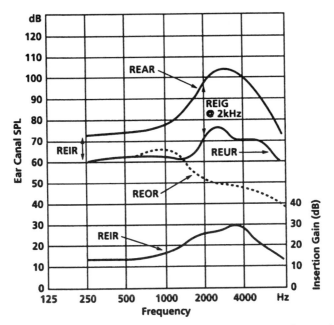

FIG. 7-7. Graphical representation of the relationships between various real-ear probe-tube measurement responses. [Reprinted with permission (29).]

Real-Ear Insertion Response

Real-ear insertion response (REIR) is the difference between SPLs measured across a range of frequencies with a probe-tube microphone placed in the ear canal with and then without a hearing instrument in place (Fig. 7-7). The REIR is a measure of the increase in the SPL in the ear canal as produced by the insertion of a hearing instrument. It is the mathematical difference between the REAR and the REUR. Because REIG and REIR are relative measures that compare the aided condition to the unaided condition, it is extremely important to locate the probe-tube at the same position for both the REIR and the REUR measurements. Measurement of the REIR is much faster and more accurate than functional-gain measurements.

Real-Ear Occluded Response

Real-ear occluded response (REOR) refers to SPLs measured across a range of frequencies with the ear occluded (Fig. 7-7). A probe-microphone is placed in the ear canal with a hearing instrument placed in the ear and turned off. By placing a plug in the ear canal, the natural amplification that occurs in a patient's unoccluded ear canal is effectively cancelled. How much and at what frequencies this amplification is reduced or shifted depends on the type of hearing instrument or earmold.

When performing real ear probe-tube microphone measurements, consistency in probe-tube placement is very important. Dirks and Kincaid (18) show that the closer a probe-tube is placed to the tympanic membrane, the more accurate the real ear measurements will be, particularly for higher frequencies. For this reason it is always good practice to place the probe-tube as close to the tympanic membrane as is practically possible. In general, if the tip of the probe-tube is placed within 5 mm of the tympanic membrane, measurements should be accurate to within 2 dB. It is also good practice to extend the tip of the probe-tube at least 5mm past the canal tip of the hearing instrument or earmold. Otherwise, measurement inaccuracies can occur in the higher frequencies (19).

THE FITTING

Target Insertion Gain

Having selected a prescriptive formula, the patient's audiogram is entered into a computerized probe-tube microphone system, and it calculates a target insertion gain. This is the desired insertion response by the hearing instrument. Unfortunately, this insertion response is the amount of gain that a hearing instrument should produce in a real ear, but manufacturers measure hearing aid performance in a metal 2-cm^3 coupler. The frequency response of a hearing aid measured in a metal 2-cm^3 coupler is different from that same instrument's response in a real ear. The difference between the 2-cm^3 coupler gain and the REIG is referred to as the real-ear coupler difference (RECD).

RECD transformations from 2-cm^3 coupler measurements to real-ear measurements vary considerably. The variability is dependent on the type of hearing instrument, the position of the microphone, and the type of earmold. Other causes of variability are the diffraction and baffle effects of the body and head when a hearing instrument is worn. Two strategies were developed to minimize this variability:

1. The Zwislocki coupler was designed to represent the actual volume and impedance of the real ear. It therefore ensures a more realistic performance by the hearing instrument.
2. KEMAR was invented to compensate for diffraction and baffle effects caused by the pinna, head, and body. KEMAR stands for Knowles Electronics Manikin for Acoustic Research, and its shape is based on the average body shapes of 5,200 men and women.

With a Zwislocki coupler mounted in KEMAR, we now have an anthropomorphic representative of the average human ear. This combination has proven invaluable in helping scientists understand the effects of venting, microphone placement, and body baffle on the average ear.

Killion and Monser (20) coined the phrase CORFIG (coupler response for flat insertion gain). The CORFIG is a set of correction factors that can be added to the prescribed insertion-gain response to determine the amount of 2-cm^3 coupler gain needed. Conversely, the GIFROC (CORFIG spelled backwards) is a set of correction factors that can be applied to the 2-cm^3 coupler gain to obtain the insertion-gain response. In general, 2-cm^3 coupler gain underestimates real-ear gain so that a given amount of 2-cm^3 gain will result in less actual insertion gain.

Hitting the Target

Following is a typical procedure for fitting a hearing instrument using insertion-gain (probe-tube) microphone measurements.

1. The patient is brought into the office and otoscopically examined for any contraindications to fitting the instrument (cerumen, infection, etc.).
2. If all is acceptable, the hearing instrument is fitted comfortably in the patient's ear.
3. If there is any discomfort, the hearing instrument shell (or earmold if a behind-the-ear instrument) is ground and polished until comfortable.
4. Having established a good comfortable fit, the patient's audiometric information is entered into the computerized probe-tube microphone equipment, which calculates a target REIR.
5. The probe-tube is placed in the unoccluded ear, with the tip of the tube placed 5 mm or closer to the tympanic membrane.
6. An REUR is conducted with an input signal of 70 dB SPL.
7. A real-ear aided measurement is taken with the hearing instrument in place. For this measurement it is crucial to keep the tip of the probe-tube in the same position as it was for the REUR.
8. The resulting REIR is compared with the prescriptive target. If the measured insertion response varies from the target insertion, electronic or acoustical adjustments are made to match the target more closely.
9. Once there is a match of the REIR to the target gain, the instrument is tested to ensure loud sounds are not uncomfortable. This can be done by turning the volume control of the hearing instrument to maximum or as high as possible before producing acoustic feedback.
10. Input signals of 70, 80, and 90 dB are then presented, and, using a modified form of Hawkin's (21) loudness growth chart, the patient gives a subjective response as to the degree of loudness each input produces (Table 7-2). As the volume of the signal increases, the patient is instructed to identify an associated category of loudness for the signal. Care should be taken not to exceed the client's discomfort level while conducting this test. If the hearing instrument is fitted properly, the instrument should not produce sounds that are uncomfortably loud.

TABLE 7-2. *Categories of loudness*

7. Uncomfortably loud
6. Loud, but okay
5. Comfortable, but slightly loud
4. Comfortable
3. Comfortable, but slightly soft
2. Soft
1. Very soft

Adapted with permission (21).

Response Adjustments

When a dispenser orders a customized hearing instrument, the manufacturer may not always be able to supply an instrument giving the response requested. There are only so many different circuits that a manufacturer can produce. Consequently, it is recommended that the dispenser order custom products with trimmers that allow adjustment of low and high frequencies and possibly output. With smaller canal instruments there is often no room to include screwdriver-adjustable trimmers. Programmable circuits therefore have an advantage with smaller products. Using a programmer or personal computer, the dispenser can instead electronically adjust numerous response settings through the hearing instrument's computer chip.

The acoustical response of a hearing instrument can be adjusted electronically using trimmers. Acoustical response changes also can be achieved through physical modification of the earmold or shell of a hearing instrument. Venting is one of the most common modifications used to adjust frequency response. Vents are used to reduce low-frequency gain. Often, newly-fitted clients complain that their voice sounds hollow, as if they were speaking in a barrel. The cause of this complaint is often due to the occlusion effect.

The Occlusion Effect

When we talk or chew crunchy food, high SPLs can be developed in our throats. Chewing crunchy tortilla chips can produce SPLs in the back of the throat as high as 140 dB in intensity. These loud SPLs cause much of the flesh and bone in the head and neck to vibrate. When the mandible and the flesh around the ear vibrate, they in turn cause the wall of the ear canal to vibrate. These vibrations produce sound waves in the canal of the ear. In the unoccluded ear this sound energy takes the path of least resistance and escapes out of the ear canal. However, in an ear occluded with a hearing instrument these sounds are trapped in the ear and directed toward the eardrum. This added sound pressure trapped in the ear causes a person's own voice to sound hollow and is referred to as the occlusion effect.

As a result of occlusion, low-frequency sounds are more amplified than are high-frequency sounds. This can be demonstrated to a patient by having the patient vocalize a closed vowel such as "ee" or "oo," first with open ears and then with ears plugged by fingers. The patient will hear the sound much louder and with more base when the ears are plugged. Conversely, having the patient vocalize a softer, high-frequency consonant sound such as "f" or "th" will produce a much smaller occlusion effect.

Because the occlusion effect is greatest in the low frequencies, drilling or enlarging a vent helps to alleviate the occlusion effect because the larger you make a vent the more you reduce the low frequencies. One drawback with this strategy is that if you make the vent too large, the hearing instrument will begin to produce feedback. This is particularly a problem for high-gain hearing instruments. Another drawback is the problem of what to do with very small hearing instruments that fit right into the canal of the ear. Because of the small size of these instruments, there is insufficient room to make a vent large enough to alleviate the occlusion effect. If venting is not feasible, the occlusion effect can often be reduced by having the hearing instrument extend deeper into the ear canal so that its tip terminates in the bony portion of the ear canal (about ⅛ inch past the second bend of the ear canal). Intuitively, one would think that plugging the ear more deeply would aggravate the occlusion effect rather than improve it. The reason that the occlusion effect is reduced by a deeper insertion of the hearing instrument into the canal has to do with the anatomy of the ear canal. The inner portion of the ear canal is surrounded by the bones of the skull, whereas the outer portion is surrounded by flesh and cartilage. Because bone is harder and much less flexible than cartilage, it will not vibrate as much. As a result, much less sound energy is produced deeper in the ear canal, and hence the occlusion effect is reduced.

Damping and Horn Effects

Behind-the-ear instruments, and some custom products, allow for the insertion of damping elements into the coupler or receiver tubing to reduce peaks in the hearing instrument's frequency response. Damping elements generally affect middle frequencies. If a hearing instrument has a large response peak, the patient may turn the hearing instrument down to avoid the uncomfortable SPLs. If the instrument is turned down, the patient will not be using the maximum available gain (Fig. 7-8). This is a particular concern for patients with a severe to profound hearing loss who require maximum output to maximize headroom (refer to glossary of definitions).

Enlarging or belling the bore of the earmold produces a horn effect that increases high-frequency gain. Lengthening the canal portion of the shell or earmold also increases high-frequency and overall gain. It also helps control feedback. Figure 7-9 provides a summary of venting, damping, and horn effects.

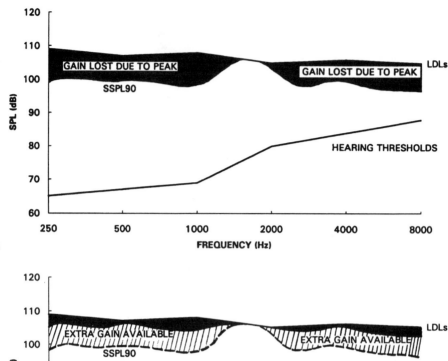

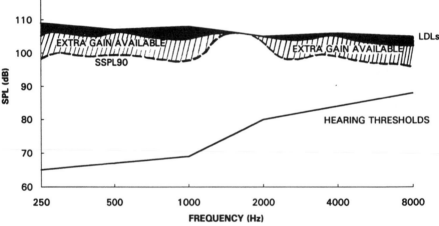

FIG. 7-8. A: Illustration of how much potential gain is lost when a hearing instrument is turned down because of the discomfort caused by a large peak in the output. **B:** Illustration of how much extra usable gain is available when a damping element is inserted into a hearing instrument to smooth out response peaks.

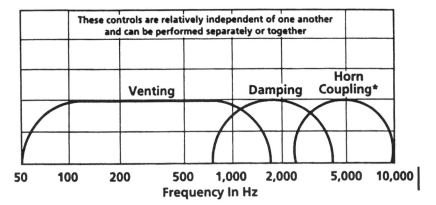

*Stepped Diameter Sound Channels

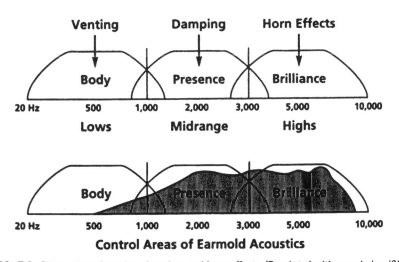

FIG. 7-9. Illustration of venting, damping, and horn effects. [Reprinted with permission (29).]

ARTICULATION INDEX

Another tool useful for measuring the potential effectiveness of different amplification systems is the articulation index (AI) (22). The AI is a calculated value
that expresses the proportion of the average range of speech cues that are audible
to a patient. The concept behind the AI is the idea that there is a division of the
speech signal into several frequency bands. Each of these bands is given a theoretical weighting as to how much it contributes to the intelligibility of speech. How
much of each of these bands a patient can hear determines the AI score. Although
AI scores do not translate directly to speech intelligibility, there is a strong correla-

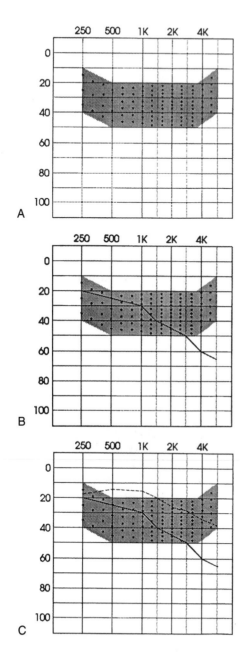

FIG. 7-10. A: The Mueller and Killion (22) count-the-dot audiogram form for calculation of the AI. This form shows 100 dots fit into the speech spectrum and laid out in a typical audiogram format. **B:** The unaided pure-tone hearing thresholds of a patient plotted on a count-the-dot audiogram. The dots below the line represent the regions of the speech spectrum that the patient can hear. The dots above the line represent regions the patient cannot hear. The AI score is determined by counting the number of dots below the line. In this example, the AI score is 0.35. **C:** The unaided and aided pure-tone thresholds of a patient plotted on a count-the-dot audiogram. With amplification, this patient's AI score increases from 0.35 to 0.80.

tion for most types of hearing losses. A score of zero indicates that the patient is unable to hear any of the speech spectrum for normal speech and will typically have very poor speech intelligibility. A score of 100 indicates that the person can hear all of the speech cues available and has excellent speech intelligibility. Put another way, the higher the AI, the better one would expect the patient's speech intelligibility to be. In the area of hearing instrument fitting, the AI can be useful in the following areas:

1. Predicting from the patient's unaided audiogram the amount of difficulty the patient may be having in understanding normal speech
2. Predicting the benefit that may be obtained from a particular hearing instrument
3. Comparing the potential benefits between one hearing instrument and another.

Many computerized probe-microphone measurement systems calculate unaided and aided AI scores and graphically display the results for the dispenser and patient to see. There are also easy-to-use count-the-dot AI forms that let you manually calculate AI scores. An example of a count-the-dot AI form and how it is used to show aided improvement is illustrated in Fig. 7-10.

POSTFITTING CARE

With all of today's new technology, it is easy to get wrapped up in the theory and science of fitting a hearing instrument and forget that you are dealing with a patient, not an ear. No matter how technically sound a fitting is, the patient who does not like the hearing instrument will return it or, worse, will keep it and not wear it. For a hearing instrument fitting to be successful, the dispenser and patient must work together in close cooperation. The dispenser must show that everything possible is being done to take care of the patient's needs. The patient, in turn, must be willing to take responsibility for the success or failure of the fitting and must be willing to work with the dispenser to achieve the best results possible.

When first fitted with amplification, a patient should be counseled that things may sound different. This is because the brain has come to accept impaired hearing as normal and anything else as abnormal. In addition to sounds not seeming normal, patients may be unable to identify the new sounds they are hearing. It appears that the brain forgets how to process sounds it has not heard for some time. When these sounds are reintroduced through amplification, the patient typically perceives them as noise. Gatehouse and Killion (23,24) have shown that it can take several weeks for the brain to rewire itself so that it can interpret meaning from all of these previously forgotten sounds. This adjustment period can be a time of great frustration. Many patients are not willing to make the effort to overcome these frustrations and they will give up on amplification and return their hearing instruments.

Sometimes an adjustment to the hearing instrument or earmold is required. To give an example, a common complaint of people with high-frequency hearing loss is that the hearing instrument sounds "tinny." This problem can be alleviated by reducing the amount of high frequencies, but this would defeat the purpose of amplification. As a compromise, the dispenser can begin with less high-frequency gain and then over a few weeks gradually increase the high-frequency gain at a tolerable rate.

HEARING HANDICAP INVENTORIES

Real-ear measurements give an objective measure of hearing instrument performance, but they tell us nothing of what the patient thinks of the hearing instrument. Because the ultimate determination of hearing instrument satisfaction rests with the patient, it is helpful to have the patient complete a self-assessment inventory that rates the effectiveness of the hearing instrument. Some, such as the Profile of Hearing Aid Benefit (25) and the Hearing Aid Performance Inventory (26), ask questions that evaluate how well a patient hears in a number of different listening conditions. Others, such as the Hearing Handicap Inventory for the Elderly (27), measure the social and emotional handicapping effects of hearing loss. These assessment inventories are typically completed by the patient both before amplification is fitted and then a few weeks after being fitted with amplification. The scores from each assessment are tallied and then compared to give an indication of how much better the patient hears with amplification. Some of these inventories also can be used to assess how well a patient hears with one hearing instrument as compared with another.

When honestly completed, these self-assessment inventories are helpful to both the dispenser and the patient alike. A significant improvement in the self-assessment inventory score in the aided condition confirms to the dispenser that an appropriate fitting has been achieved. For patients, participation in the evaluation process allows them to see for themselves how much they are benefiting from amplification. This gives patients greater confidence in the fitting than simply being told by the dispenser that it is a good fit.

With current and impending changes in health-care reform, it appears that third-party payers are going to play a much larger role in financing hearing instrument fittings. These third-party reimbursers are going to demand positive proof that a treatment has been helpful for a patient. Guidelines for what constitutes positive proof are not well defined by many of today's current third-party suppliers. This is likely to change in the near future, and self-assessment inventories may play a more prominent role in the validation of hearing instrument fittings.

THE FUTURE

Currently, a successful hearing instrument dispensing practice demands a diverse range of expertise. Today's reality is that few dispensers are experts at everything or have all the necessary resources in-house. As a result, most dispensers limit the products and services they offer. These limitations are usually dependent on the dispenser's knowledge, skills, equipment, and experience.

In the future, successful dispensers will rely heavily on partnerships and the sharing of information with outside specialists. Manufacturers and distributors of hearing-related products will likely provide the bulk of the support. However, stronger relationships with other members of the hearing health team will be a key element in the future dispenser's success. This team consists of the family physician, the otolaryngologist, the audiologist, and the hearing instrument specialist. Cooperation and the free exchange of information between these hearing healthcare professionals will be critical factors in the demand for higher levels of patient satisfaction.

Tomorrow's hearing instrument dispensers will need to commit more time to upgrading in the following areas:

1. Training: Continual improvements and changes in hearing instrument technology; testing/dispensing equipment and operating software will demand constant upgrading.
2. Education: New research and discoveries in the human central and peripheral auditory system, microcircuitry, digital processing, and the like will demand a higher level of knowledge through further education.
3. Marketing/promotion: Future dispensers will have to contend with a much higher level of competition. The main source of this competition will come from their peers and the ever-growing number of national dispensing firms.
4. Information highway: Information from a plethora of sources offers an abundance of possibilities. Future dispensers will need to know how to access this information and how to separate the relevant from the irrelevant. They will have to be computer literate and be comfortable keeping up to date with new software programs.

The potential of hearing instrument technology staggers the imagination. The hearing instrument industry currently produces circuits that are multiprogrammable and multichannel, have multiband compression, and are so small that they can be hidden deep within the ear canal. Many of these new circuits are operated by remote control. The hearing instrument of tomorrow will press the limits of our present paradigm. This industry has never before seen such exciting times.

CONCLUSION

The challenge facing today's hearing instrument dispensers is to successfully select, fit, and adjust hearing instruments using myriad complex systems, equipment, and technology. They must maintain rigorous quality-control standards and flawless examination and testing protocols for patients. Efficient office systems and procedures, coupled with friendly and well-trained staff, are critical to patient satisfaction and loyalty. To achieve a high level of patient satisfaction, dispensers must use the education and knowledge of their certification and the skills of a master technician, in addition to the sensitivity and caring of a hearing health-care provider dedicated to excellence. To retain satisfied patients, dispensers must be vigilant in their postfitting follow-up care. Their services should offer scheduled after-purchase maintenance visits to prevent unforeseen hearing instrument problems and patient complaints. A satisfied patient will tell many others, thus loudly hailing the benefits of amplification. It is estimated that 10% of the population, about 28 million Americans and Canadians, have a loss of hearing. However, only about 20% of these 28 million people are wearing amplification. The continual improvements in hearing-related products and services are contributing to a gradual improvement in these statistics. Yet it is obvious to all those who serve the hard of hearing that there is much to overcome. With the technological innovations already available, the potential is there to increase patient satisfaction and make hearing instruments as widely used as eyeglasses or contact lenses.

REFERENCES

1. Duhamel G, Yoshioka P. Subjective listening techniques for assessing hearing aid function. In: *The Unitron Report*. Kitchener, ONT: Unitron Industries Ltd; 1984.
2. American National Standards Institute (ANSI). *American national standard: specification of hearing aid characteristics*. Publication no. S3.22. New York: Acoustical Society of America; 1987.
3. Byrne D. The speech spectrum: some aspects of its significance for hearing–aid selection and evaluation. *Br J Audiol* 1977;11:40–46.
4. Byrne D, Tonisson W. Selecting the gain of hearing aids for persons with sensorineural hearing impairments. *Scand Audiol* 1976;5:51–59.
5. Byrne D. Hearing-aid selection formulae: same or different? *Hear Instrum* 1987;38:5–11.
6. Humes LE. An evaluation of several rationales for selecting hearing aid gain. *J Speech Hear Disord* 1986;51:272–281.
7. Sullivan JA, Levitt H, Hwang JY, Hennessey AM. An experimental comparison of four hearing aid prescription methods. *Ear Hear* 1988;9:22–32.
8. Crammer KS. 1992 Hearing instruments dispenser survey results. *Hear Instrum* 1992;43:8–9, 12–15.
9. Berger K, Hagberg N, Rane R. A re-examination of the half-gain rule. *Ear Hear* 1980;1:223–225.
10. Berger KW, Hagberg EN, Rane RL. *Prescription of hearing aids: rationale, procedures and results*. 5th ed. Kent, OH: Herald; 1989.
11. Libby ER. The ⅓–⅔ insertion gain hearing aid selection guide. *Hear Instrum* 1986;37:27–28.
12. Byrne D, Dillon H. The National Acoustic Laboratories' (NAL) new procedure for selecting the gain and frequency response of a hearing instrument. *Ear Hear* 1986;7:257–265.
13. McCandless GA, Lyregaard PE. Prescription of gain/output (POGO) for hearing aids. *Hear Instrum* 1983;34:16–21.
14. Dillon H, Murray N. Accuracy of twelve methods for estimating the real ear gain of hearing instruments. *Ear Hear* 1987;8:2–11.
15. Tecca JE, Woodford CM. A comparison of functional gain and insertion gain in clinical practice. *Hear J* 1987;40:18–20.
16. Zemplenyi J, Dirks D, Gilman S. Probe-determined hearing-aid gain compared to functional and coupler gains. *J Speech Hear Res* 1985;28:394–404.
17. Mueller HG. Insertion gain measurements. In : Mueller HG, Hawkings DB, Northern JL. *Probe microphone measurements: hearing aid selection and assessment*. San Diego: Singular Publishing; 1992.
18. Dirks D, Kincaid G. Basic acoustic considerations of ear canal probe measurements. *Ear Hear* 1987;8(suppl 5):60–67.

19. Burkhard M, Sach R. Sound pressure in insert earphone couplers and real ears. *J Speech Hear Res* 1977;20:799–807.
20. Killion MC, Monser EL. CORFIG coupler response for flat insertion gain. In: Studebaker GA, Hochberg I, eds. *Acoustical factors affecting hearing aid performance.* 2nd ed. Boston: Allyn & Bacon; 1993.
21. Hawkins DM, Walde BE, Montgomery AA, Prosek R. Description and validation of an LDL procedure designed to select SSPL90. *Ear Hear* 1987;8:162–169.
22. Mueller HG, Killion MC. An easy method for calculating the articulation index. *Hear J* 1990; 43:14–17
23. Gatehouse S. The time course and magnitude of peripheral acclimatization to frequency responses: evidence from monaural fitting of hearing aids. *J Acoust Soc Am* 1992;92:1256–1268.
24. Gatehouse S, Killion MC. HABRAT: "Hearing Aid Brain Rewiring Accommodation Time." *Hear Instrum* 1993;44:29–32.
25. Cox RM, Gilmore C. Development of the profile of hearing aid performance (PHAP). *J Speech Hear Res* 1990;33:343–357.
26. Walden BE, Demorest M, Hepler EL. Self-report approach to assessing benefit derived from amplification. *J Speech Hear Res* 1984;27:49–56.
27. Ventry I, Weinstein BE. The hearing handicap inventory for the elderly: a new tool. *Ear Hear* 1982;3:128–134.
28. Pascoe DP. Clinical measurements of the auditory dynamic range and their relation to formulas for hearing aid gain in presbyacousis and other age related aspects. *Proceedings of the 13th Danavox Symosium.* 1988:129–147.
29. Wilson PV, Kramar CE, eds. *Training manual for professionals in the field of hearing instrument sciences.* Livonia, MI: National Institute for Hearing Instruments Studies; 1993.

HEARING AIDS: A MANUAL FOR CLINICIANS,
edited by Robert A. Goldenberg
Lippincott–Raven Publishers, Philadelphia © 1996

C H A P T E R   ✦ 8 ✦

Using the Hearing Aid

Donna S. Wayner

The Hearing Center, Albany Medical Center, Albany, New York

Key Points

Development • instructions for care, maintenance, and safety precautions • gradual adjustment schedule • using a telephone with a hearing aid • information about hearing aid insurance/self-help groups.

Having a hearing loss means much more than just not being able to hear well. It can bring many experiences that change how a person interacts with family, friends, and fellow workers. It can affect how an individual feels about him/herself.

The information in this chapter has been compiled to help you help your patients and their families as they do something to learn how to hear better and therefore communicate more effectively. Experience indicates that those persons who follow a guided, gradual adjustment and training program to hearing aids realize a smoother, more satisfactory transition to better hearing.

Some may consider the hearing aid as the end process in coping with a hearing loss. Our experience shows that this is far from the truth and that diligent practice with the instruments, proper training regarding their use and care, hearing therapy, and a positive attitude are essential components to improved auditory function and more effective communication. Specific guidelines and curriculum outlines are provided as a means to achieve such success.

Remind patients that their new hearing aid(s) have been prepared to meet their special needs. The instruments are being carefully fit, and now they will begin their adventure in learning to use them to their maximum advantage. Although it takes a little time, practice, and patience, it is worth it.

The Orientation to Hearing Aids Program has been designed to assist patients use their hearing aids most effectively by:

1. guiding them to evaluate the effect of hearing loss on their communication ability.
2. providing a gradual adjustment schedule to using hearing aid(s).

193

3. reviewing how to insert and operate their new hearing aid(s).
4. reviewing information about easy maintenance and troubleshooting tips.

To begin, prepare appropriate handouts for the patients scheduled using the samples included in this chapter. After the patients' arrival and comfortable seating, take time to go over the following points:

1. List the class plan and review the goals and objectives.
2. Periodically check if patients have any questions. This is true for the accompanying parties as well.
3. Be certain to encourage the patients to let you know if they are having any difficulty hearing you at any time during the session. Tell them to ask for repetitions if they do not understand. Let them know that it is their responsibility to request that the person speaking needs to speak louder, softer, or more slowly. This is important to encourage patients to become more assertive in this area and this is an excellent place for them to begin.

Provide information but importantly counsel patients in making a gradual but steadily increasing adjustment to amplification. Assist in their learning to make sense out of the new experiences connected with amplification. You are helping the patients to learn to hear again, this time somewhat differently than they have been accustomed to hearing. Help them realize that such an adjustment takes time. Tailor the sessions to each individual's needs and capabilities.

SAFETY RULES AND WARNINGS

It is useful and important to review the information about safety regarding hearing aids and batteries. Having a handout of these materials for the patient is strongly recommended. We have found it best to hold back handouts until after the material is verbally presented so that the person with hearing loss is not visually distracted while information is explained.

Hearing Aids and Batteries Can Be Dangerous if Swallowed or Improperly Used and Can Result in Severe Injury or Permanent Hearing Loss and Can Even Be Fatal

Become familiar with the following general warnings and the full contents of the user booklet before using the hearing aid.

1. Hearing aids should be used only as directed and adjusted by the hearing aid dispenser. Misuse may result in sudden and permanent hearing loss.
2. Hearing aids, their parts, and batteries are not toys and should be kept out of reach of anyone who might swallow these items or otherwise cause themselves injury.

3. Never change the battery in front of infants, small children, or persons of mental incapacity. Discard batteries carefully in a place where they cannot be reached.
4. Always check medication before swallowing because batteries have been mistaken for tablets.
5. Never put the hearing aid or batteries in your mouth for any reason because they are slippery and may be swallowed.
6. Never allow others to wear your hearing aid because it could be misused and permanently damage another person's hearing.
7. Hearing aids may stop functioning, for instance if the battery goes dead. You should be aware of this possibility, particularly when you circulate in traffic or otherwise depend on warning sounds.
8. In case batteries of a hearing aid are swallowed, see a doctor immediately and call the National Button Battery Hotline collect at (202) 625-3333.

BEGINNING TO USE HEARING AIDS

Begin the Orientation to Hearing Aids Program by reviewing the following introductory guidelines with the patients. Encourage them to:

1. Start wearing the aids at home, where the noise level is low.
2. Find a comfortable volume starting at a low level and slowly increase the volume until they have reached a satisfying listening setting.
3. Discover those sounds in their home that they may not have heard before or have heard but that now sound louder or have a different quality (e.g., crackling paper, footsteps, door bell, squeaky chair).
4. Listen to their voice. Initially, it may sound louder. Have them ask family members or friends to compare their voice volume with the aid on and with the aid off. They should try reading aloud from a newspaper or book. This will help them get used to their voice.
5. Not overtire themselves. They can begin wearing the aid for 2 hours three times each day (morning, afternoon, and evening) and slowly increase their wearing time by 1 hour each day so that within 7 to 10 days they are able to wear the hearing aid all of their waking hours.
6. Be patient. As they become more adjusted to listening with the hearing aid, noise and meaning will slowly sort themselves out.

THE ORIENTATION TO HEARING AIDS PROGRAM

Outlining the goals and objectives of the program helps to set the stage for the information to be presented, allowing the participants an awareness of what to expect.

The goals of the program are:

1. To learn (a) about the effects of hearing loss on communication ability, (b) a gradual adjustment schedule to hearing aid use, (c) insertion and removal of the instruments, (d) care and cleaning of hearing aids, and (e) how to operate them effectively.
2. To practice using the telephone with a hearing aid.
3. To review easy maintenance and troubleshooting tips for hearing aid(s).

The objectives of the program are:

1. To assess the patient's and accompanying person's Communication Performance Ability.
2. To assist them to learn how to put on and take off earmold(s) and hearing aid(s).
3. To practice the necessary steps for the proper cleaning and care to maintain the earmold and hearing aid.
4. To teach about batteries and how to perform a battery check.
5. To help them to learn how to listen with new hearing aid(s).
6. To discover the steps to being a good hearing aid user and a good communicator.
7. To practice using the telephone with a hearing aid.
8. To help them learn about troubleshooting hearing aid(s) problems.
9. To know what to do about earwax.
10. To review information about hearing aid insurance and self-help groups.

Assess the Patient and Accompanying Person's Communication Performance Ability

The Communication Performance Assessment (CPA) (Table 8-1) is a questionnaire to help the patient evaluate his or her hearing function. Read the statements out loud and ask the patient to decide how he or she feels regarding each statement. Have them put an (X) on the scoring sheet under the number they have chosen. An index card may be used as a guide to help keep place on the scoring sheet. It is a good idea to involve family members in this assessment process and invite them to write their responses as well, making their best guess as to how the new hearing aid user is responding to the questions. The CPA is an excellent tool to better understand the effects of the hearing loss on the patient's daily life. It also provides many topics for discussion with the patient and family members. Remember to reverse the count when scoring questions 3, 6, 11, 12, 26, 27, and 28. It is useful to repeat the CPA after the hearing aids have been worn for at least 1 month to check how the patient's communication function has changed with the new hearing instruments.

TABLE 8-1. *Communication performance assessment*

	5	4	3	2	1					1	2	3	4	5
1.								1.						
2.								2.						
3.								3.						
4.								4.						
5.								5.						
6.						5 = always	5 = always	6.						
7.						4 = usually	4 = usually	7.						
8.						3 = sometimes	3 = sometimes	8.						
9.						2 = rarely	2 = rarely	9.						
10.						1 = never	1 = never	10.						
11.								11.						
12.								12.						
13.								13.						
14.								14.						
15.								15.						
16.								16.						
17.								17.						
18.								18.						
19.								19.						
20.						Self	(1–8)	20.						
21.						Family	(9–13)	21.						
22.						Func. Hg.	(14–25)	22.						
23.						Vocational	(26–30)	23.						
24.								24.						
25.						Pretest	Posttest	25.						
26.						total: _____	total: _____	26.						
27.								27.						
28.						Date: _____	Date: _____	28.						
29.								29.						
30.						Name: _____		30.						

Communication Performance Assessment

1. I get upset if I cannot hear or understand a conversation.
2. Since I have trouble hearing, I hesitate to meet new people.
3. I admit that I have a hearing loss to most people.
4. I take less of an interest in things because I have a hearing problem.
5. Having a hearing problem causes me to feel less capable.
6. I feel that people understand what it is like to have a hearing loss.
7. I am not an "outgoing" person because I have a hearing loss.
8. I feel self-conscious when asking others to repeat what they have said.
9. My family and friends are annoyed with my loss of hearing.
10. Sometimes my family and friends leave me out of conversations or discussions.
11. My family and friends understand what it is like to have a hearing loss.
12. Members of my family and friends speak loud and clear.
13. My hearing loss has affected my relationship with my spouse and family.

14. I feel that people avoid talking to me because of my hearing loss.
15. Listening to conversations requires a lot of concentration and effort for me.
16. Because of my hearing problem, it is easier to avoid social situations.
17. My hearing loss interferes with my participating in activities I enjoy.
18. When people talk from behind me or from another room, I miss what they say.
19. I have difficulty understanding if I cannot see the speaker's face.
20. People act annoyed when I cannot hear and understand them.
21. I do not hear important sounds around me like a doorbell or the phone.
22. I avoid going to movies or plays because of my hearing loss.
23. I avoid going to restaurants because of my hearing loss.
24. Does a hearing problem cause you to visit friends, relatives, and neighbors less often than you would like?
25. Do you listen to television or radio less often because of your hearing loss?
26. I admit that I have a hearing loss to my employer and coworkers.
27. My coworkers speak loud and clear.
28. The people I work with understand what it is like to have a hearing loss.
29. I feel pressure at work because of my hearing loss.
30. I feel that my hearing loss has interfered with my job performance.

Learn How to Put On and Take Off Earmold(s) and Hearing Aid(s)

Review the components of the patient's hearing aids with them. Ask them to remove one of their hearing aids and review this component information with them. Share the information with family as well. Become comfortable with conveying instructions for removal and insertion for the different types of hearing aids. This includes the following general tips:

1. Always turn the volume all the way down when removing an in-the-ear (ITE), low-profile in-the-ear (LP/ITE), or in-the-canal (ITC) aid to avoid feedback. For the behind-the-ear (BTE) instrument, switch the aid off.
2. Manipulating the auricle may assist in the insertion process.
3. Be certain the earmold or aid is clean and free of wax buildup before inserting into the ear.
4. Be sure never to remove the earmold of the BTE aid by the tubing.

The specific procedures for inserting earmolds and ITE and LP/ITE hearing aids are as follows:

1. Hold the earmold or hearing aid in an upright position, i.e., the canal nib with hole should be pointed downward in the direction of the ear canal and the helix tip should be pointed upward.
2. Direct the nib into the ear canal, settling it in snugly.
3. Rotate the helix tip backward, like turning a key.
4. Move helix tip forward, tucking the rotated tip behind the upper ridge of the ear.

5. Press and be certain that the earmold or aid is set comfortably in the ear.
6. For the ITE or LP/ITE, turn the aid on and set volume
7. For the BTE fitting, lift and place the aid upward and then around behind the ear.
8. Being certain that the BTE aid is comfortably in place, turn on switch to "M" and adjust volume to the most comfortable listening level.

Practice the Necessary Steps for the Proper Cleaning and Care of the Earmold and Hearing Aid

It is advisable to review methods for cleaning the earmold and aid and the equipment available to facilitate this (Table 8-2). If the patient has a BTE hearing aid, review the information describing how to clean the earmold. Review the information pertaining to maintenance checks, visual checks, and listening checks specific to each type of hearing aid. Review the information about feedback so that the patient will learn that feedback is a natural way to check battery function and is not usually caused by an internal problem. Some hearing aids are equipped with wind guards, vents, and/or vent plugs; review the function of these features. Share copies of the information with the patient.

Equipment Used with Hearing Aids

Become familiar with the items available to keep hearing aids operating well so you can demonstrate them to your patients.

The Dri-Aid Kit

This kit is highly recommended as an overnight storage device for ensuring that humidity, moisture, or perspiration is regularly removed from hearing aids. A con-

TABLE 8-2. *Maintenance check: behind-the-ear hearing aid*

Every day	1. Wipe off aid with a dry cloth 2. Test battery 3. Check earmold opening for wax
Every night	1. Store hearing aid in a dry, cool place 2. Turn aid off and open the battery compartment
Every year	1. Have hearing and hearing aid checked by the hearing aid dispenser 2. Replace plastic tubing (if necessary)
As needed	1. Change battery 2. Wash earmold 3. Check for moisture 4. Replace earmold 5. Replace aid

See also Fig. 1.

tainer of silica gel crystals is placed with the aid(s) into a plastic bag and sealed. If it is more convenient, the metal container housing the silica gel can be placed into a shallow glass jar or a sealable plastic container. The silica gel crystals visible through the window of the metal container should be blue. They will turn pink as an indicator that moisture has been absorbed and that they need to be dried out. They can be regenerated (turned blue again) by drying in the oven and can be reused. Instructions are clearly indicated on the Dri-Aid Kit box.

The Super Dri-Aid Kit

The Super Dri-Aid Kit may be recommended for those patients who come into contact with excessive moisture because of climatic living conditions, work situations, or excessive perspiration. Instructions for regenerating these crystals are clearly noted on the jar, and patients should be instructed to follow them.

Air Blower

This device is used to remove moisture from the tubing and earmold of BTE aids after washing. Describe clearly the cleaning procedure for BTE aids. Patients, parents, or care-givers should know that the tubing must be detached from the hearing aid before washing because moisture will damage the hearing aid. Patients should be instructed to soak the earmold and tubing in soapy water for a few minutes about once a week or as needed. Then the tubing and earmold must be dried with a tissue and with the air blower. The earmold can be air dried should they choose, but in either case patients must be sure that there is no moisture in the tubing before reattaching and using the hearing aid. The air blower also may be useful to dry out the small recesses of the ITE, LP/ITE, and ITC aids. Demonstrate its use by inserting the tip into the opened battery drawer and aerating.

Battery Tester

Encourage patients to use a battery tester to determine if their battery is weak. Demonstrate and practice its use as follows. Place the battery on the small metal strip at the bottom of the tester face. Take the wire and place the metal tip on the top side of the battery, holding it firmly. The needle should move to 1.4 on the dial. If it registers below 1 volt, it is recommended that the battery be replaced. (Note: the battery tester malfunctions if placed on a metal desk or surface.) It is especially recommended that a battery tester be used by parents and teachers monitoring hearing aid function of children and for care-givers of the elderly.

Wax Loop Remover

Most ITE and ITC aids come with their own wax loop remover, a small plastic handle with a thin wire loop tip. This tip is inserted into the canal nib opening to clean out any wax accumulation. This needs to be checked daily. Wax loop removers come in variable sizes to fit different hearing aids; be sure that the wearers use only the correct size for their aid. Earmold openings of BTE aids may be carefully cleaned using the wax loop remover or carefully with a straight pin. A toothpick is not recommended as it can easily break off, possibly leaving residue in the openings.

Aura-Clean

This is a cleaning and disinfecting solution available for ITE, LP/ITE, and ITC hearing aids. It is not essential, but it can be useful and sanitary. It is available from Hal-Hen.

Clean Aid

This is a cleaning and disinfecting solution available, but not essential (unless your patient has frequent ear infections), for cleaning the earmolds of BTE or body aids. It is available from Hal-Hen also.

Use a brightly colored terry cloth washcloth as a protective covering over the table upon which patients may place their hearing aids when removed during training. This will keep the aids from being damaged on a hard surface. The bright, contrasting color also creates a back-drop for ease of visibility. Similar protection should be encouraged for their home setting.

Cleaning and Care of an Earmold (Table 8-3)

On A Daily Basis

1. The earmold should be wiped off with a dry cloth (tissue) each time it is removed from the ear.

TABLE 8-3. *Maintenance check: in-the-ear/in-the-canal hearing aid*

Every day	1. Wipe off aid with a dry cloth 2. Test battery 3. Check earmold opening for wax
Every night	1. Store hearing aid in a dry, cool place 2. Turn aid off and open the battery compartment to store
Every year	1. Have hearing and hearing aid checked by the hearing aid dispenser
As needed	1. Change battery 2. Replace aid

See also Figs. 8-2 and 8-3.

2. The earmold opening should be checked for wax daily. If wax is seen in this opening, gently remove it (using a pipe cleaner or wax tool). Do not poke the earmold. Simply remove whatever wax is present. Do not use a toothpick.

Weekly or as Needed

Occasionally, the earmold will need to be washed.

1. Remove the earmold and tubing from the hearing aid.
2. Use warm, sudsy water to wash the earmold. An earmold deodorizing cleaner also may be used.
3. Carefully dry the earmold and use a forced-air earmold cleaner to remove moisture from the tubing.
4. Allow earmold and tubing to dry out overnight, then reattach to the hearing aid the next morning or use a hearing aid dehumidifier to store the aid.

Equipment to Help Care for your Earmold/Hearing Aid

Forced-air earmold cleaner
Cetycide earmold deodorizer and cleaner
Wax remover tools
Hearing aid dehumidifier

CARE OF THE HEARING AID

1. Excessive heat and cold may damage the hearing aid. Never leave it on a radiator, near a stove, in a sunny window, or in any other hot place, e.g., an oven or clothes dryer.
2. Do not wear the aid when using a hair dryer, either at home or at the hair dresser.
3. Do not apply hair spray when wearing the aid. It may damage the microphone.
4. In extreme cold, or wet and rainy weather, be particularly careful when wearing the hearing aid outdoors.
5. Never wear the aid while taking a bath or shower or while swimming.
6. If perspiration is excessive, avoid wearing the hearing aid during strenuous activity and in hot weather. A protective wrapping material is available for BTE hearing aids.
7. For best results in prolonging the life of a hearing aid, store the instrument overnight in a tightly closed container with a silica gel packet to absorb moisture. Silica gel is a chemical material that absorbs moisture. It is inexpensive and can be found packaged with boxes containing electrical instruments, stereos, clocks, amplifiers, etc. When storing the hearing aid with silica gel crystals, be sure to remove the battery before doing so.
8. Do not be caught without a fresh battery. Always carry a spare fresh battery.

9. Battery contacts may be dried with a dry cotton swab in case of humid weather or heavy perspiration.
10. Dogs and cats may chew on hearing aids. Safely store your hearing aid away from animals when not in use.
11. Avoid wearing the aid when using a sun lamp or during diathermy therapy. (Diathermy is a medical treatment in which heat is produced in the tissues beneath the skin by a high-frequency electric current.)
12. Do not attempt to open up a hearing aid. This voids the warranty.

Learn about Batteries and How to Perform a Battery Check

It is useful for the patient to learn how to operate a simple battery tester. Zinc air batteries last at least twice as long as mercury batteries (which are no longer being manufactured because of environmental reasons). It is useful to encourage the patient to keep track of battery life by placing the tab which comes on the battery onto a calendar when inserted. This allows them a means of keeping track. With zinc-air batteries, remind the patient that they will get little warning when they are out of power. The battery will work at full capacity and then simply stop. It is therefore advisable that they carry spare batteries. The battery life is related to the size of the battery, the degree of hearing loss, the number hours the instrument is worn, and the volume at which it is set. On average, zinc-air batteries last anywhere from 1 to 4 weeks depending on the variables mentioned above.

Learn How to Listen with New Hearing Aid(s)

It is useful to proceed gradually in adjusting to hearing aid use. Use judgment about how carefully each step of the hierarchies on the handouts need to be reviewed. Some people require a great deal of adjustment time to amplification, whereas others can move quickly. Encourage the patients to take some notes of their experiences as they practice with amplification. A comment section should be included on the handouts.

Hierarchy of Listening Experiences with Your New Hearing Aids

The following items are listed in order of increasing difficulty.

1. A good place for beginning might be a quiet living room. One person should talk about familiar, everyday things. Practice listening with the sound source in different positions and at varying distances.
2. Move to the kitchen, where acoustics are not quite so good. Listen to one person talking or to water running at different levels, but not too loud.

3. Try listening to television in a quiet room. Begin with easier situations (the news, etc.). Try listening to the radio and television when it has been adjusted to a comfortable loudness level by a person with normal hearing.
4. Wear at a quiet dinner table.
5. Engage in conversation in a quiet room with two, then three or four other people.
6. Wear outside in a quiet place (back yard). The goal is to become accustomed to wind noise.
7. Walk along the street in a quiet neighborhood.
8. Try using the hearing aid at church, a lecture, or a play. The first time, sit as close to the speakers as possible. Next time try listening at a distance.
9. Try the hearing aid while driving. Listen to the background noises. Try opening the window and listen.
10. Try a shopping trip.
11. Try wearing the aid at a party or in a room where a number of people are talking.

Listening Tips to Share with the Patient and Family Members

Encourage them to:

1. Relearn the trick of concentration. Pay attention. Listen.
2. Avoid pretending that they have understood what was said. It will only confuse things later.
3. Not be afraid to ask people to repeat or speak up louder.
4. Not to hesitate to inform the speaker that they have a hearing impairment and suggest what he or she can do to help you hear better.
5. Remind people to speak *to* them.
6. Carefully watch the speaker and pay attention to the lips, facial expressions and gestures, and body language.
7. Position themselves to take advantage of good lighting. Have the light come from behind them, rearranging their position if they find that there is a glare on the speaker's face. This will assist them in using all nonverbal clues.
8. Try to limit the number of people they speak with at one time. One-to-one conversations are easier than group conversations.
9. Realize that hearing in noisy places is a problem for all listeners. At parties, meetings, theater, movies, and church, practice will help them learn to separate speech from background noise.
10. Recommend the use of public address systems at meetings or at church, when they are available.
11. Try to arrive early at large group functions so that they can have the option of sitting close to the speaker(s), positioning themselves in the best situation to hear as well as see.

12. Use the "T" switch and place the receiver close to the microphone, then listen over the telephone.

Discover the Steps to Good Communication and Good Hearing Aid Use

Communication Strategies

Review the strategies and tips for good communication listed below with the patients by encouraging them to:.

1. Make it a habit to watch the speaker even if listening is not difficult. It is good to get in the habit of paying attention.
2. Not interrupt the speaker before he or she finishes a sentence because they may not understand the beginning, but may catch the end.
3. When they are aware that they missed something that was said, ask for it to be repeated.
4. Summarize what they did hear so that the communication partner knows what to fill in.
5. Learn the topic being discussed. When they know what a person is talking about, it is easier to follow the conversation.
6. Learn to look for ideas rather than isolated words.
7. Keep alert for key words in sentences in order to follow ideas.
8. Use the clues from the situation to help get meanings. The idea is often spelled out by the actual situation. They may be able to anticipate words or phrases that will probably be used.
9. Not be afraid to guess using situational and contextual clues.
10. Keep informed of their friends' interests. If they and their friends have favorite topics, this limited content makes understanding easier.
11. Stay aware of current events. When they know something about a topic they can more readily recognize key words, names, and so forth. It will be helpful to read the daily newspaper and to be aware of the programs many people may watch, even if they do not regularly watch television.
12. Ask family members to keep them informed about things that are happening in their community and neighborhood and about events in the lives of people they know.
13. Keep their sense of humor.

Tips for Communicating with Persons with Hearing Impairmentment

1. If necessary, speak a bit louder, but do not shout.
2. Speak clearly and slowly.

3. Speak at a distance of between 3 and 6 feet.
4. Stand in clear light facing the person with whom they are speaking for greater visibility of lip movements, facial expressions, and gestures.
5. Do not speak to the hearing-impaired person unless visible to him or her, e.g., not from another room or while he or she is reading or watching television.
6. Move away from background noise.
7. If the hearing-impaired person does not appear to understand what is being said, rephrase the statement rather than simply repeating the misunderstood words.
8. Do not overarticulate. Overarticulation not only distorts the sounds of speech, but also the speaker's face, making the use of visual clues more difficult.
9. Do not obscure the mouth with a cigarette or hands and do not chew food while speaking.
10. Arrange the room (living room or meeting room) where communication will take place so that no speaker or listener is more than six feet apart and all are completely visible. Using this direct approach, communication for all parties involved will be enhanced.
11. Include the hearing-impaired person in all discussions about him or her. Persons with hearing impairment sometimes feel quite vulnerable. This approach will aid in alleviating some of those feelings.
12. Ask the person what might make conversation easier.
13. In meetings or any group activity where there is a speaker presenting information (church meetings, civic organizations, etc.), make it mandatory that the speaker(s) use the public address system.

Practice Using the Telephone with a Hearing Aid

The first thing to do is to determine which ear each patient regularly uses for the telephone. Even if they use an unaided ear, provide them with the basic information described because they may prefer the sound quality using their new hearing aid.

Determine whether the patients have a "T" switch or a telephone setting on their hearing aids. If they do, you will need to demonstrate and explain how it is used. They should know that the "T" switch also can be used with an audio loop and other public amplification systems as well as for the telephone. Demonstrate these devices (audio loop, FM system), if available.

Make certain to stress that the "T" switch must always be returned to the normal setting once they are finished using it in the "T" position. Patients need to know that the telephone receiver must physically contact the hearing aid when using the "T" switch and that the volume setting must often be increased, many times to full on, for optimum telephone function. Demonstrate operation of the "T" switch using a telephone with a normal ear piece (no foam pad). Work and practice with the patients to ensure that they can manipulate the switch and set it correctly. Explain the purpose and availability of the telephone foam pad. Allow the patients an opportunity to try their hearing aid with the "T" switch in the normal setting, using the telephone foam pad. Invite their evaluation as to which method is best for them.

During the instruction regarding use of the "T" switch, you may wish to include information regarding assistive listening systems and other convenience devices to alert and assist. If possible, equip your facility with an audio loop system. Demonstrate this system and advise patients that many public facilities such as churches and theaters now use such supplementary listening systems. Demonstrate an FM system (if available) and, depending upon the needs of the patients, describe the availability of the other devices.

Learn about Checking and Troubleshooting Hearing Aid(s)

It can be expected that at one time or another the patient may have some problems with their hearing aid. Because they are already familiar with the different parts of their hearing aid, they are now in a position to better understand the problem with their instrument as they troubleshoot.

The following charts list ways to check the instruments and the common problems associated with hearing aid use, as well as their possible causes and solutions.

If the hearing aid still does not work properly after checking possible causes and solutions, instruct them to contact you.

Checking the Hearing Aid

A hearing aid is a complex and delicate instrument that needs attention to ensure good operation. Before putting the hearing aid on, it should be given a quick, thorough visual inspection and listening check.

Use the following checklist.

Behind the ear (BTE) (Table 8-4)
Visual inspection (Fig. 8-1)

1. Check all switches (on-off, M-T-O, NS-O-M) to make sure they are not broken.
2. Is the input selection switch on "M" or "NS" and not "T"?
3. Is the tone control setting (if movable) in its correct position?
4. Are the battery contacts clean?
5. Use a fresh battery for the hearing aid check.
6. Check the battery using a battery tester if you have one.
7. Is the battery inserted properly? Match "+" on battery to "+" on battery compartment.
8. Is the compartment clicked shut all the way?
9. Is the tubing free of twists, cracks, or holes?

TABLE 8-4. *Troubleshooting the behind-the-ear hearing aid*

Problem	Causes	Solutions
"Dead" hearing aid (no sound at all)	1. Battery is weak	1. Put in new battery
	2. Battery is inserted in hearing aid incorrectly	2. Put battery in aid correctly
	3. Wrong type of battery	3. Replace with right type of battery
	4. Battery contacts corroded	4. Check with audiologist
	5. "M-T-O" switch on "T" or "O"	5. Turn "M-T-O" switch to "M"
	6. Earmold canal plugged with wax	6. Remove wax with a pipe cleaner, wash and dry mold using forced air blower
	7. Disconnected tubing	7. Push tubing firmly onto aid
	8. Twisted or kinked tubing	8. Straighten tubing
	9. Plugged tubing	9. Clean tubing with a pipe cleaner, wash and dry with forced air blower
	10. Moisture in tubing	10. Use forced air blower to dry
Distortion of sound	1. Battery almost dead	1. Put in new battery
	2. Battery contacts corroded	2. Check with audiologist
	3. Earmold canal plugged	3. Remove wax or dirt from earmold canal with a pipe cleaner and wash earmold
	4. Volume control turned to full-on	4. Turn down volume control to correct volume setting
	5. Microphone opening dirty or covered	5. Remove dirt, food, etc. from microphone and be sure microphone is left uncovered (sometimes cleaning must be accomplished by the audiologist)
	6. Moisture in earmold and/or tubing	6. Dry earmold and tubing well after washing, using forced air blower
	7. Tubing collapsed or twisted	7. Untwist and open tubing
Intermittent sound (aid goes on and off)	1. Battery almost dead	1. Put in new battery
	2. Battery contacts corroded	2. Check with audiologist
	3. Bad volume control switch	3. Check with audiologist
	4. Moisture in tubing	4. Use forced air blower
	5. Moisture in aid	5. Use dehumidifier overnight; if problem persists, check with audiologist
Feedback (whistling)	1. Earmold not put into ear correctly	1. Put earmold carefully into the ear so it fits snugly
	2. Earmold does not fit well (too big or too small)	2. Check with hearing aid dispenser
	3. Aid not firmly attached to earmold or tubing	3. Push earmold or tubing firmly together with hearing aid
	4. Volume control turned too high	4. Turn down volume (but not below its normal setting)
	5. Internal feedback inside the hearing aid case because of defect in aid (see "Listening Check")	5. Check with hearing aid dispenser
	6. Tubing cracked or has hole in it	6. Have tubing replaced

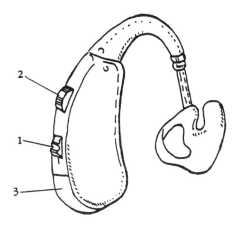

FIG. 8-1. Components of a be-hind-the-ear hearing aid: 1, on = off switch; 2, volume control; 3, battery.

10. Does the tubing fit snugly onto the aid?
11. Is the earmold channel free of wax and moisture?

Listening check

1. Set hearing aid to "O."
2. Turn volume control completely down.
3. Put on the hearing aid.
4. Turn the M-T-O or NS-T-M switch to "M."
5. Move the volume control up slowly to check if the sound gets louder as you increase the volume wheel and softer as you decrease the wheel.
6. Are there any sudden jumps in loudness as you turn the wheel?
7. Does the wheel itself turn smoothly?
8. Is the sound scratchy as you turn the volume control?
9. Check for feedback.

Feedback
Feedback is a whistling, high-pitched sound that may occur:

1. When the earmold is not in your ear properly.
2. When the volume control is turned on maximum.
3. When a hand is placed over the aid, causing an acoustic baffle.
4. When there is a hole in your earmold tubing.
5. When the hearing aid itself malfunctions.

If you have checked the above and are sure it is not caused by items 1–4, take off the hearing aid and turn it up all the way and check the sound output.

1. Is there a squealing sound? There should be.
2. Are there clicks or buzzing? There should not be.
3. Can the squealing be stopped by putting a finger tightly over the end of the ear-mold(s)? It should.

If not, remove the tubing and earmold from the aid and hold a thumb over the sound outlet. If there is no whistling now, the cause of the leak is in the tubing or its connection. If whistling persists, the aid may have internal feedback and should be serviced.

In the ear/in the canal (ITE/ITC) (Table 8-5)
Visual inspection (Figs. 8-2 and 8-3)

1. Use a fresh battery for the hearing aid check.
2. Check the battery using a battery tester if you have one.
3. Is the battery inserted properly? Match "+" on battery to "+" on battery compartment.
4. Is the compartment clicked shut all the way?
5. Is the canal opening free of wax?

TABLE 8-5. Troubleshooting the in-the-ear/in-the-canal hearing aid

Problem	Causes	Solutions
"Dead" hearing aid (no sound at all)	1. Battery is weak	1. Put in new battery
	2. Battery is inserted in hearing aid incorrectly	2. Put battery in aid correctly
	3. Wrong type of battery	3. Replace with right type of battery
	4. Openings in nib plugged with wax	4. Remove wax with a wax removal tool and clean vent with a pipe cleaner (never use a toothpick)
Distortion of sound	1. Battery almost dead	1. Put in new battery
	2. Opening in nib plugged	2. Remove wax or dirt from nib with a wax removal tool
	3. Volume control turned to full-on	3. Turn down volume control to correct volume setting
	4. Microphone opening dirty or covered	4. Remove dirt, food, etc. from microphone and be sure microphone is left uncovered (sometimes cleaning must be accomplished by the audiologist/dispenser)
Intermittent sound (aid goes on and off)	1. Battery almost dead	1. Put in new battery
	2. Bad volume control	2. Check with hearing aid dispenser
	3. Moisture in aid	3. Use dehumidifier overnight; if problem persists, check with audiologist/dispenser
Feedback (whistling)	1. Hearing aid not put into ear correctly	1. Put hearing aid carefully into the ear so it fits snugly
	2. Hearing aid does not fit well (too big or too small)	2. Check with audiologist/dispenser
	3. Volume control turned too high	3. Turn down volume (but not below its normal setting)
	4. Internal feedback inside the hearing aid case because of defect in aid (see "Listening Check")	4. Check with audiologist/dispenser

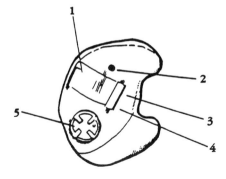

FIG. 8–2. Components of an in-the-ear hearing aid: 1, battery; 2, microphone; 3, amplifier; 4, receiver; 5, volume control.

Listening check

1. Turn volume control completely down.
2. Put on the hearing aid.
3. Move the volume control up slowly to check if the sound gets louder as you increase the volume wheel and softer as you decrease the wheel.
4. Are there any sudden jumps in loudness as you turn the wheel?
5. Does the wheel itself turn smoothly?
6. Is the sound scratchy as you turn the volume control?
7. Check for feedback.

Feedback

Feedback is a whistling, high-pitched sound that may occur:

1. When the hearing aid is not in your ear properly.
2. When the volume control is turned on maximum.
3. When a hand is held over the aid, causing an acoustic baffle.
4. When the hearing aid itself malfunctions.

If patients have checked the above items and are sure the problem is not caused by items 1–3, take off the hearing aid and turn it up all the way and check the sound output.

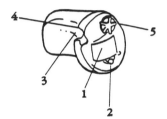

FIG. 8–3. Components of a canal hearing aid: 1, battery; 2, microphone; 3, amplifier; 4, receiver; 5, volume control.

1. Is there a squealing sound? There should be.
2. Are there clicks or buzzing? There should not be.
3. Can the squealing be stopped by putting a finger tightly over the ear canal opening? It should.

If whistling persists, the aid may have internal feedback and should be serviced.

Learn What to Do about Earwax

Because earwax can be a contributing problem to good hearing aid function, reviewing the following information could save the dispenser and the patient a good deal of trouble in keeping the instruments working at their optimum level.

Earwax and a Hearing Aid

Earwax is formed near the outer part of the ear canal, not deep in the canal near the eardrum. It is healthy in normal amounts and serves to coat the skin of the canal serving as a temporary water repellent. The absence of earwax results in dry, itchy ears. Most of the time, ears are self-cleaning because there is a slow and orderly migration of the ear canal skin from the eardrum to the ear opening. Old earwax is constantly being transported from the ear canal to the ear opening where it usually dries, flakes and falls out. Under ideal circumstances, it should never be necessary to clean one's ear canals; however, this is not always the case.

The use of an ITE or ITC hearing aid or earmold with a BTE hearing aid tends to prevent the natural airing of the ear canal and cleansing of earwax. The instrument may push earwax further back into the canal and cause it to become impacted or hardened. This may result in discomfort when worn or may cause feedback.

Some people need to have their ears professionally cleaned every 3 to 6 months (especially if they wear hearing instruments), whereas others never need to have the earwax removed with special instruments or by washing or suctioning. The production of earwax can increase as one gets older.

For good ear hygiene, remind the patient never to put anything smaller than their elbow into their ear. They should not use cotton-tipped applicators, bobby pins, pencils, matches, or twisted napkin corners because these tend to push the earwax deeper toward the eardrum. They can wash their ears regularly with a wash cloth and dry them well before putting on their hearing aids. Periodically, they may find it useful to soften any accumulation of earwax by putting a few drops of mineral oil on a small piece of cotton and placing it into each ear before going to sleep. Note that placing a dry piece of cotton on top keeps the pillow clean. Repeat this for 2 or 3 nights, washing the ears with a wash cloth each morning. If they feel there is a wax blockage remaining, they should see their family physician or ear, nose, and throat specialist.

Often people experience itching in the canal due to reactions to soap, shampoo, hair spray, or perspiration more frequently if hearing aids are worn. Lubricating the skin with a lotion, mineral oil, olive oil, or over-the-counter lubricant for the ears can decrease this problem. The lubricant is best applied at night so that it can absorb into the skin and so it does not get into the working components of the ITE or ITC hearing aids. The person wearing a BTE instrument may apply a small amount of lubricant to the earmold before inserting to help reduce dry ears. To reduce perspiration, a small amount of corn starch or nonscented Shower to Shower powder (Johnson & Johnson) can be placed in the concha before the hearing aid is inserted.

Learn about Hearing Aid Insurance and Self-Help Groups

Review the specific information regarding the warranty and the type and period of coverage. All new hearing aids are warranted for at least the first year for repairs. After the warranty expires, there is a charge for repair. Some manufacturers make available an extended warranty. Some manufacturers also cover the instruments for loss, and patients might be advised to check if they can add a rider to their homeowner's insurance to provide loss coverage. In addition, distribute brochures about independent companies that provide a hearing instrument insurance plan protecting for loss, theft, and damage. Charges vary per year per hearing aid.

Providing each patient information about the availability of local and national self-help groups for people with hearing loss is a good idea. Contact the following groups for brochures to distribute to patients.

Alexander Graham Bell Association for the Deaf
3417 Volta Place, N.W.
Washington, DC 20007
(202) 337-5220, FAX: (202) 337-8314

American Tinnitus Association
P.O. Box 5
Portland, OR 97207
(503) 248-9985, FAX: (503) 248-0024

Meniere's Network
The Ear Foundation
2000 Church Street
Box 11
Nashville, TN 37236
(615) 329-7809

National Association of the Deaf
814 Thayer Avenue
Silver Spring, MD 20810
(301) 587-1788 (voice), (301) 587-1789 (TTY), FAX: (301) 587-1791

Self Help for Hard of Hearing People, Inc.
7910 Woodmont Avenue, Suite 1200
Bethesda, MD 20814
(301) 657-2248 (voice), (301) 657-2249 (TTY), FAX: (301) 913-9413

SUGGESTED READINGS

Alpiner JG, McCarthy P. *Rehabilitative audiology.* Baltimore, MD: Williams & Wilkins; 1987.
Chermack GD. *Handbook of audiological rehabilitation.* Springfield, IL: Charles C. Thomas; 1981.
Davis J, Hardick EJ. *Rehabilitative audiology for children and adults.* New York: Wiley; 1981.
Helleberg MM. Your hearing loss: how to break the sound barrier. Chicago: Nelson-Hall; 1979.
Kaplan H, Ball S, Garretson C. *Speechreading, a way to improve understanding.* Washington, DC: Gallaudet College Press; 1985.
Sandlin RE. *Handbook of hearing aid amplification.* Vol. I & II. Boston: College Hill Press; 1988.
Schow RL, Nerbonne MA. *Introduction to aural rehabilitation.* Baltimore, MD: University Park Press; 1980.
Wayner DS, Goldstein JC. Sensorineural hearing loss: medical rehabilitation. In: Gates GA, ed. *Current therapy in otolaryngology/head and neck surgery.* Philadelphia: B.C. Decker; 1984:54–62.
Wayner DS. Assistive listening devices for improved communication and greater independence. *Hear Instr* 1986;37:21–24.
Wayner DS. *The hearing aid handbook: clinician's guide to client orientation.* Washington, DC: Gallaudet University Press; 1990.
Wayner DS. *The hearing aid handbook: user's guide for adults.* Washington, DC: Gallaudet University Press; 1990.
Wayner DS. *The hearing aid handbook: user's guide for children.* Washington, DC: Gallaudet University Press, 1990.

HEARING AIDS: A MANUAL FOR CLINICIANS,
edited by Robert A. Goldenberg
Lippincott–Raven Publishers, Philadelphia © 1996

C H A P T E R ✦ *9* ✦

Hearing Aids for Children

Patricia A. Chase and Judith S. Gravel

Division of Hearing and Speech Sciences, Vanderbilt University School of Medicine, Nashville, Tennessee; and Department of Otolaryngology and Pediatrics, Albert Einstein College of Medicine, Montefiore Medical Center, Bronx, New York

Key Points _____

Need for early identification in children • importance of hearing for speech development • methods of testing unique to children • use of specific pediatric prescriptive formulae • dynamic process of evaluation.

The selection, evaluation, and long-term management of amplification for children has become more challenging due to the increasing emphasis, both on the local and national level, on early hearing loss detection. Neonatal hearing loss identification initiatives (newborn hearing screening programs) have increased the number of infants (babies whose hearing loss has been diagnosed before the end of the first year of life) referred for amplification. Although many infants do not undergo a hearing screening in the neonatal period, the importance of early hearing loss identification has been supported jointly by professional organizations and public health agencies (1,2). Thus, we are faced with an increasing number of infants and young children who require speech signal amplification in order to afford them the opportunity to develop optimal aural/oral communication abilities. Moreover, older children who have been previously fitted with hearing aids can now benefit from the advent of new technologies and procedures that will further improve the amplification arrangements they use both at home and in the classroom.

This chapter provides clinicians with an overview of the procedures and considerations involved with providing amplification to the pediatric population. The important components of selection, evaluation, verification, and management of amplification for infants and children with hearing loss are also reviewed. The following issues are explored:

Candidacy for amplification
Audiologic assessment

Amplification selection and evaluation
Verification of aided auditory function
Counseling and follow-up
Interdisciplinary roles

Hearing aid assessment, selection, and management is the responsibility of an audiologist who has experience in pediatric hearing assessment, as well as a thorough knowledge-base in infant and child development, developmental psychoacoustics, and family-centered management strategies.

AMPLIFICATION CANDIDACY

Many more children are candidates for one or several amplification options than has heretofore been appreciated. This realization stems from the increasing understanding of the importance of hearing to child development. The needs of children with hearing loss differ significantly from those of adults. Thus, audiometric criteria used for adults to determine hearing aid candidacy cannot be applied arbitrarily to children. Infants born with hearing loss are at a greater disadvantage than are adults who acquire hearing loss gradually and after having established an aural/oral communication system. Infants who do not hear a complete auditory signal will not establish an accurate representation of the auditory–linguistic aspects of their native language.

Deficits in auditory input during early childhood can result in consequences for both communication acquisition and later academic performance. Although most people would not question the importance of amplifying the speech signal for children with moderate to profound hearing losses, lesser degrees of hearing loss (sometimes conductive and transient in nature) also can adversely affect a child's development. Hearing losses that often have been considered minimal (inconsequential) are now known to have deleterious consequences for some children. Often developmental sequelae are unpredictable by cursory examination of an audiogram alone. There is no consensus regarding the degree of hearing loss that determines whether a child needs amplification. Conservatively, however, developing children are at high risk for difficulties in perceiving all the acoustic features of conversational-level speech when hearing thresholds are found to be 25 dB hearing level (HL) or poorer (3).

Unquestionably, children with permanent bilateral peripheral hearing loss need hearing aids in order to function optimally. However, some children with unilateral loss, high-frequency hearing loss with normal low and mid-frequency thresholds, rising audiometric configurations, or hearing loss associated with persistent otitis media with effusion (OME) may be candidates for some form of amplification. Children with minimal or mild bilateral sensorineural hearing losses and those with unilateral sensorineural hearing losses (normal hearing in one ear only) have difficulties understanding speech, particularly in adverse listening environments. Bess and colleagues demonstrated that 30% of children with unilateral hearing loss failed a grade in school or required some type of academic support services. Many were reported to have attentional-behavioral problems in the classroom (4). Moreover, some children who have, or experienced in early childhood, hearing loss secondary to chronic OME also have been shown to be at risk for early problems in speech–language development and later difficulties in the academic environment.

AUDIOLOGIC ASSESSMENT

Determining amplification candidacy always requires that the audiologist obtain a reliable and comprehensive assessment of auditory function. The pediatric audiologic assessment requires the clinician to have available a plethora of evaluation techniques suitable for use with children across a wide developmental (age) range. Fundamentally, the audiologic assessment should delineate the type, degree, configuration, and symmetry of any existing hearing impairment. The audiometric findings (a) serve as the basis for medical/otolaryngological referral and treatment; (b) allow the clinician to monitor the hearing loss stability; (c) form the basis for the amplification's initial electroacoustic characteristic selection through prescriptive fitting formulas; and (d) provide direction and expectations for the initial stages of aural habilitation/intervention. Because of the multiple test procedures and the knowledge of necessary child development, an audiologist trained and experienced with young children is the best qualified professional to complete the pediatric hearing assessment.

The Guidelines for the Audiologic Assessment of Children from Birth through 36 months of Age (5) developed by the American Speech-Language-Hearing Association (ASHA) provides an overview of the pediatric audiologic evaluation's minimum components. The 1991 Guideline's (5) core principles include the need for the following elements: (a) an individualized, timely audiologic assessment; (b) frequency-specific test stimuli for threshold acquisition; (c) ear-specific assessment; and (d) determination of middle ear status using aural acoustic immittance and bone conduction measures.

Figure 9-1 (5,6) details the assessment techniques recommended for determining the hearing status of the infant and young child. The recommended procedures have been divided according to age (or developmental level). Evoked otacoustic emissions (EOAEs; and transient EOAEs and distortion product EOAEs) are currently contributing important information in the audiologic assessment of infants and young children. As such, they have been incorporated into the audiometric procedures appropriate for young children (Fig. 9-1). Regardless of new technologies, multiple measures (i.e., a test battery approach) rather than a single test instrument or procedure should be used to determine the hearing status of young children. Results obtained from the test battery as well as case history information, parent/care giver reports, and behavioral observations are used to substantiate the audiologist's clinical impressions of the hearing loss characteristics and the child's current auditory abilities. Audiologic assessment should be regarded as a continu-

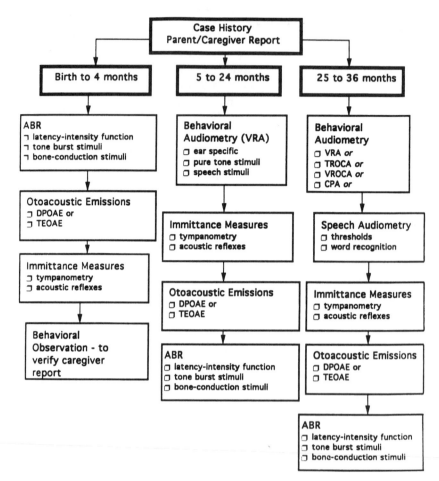

FIG. 9-1. Schematic diagram of the components of the pediatric audiologic assessment test battery according to three age categories: birth to 4 months, 5 to 24 months, and 25 to 36 months of age. Procedures recommended are based on those evaluation tools that are developmentally appropriate for the child and provide the most reliable and efficient means of obtaining audiometric test information. The figure was based on the ASHA guidelines for the audiologic assessment of children from birth through 36 months of age (1991). DPOAE, distortion product otoacoustic emission; TEOAE, transient evoked otoacoustic emission. [Reprinted with permission (6).]

ous process. Behavioral visual reinforcement audiometry (VRA), tangible reinforced operant conditioning audiometry (TROCA), visually reinforced operant conditioning audiometry (VROCA), and conditioned play audiometry (CPA), electrophysiologic auditory brainstem response (ABR), aural acoustic immittance, and EOAE results are integrated and combined with otolaryngological, medical, and parent/caregiver input to verify auditory function and determine some of the subsequent amplification requirements. Intervention should be initiated even when the audiological data may be incomplete; results may still be sufficient to begin the habilitative process.

SELECTION, EVALUATION, AND VERIFICATION OF AMPLIFICATION

General Considerations

Our challenge is to fit a child with comfortable, versatile, and safe amplification that provides audibility of the full speech spectrum in all the environments in which listening and learning occur. As soon as an infant or young child is determined to be an amplification candidate, the selection of the child's personal hearing aid characteristics and features begins. The guiding premise of hearing aid selection is to make all components of speech audible to the child. The amplified speech signal must be detectable (i.e., above the threshold of hearing) and at a sufficient level for the child to have access to the dynamics and breadth of the input signal's frequency range. The amplified signal delivered to the child's ear must always be below his or her loudness discomfort level. Thus, the hearing aid's selected electroacoustic characteristics must place the amplified speech within a range of best listening such that the speech signal's acoustic features are audible and, when combined with experience and training, can serve as the basis for language acquisition. Although this premise is basic, accomplishing the task is a major challenge.

A knowledge of the array of amplification devices currently available is also important. The reader is referred to the numerous chapters in this text that detail wide varieties of both conventional amplification arrangements, newer hearing aid technology, and assistive listening devices. An in-depth appreciation of the benefits and limitations of these systems, together with an understanding of the young hearing-impaired child's needs, form the requisite basis for the selection process to begin. The hearing loss, the various acoustic environments in which the child spends his or her waking hours, and the demands of normal listening must be considered. Appreciation of any cognitive or physical disabilities, family history and expectations, and the support systems available to the child in both the home and educational environment are all important factors in the amplification selection and evaluation processes.

There are several fundamental considerations regarding the fitting and selection of amplification. First, the goal should always be to provide the young child with hearing loss with the advantages of binaural hearing. Generally, this means that two hearing aids should be recommended unless there is a specific contraindication to the fitting (as in the case of a unilateral profound hearing loss or a complete unilateral atresia). Even in those cases in which test results indicate audiometric asymmetry between ears, binaural amplification should be provided unless there is behavioral and audiometric evidence that substantiates decreased performance when amplifying the poorer ear. The importance of a binaural advantage should never be underestimated. In cases in which binaural amplification is not recommended, another form of assistive listening device may be necessary (3).

Second, there are substantial physical differences between infant and adult external ears. The outer ear structures (pinna and ear canal) serve as transducers; their size and shape modify the acoustic characteristics of any signal arriving at the child's eardrum. The physical characteristics of these transducers are obviously not static but change with development. For example, as an infant matures there is a significant shift in the primary resonance frequency of the unoccluded ear canal. In the newborn, a resonance peak can be measured at approximately 6,600 Hz. This primary resonance peak progressively shifts downward, reaching adult values of 2,500 to 3,000 Hz by the time children are about 3 years of age (7).

A third consideration relates to the relationship between the volume of a closed space and the measured sound-pressure level (SPL). The electroacoustic response characteristics of hearing aids are typically examined in a standard, 2-cm^3 hard-walled coupler. The coupler volume approximates the typical volume of an occluded adult ear canal. When the ear canal is occluded with a hearing aid earmold, however, the volume of space between the earmold tip and the eardrum may actually be smaller, varying by both the size of the ear canal and the depth of the earmold's insertion. Any decrease in volume (<2 cm^3) in the real ear would result in an increase in the SPL of a signal that was originally specified (measured) in the standard 2-cm^3 test cavity. For example, if the volume is halved, the same input level that resulted in an output of 130 dB SPL in the 2-cm^3 coupler would measure 136 dB SPL in a 1-cm^3 cavity (halving the volume results in a 6-dB increase). For infants and young children, occluded ear canal volumes of less than 1 cm^3 are not uncommon. In our example, the same input signal that resulted in a 130-dB SPL output in the 2-cm^3 cavity would measure 142 dB SPL in a 0.5-cm^3 cavity, clearly an unacceptable circumstance. Indeed, real ear-to-coupler differences (RECD) range from 5 to 25 dB in children, depending on the frequency (8). RECD values are significantly larger and more variable in children than in adults. SPLs that exceed comfortable listening levels can cause the child to reject or markedly reduce the volume control of the hearing aid. In both cases the hearing aid cannot provide optimal amplification. In the worse-case scenario, exposure to unsafe sound pressure levels may cause further damage to the child's hearing.

These factors suggest that the characteristics of the amplified input arriving at the child's ear can be highly dynamic, particularly in the early years of life. Such factors, among others described below, support the importance of careful and frequent hearing aid response monitoring that includes measuring the hearing aid's characteristics as actually worn by the child (i.e., real-ear measurements). Figure 9-2 illustrates the use of probe microphone techniques to directly measure amplified sound pressure levels in an infant's ear canal (9).

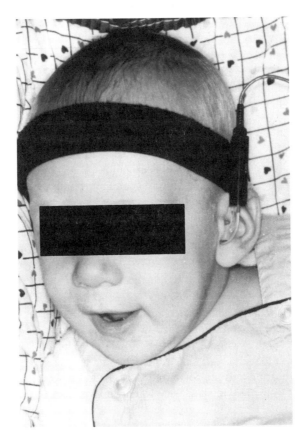

FIG. 9-2. Real-ear probe microphone measurement being conducted on an infant. A small probe tube is placed in the infant's ear canal. Both unaided and aided responses are used in prescriptive hearing aid selection and evaluation procedures. [Reprinted with permission (9).]

OTHER PRACTICAL CONSIDERATIONS

Because the hearing aid selected for a young child must be useful across a broad developmental range, instrument flexibility is a key consideration in the selection process. A flexible hearing instrument allows the hearing aid's gain, output, and frequency to be adjusted as new audiologic test results or real-ear measurement data warrant (3). In order for the child to access the telephone and current assistive device technology, the hearing instrument must include both a telecoil option (T-switch) and direct audio input capability for coupling to assistive listening devices such as frequency-modulated (FM) systems. A microphone telecoil option allows the child access to both the environmental microphone signal as well as telecoil input.

Safety features such as tamper-resistant battery compartments and volume controls are also important considerations at the youngest ages, before children can become responsible users and maintainers of their own amplification (3). A waterproof hearing aid recently has been developed that enables the child to hear important instructions or warnings while in the water.

Behind-the-ear (BTE) hearing aids are appropriate for most young children. Today's BTE hearing aids can usually provide sufficient power to meet the needs of children with severe or even profound hearing loss. BTE hearing aids offer several advantages over other styles. They afford sound reception at ear level. This allows the child to take advantage of naturally occurring binaural cues (at ear level, separated by the head) for localization of sound and improved listening in background competition. BTE hearing aids are also more cosmetically appealing than body-worn instruments. The importance of appearance in gaining parent and child acceptance of hearing aids cannot be overlooked.

The disadvantage of BTE hearing aids for use with children, particularly those with profound hearing loss, is that acoustic feedback problems frequently arise. It is sometimes difficult to achieve an acoustic seal of the external ear canal with the custom earmold that is sufficient to allow the BTE hearing aid to be worn at the recommended volume without feedback. Sometimes the BTE hearing aid's size makes it difficult to maintain the instrument behind the pinnae of small babies.

Body-worn hearing aids are sometimes advocated for short periods of time during the initial fitting of infants and very young children. The separation of the hearing aid microphone from the receiver reduces the possibility of acoustic feedback. However, it may be difficult to achieve sufficient separation of the microphones for a binaural body-worn arrangement, compromising true binaural hearing. Body-worn microphones also increase low-frequency energy due to the body baffle effect. This may or may not be desirable; however, it is important for the clinician to realize the possibility of this occurrence.

In-the-ear (ITE) hearing aid styles may be considered for children 8 to 10 years of age when ear growth has stabilized and the child can be responsible for the instrument (3). The disadvantage of ITE hearing instruments for children center around flexibility, the lack of coupling options for assistive device technology, an increased possibility of damage, and sometimes insufficient gain for degree of hearing loss. Manufacturers often are willing to provide innovative fitting options for the child who desires to use ITE hearing aids. Certainly, other than the disadvantages discussed above, ITE instruments offer the same acoustic and cosmetic advantages for children as are realized by adult users. Fitting flexibility in a child's hearing aid should never be sacrificed for size without a thorough understanding of the constraints of such a fitting. However, some older children are satisfied "part-time" ITE users, selecting them as their amplification choice outside the classroom situation.

It is always important to be sensitive to casing and earmold color when selecting a personal hearing aid for the child. The color should be chosen in accordance with the child's natural skin tone. Earmolds fabricated of soft materials are usually more comfortable for the child and are less likely to cause injury when infants and young children fall than are those made of hard materials. Devices that help to retain BTE hearing aids behind the ears of infants and young children are often used. Headbands generally are used only to maintain a bone oscillator on the mastoid when a bone-conduction style of hearing aid is recommended (as in the case of bilateral atresia/severe microtia). Air-conduction hearing instruments are always the option of choice. It is necessary for the clinician to work particularly closely with the otolaryngologist in more difficult cases (i.e., children with chronic ear drainage) in which otologic considerations for hearing instrument/earmold style are of concern.

FITTING OPTIONS OTHER THAN THE TRADITIONAL HEARING AID

Some children need amplification devices beyond traditional hearing aids to optimize development of aural/oral communication abilities. These options include FM hearing systems, frequency transposition hearing aids, or, in some cases, cochlear implants.

FM systems have been advocated for use as personal amplification. This is sometimes considered the option of choice for children with severe and profound hearing loss. FM systems provide the child with a signal-to-noise advantage for both distance listening and in adverse acoustic environments. However, full-time use of these systems requires the child to switch between FM and regular environmental microphones and makes it necessary to pass the FM transmitter each time the speaker changes. FM receivers are also accessible with low gain and output for children with milder degrees of hearing loss and those who have difficulty attending in the classroom.

FM systems are now available as completely ear level instruments; that is, all components are housed in a BTE case, including the receiver and antenna without the need for a body-worn receiver or cords. The BTE FM unit can operate in an FM as well as a conventional amplification mode. With these newer instruments, the advantage of the FM option may be more fully realized. All FM hearing systems, whether body-worn or ear level, improve a child's ability to understand speech in background noise, in reverberant environments, and when distance separates the speaker and the child. Fitting these devices requires that the audiologist work closely with school personnel and conduct evaluations of the acoustic environment of the classroom (10). Additional information regarding FM systems and cochlear implants is available in other chapters of this text.

AMPLIFICATION SELECTION
AND EVALUATION PROCEDURES

Pediatric hearing aid selection procedures have historically been modeled on the traditional comparative approaches used with adults. One of the major difficulties with such approaches is that children are often unable to provide the subjective judgments necessary for decisions such as comfortable and uncomfortable listening levels and sound quality differences among hearing instruments. Also, comparative approaches use measures of speech recognition ability (percentage correct repetition of monosyllabic words) in the selection of the most appropriate hearing aid for an individual. Moreover, comparative methods usually incorporate aided threshold response measures in order to examine the functional gain provided by the hearing aid. Numerous limitations of such aided functional gain measures are described elsewhere in this text. Clearly, comparative hearing aid selection and evaluation methods that require subjective, detailed responses, use speech intelligibility measures, and require a prolonged test time have limited utility for use with young children.

Recently, prescriptive hearing aid selection and evaluation procedures have afforded audiologists more objective methods to circumvent some of the limitations of the traditional comparative approach. Most prescriptive procedures use the behavioral audiogram and listener judgments of most comfortable and uncomfortable listening levels for speech as well as frequency-specific signals. In some procedures, real-ear measures of the individual's unaided responses also are obtained. Selecting a hearing aid's electroacoustic characteristics depends on the audiometric and, frequently, real-ear data. After fitting, whether the hearing aid meets the prescribed amplification requirements is verified via real-ear measurements. Several prescriptive fitting procedures, which are covered elsewhere in this text, are currently widely used with adults.

The prescriptive procedure known as the Desired Sensation Level (DSL) approach (11) has recently begun to receive recognition because it addresses many of the problems with selecting and evaluating hearing aids of children. The DSL, developed specifically for use with children by Seewald (11) and coworkers (12), recognizes that threshold data are often limited or unavailable and that reliable judgments of comfort and discomfort levels are nearly impossible to obtain from infants and young children. Thus, the DSL requires only that the audiologist obtain frequency-specific thresholds from the child, preferably from each ear independently. The optimum frequency-gain characteristics for the hearing aid are calculated from the threshold values.

The DSL's premise is that for any given degree of hearing loss the speech signal is most useful for aural language acquisition when it is made available in a range of best listening. Because this range varies as a function of degree and configuration of hearing loss, the individual DSL targets are those that place the amplified speech spectrum at a particular sensation level above threshold. This level is useful for speech understanding and does not exceed the child's loudness discomfort level. The DSL prescriptive procedure provides individually determined desired sensation levels for the amplified average speech range (250–8,000 Hz). These levels form the basis of the series of amplification targets that the audiologist attempts to achieve by manipulating the hearing aid's gain and frequency response characteristics.

Additionally, the DSL provides large values for the hearing aid's maximum output (SSPL90). It is essential to set the output limiting characteristics of the child's hearing aid in order to prevent the child from experiencing loudness discomfort and avoid possible hearing damage from amplified sounds. Output limiting levels are determined by direct measurements of the real-ear saturation response and through the use of previously published values from adults and older children. Figure 9-3 illustrates DSL usage to make aided speech input both audible and com-

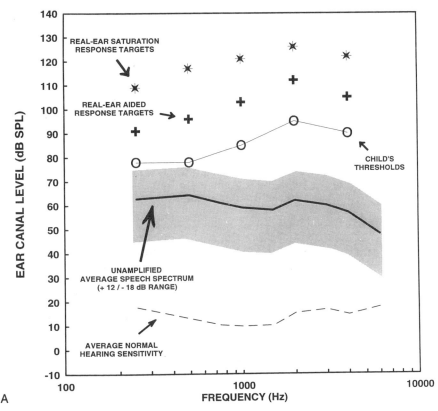

FIG. 9-3. Schematic representations of the basic principles of the DSL prescriptive hearing aid selection and evaluation approach (11). Depiction of the method for selecting the child's individualized DSL targets in the unaided condition (**A**) and evaluating or verifying how closely the prescription has been achieved in the aided condition (**B**). (Reprinted with permission of the author, R. Seewald.)

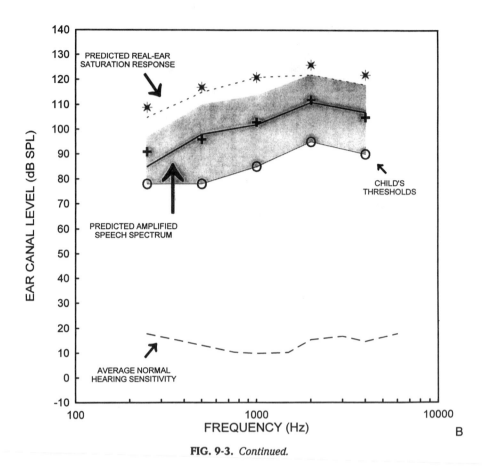

FIG. 9-3. *Continued.*

fortable for a child with severe hearing loss. Using systematic prescriptive hearing aid fitting procedures does not guarantee safe hearing aid output levels; frequency-specific output measures should be obtained routinely whenever possible. When children become capable of providing reliable loudness judgments, these also can be incorporated into the DSL prescriptive procedure (13).

Real-ear measurement is an important component of the DSL procedure because these values are used to calculate individualized amplification targets. In cases in which probe microphone measurements are not possible, age-appropriate RECD values can be used to predict amplification targets. However, the individual real-ear measurements are the only way to ensure that the targets provided by the DSL program are specific to the individual child and to verify that the amplification targets have been achieved.

The DSL prescriptive procedure eliminates the need to obtain any measures beyond threshold measures that delineate the degree and configuration of the hearing loss and (ideally) real-ear unaided response from the youngster. Thus, the process of selecting the individual hearing aid, setting the gain and output characteristics, and determining the volume control position can all be set in a hearing aid test box before evaluating them on the child.

VERIFICATION PROCEDURES

After hearing aid electroacoustic parameters have been predicted, verification of aided responses is completed using the child's own custom earmolds. Probe microphone measurements of real-ear hearing aid performance are preferred in the verification process. Real-ear aided response measures (whenever possible) verify the selection characteristics. Any necessary adjustments can then be made.

Functional-gain targets (aided sound-field threshold response values) also are provided in the DSL approach. However, because numerous factors influence aided functional gain measures, these are the least desirable measures for verifying that the selected targets and electroacoustic response parameters have been achieved. Verifying the frequency-gain characteristics of a child's hearing aid should incorporate individual probe microphone measures or the default RECD values to avoid problems associated with aided sound-field threshold measurements. These problems include lengthy test times, the need for extensive cooperation/attention from the child, and poor test–retest reliability.

The DSL prescriptive procedure recently was incorporated into one commercially available probe microphone system. Calculations also can be made via simple paper and pencil techniques using published tables. Perhaps the most useful and convenient method of determining DSL is the DSL computer software program, which can be readily used on any personal computer.

VALIDATION OF AIDED FUNCTION

Validation of aided auditory function is critical to the pediatric amplification process. It is important for the audiologist to demonstrate the benefits and limitations of a particular child's aided auditory abilities for the perception of speech. The pediatric audiologist integrates the directly obtained measurements of the child's aided auditory performance with input from parents and others to validate that the child is receiving an audible, comfortable speech signal.

A variety of functional performance measures are available for use with children. Speech awareness, discrimination, and identification measures are used to provide evidence that the child is learning an auditory–linguistic code that is useful for communication purposes. This validation of aided auditory performance is an ongoing process of measurements and direct observations made over a considerable period of time. If the child's performance with hearing aids does not meet expectations, then either additional hearing aid assessment and selection procedures are considered, or a supplemental form of amplification is considered (see above).

COUNSELING AND FOLLOW-UP

Counseling families of children with hearing loss requires professional cooperation to convey essential information to everyone involved with the child. Parents
who are actively involved throughout the hearing aid selection and evaluation process more effectively use this knowledge to advocate on behalf of their children.
Parental concerns and expectations guide the management process, reinforcing the
importance of the parent as a collaborative team member.

With regard to pediatric amplification, Thibodeau (14) reports that audiologists
generally provide both informational counseling and interpersonal counseling. Informational counseling focuses on hearing and hearing loss, amplification candidacy and selection, speech audibility and communication skills development, and
hearing aid adjustment issues. Interpersonal counseling focuses on how parents
use this information to help their child accept hearing aids and be responsible for
them, as well as advocate for their own hearing needs as they grow and develop.

Systematic monitoring of all children with sensorineural hearing loss is critical.
Cases of hearing loss exacerbated by recurrent otitis media, or progressive or de-
layed-onset sensorineural hearing loss, require even more frequent monitoring of
hearing status. Infants and young children should have their hearing and hearing
aids assessed at least every 3 months for the first year after amplification fitting.
Earmolds need to be remade every 3 months initially, and then usually every 6
months thereafter. Length of time between hearing status and amplification assessments can gradually be increased during the preschool years at intervals of 3 to 6
months. School-age children need their hearing and hearing aids checked at least
annually; other amplification systems used by these children (e.g., FM systems)
also should be included in this monitoring process.

It is important that professionals realize that counseling regarding amplification
is required beyond the initial period of first fitting. Children's amplification needs,
as well as technology, change with time. Parents must remain informed and current
with regard to their child's hearing aids and the options that are available for them.
In turn, this provides the basis for encouraging children to become educated con-
sumers and advocates for their own amplification needs.

THE INTERDISCIPLINARY TEAM

Interdisciplinary collaboration and teamwork are vital to successful management of every child with hearing loss. Public laws such as 94-142 and 99-457 underscore the essential nature of a family-centered, multidisciplinary team approach
to optimize outcomes. An audiologist experienced in the assessment and management of infants and children with hearing loss is the professional qualified to
select and fit amplification for children, including hearing aids, FM systems, and
other assistive listening devices (3). In addition to the audiologist, the child's
parents/caregiver, and the otolaryngologist, the team often includes the pediatri-

cian or family physician, the speech–language pathologist, and the teacher. Other specialists who may be consulted include a social worker, a pediatric nurse, a psychologist, an occupational therapist, a physical therapist, a special educator, a pediatric ophthalmologist, a pediatric neurologist, a geneticist, and a child psychiatrist (15).

SUMMARY

Infants and young children with hearing loss must hear speech comfortably and consistently in order to develop aural/oral communication. Today, children with permanent bilateral sensorineural hearing loss, unilateral hearing loss, high-frequency hearing loss, and hearing loss associated with otitis media all may be candidates for amplification. In addition to personal hearing aids, amplification options include FM systems, frequency transposition hearing aids, cochlear implants, and other assistive listening devices.

The audiologist is the professional qualified to select, evaluate, and manage amplification for infants and young children with hearing loss. Interdisciplinary collaboration and a family-centered approach optimize outcomes for children and their families. Primary caregivers, pediatricians or family physicians, speech–language pathologists, preschool teachers, and otolaryngologists are essential team members for every child with hearing loss.

Audiologic assessment of young children is an ongoing process of assimilating behavioral, electrophysiologic, and acoustic immittance data. No single test is used to determine hearing status. Intervention must often be initiated before precise frequency-specific information is available. Hearing aids for children must be flexible in tone, gain, and output-limiting characteristics. Binaural BTE hearing aids with tamper-resistant battery and volume controls are appropriate for most young children.

Prescriptive rather than comparative approaches are preferred for selecting and evaluating hearing aids. The DSL method, developed specifically for children, requires only frequency-specific thresholds, preferably from each ear. Target gain and output-limiting parameters are calculated in the DSL approach incorporating probe-microphone measurements. Hearing aid performance is verified through probe-microphone measures or the use of age-appropriate RECD correction values. Subjective frequency-specific comfort levels should be determined as children mature enough to respond reliably.

Aided auditory function is validated over time using functional performance measures in conjunction with parent and teacher input. Additional assessment and selection procedures are indicated when aided performance does not meet expectations based on the integration of audiologic data, parent/caregiver reports, and the individual child's physical and cognitive abilities. Parents become advocates for their child with a hearing loss as a result of their participation throughout the hearing aid selection and management process. Children with hearing loss learn from their parents the importance of accepting responsibility for their amplification and, in turn, become their own best advocates.

REFERENCES

1. National Institutes of Health. *Early identification of hearing impairments in infants and young children.* Bethesda, MD: National Institutes of Health; 1993.
2. Joint Committee on Infant Hearing. 1994 Position statement. *Audiol Today* 1994;6:6–9.
3. The Pediatric Working Group of the Conference on Amplificiation for Children with Auditory Deficits. Amplification for infants and children with hearing loss. *Am J Audiol* 1996;5(1):53–68.
4. Bess FH, Tharpe AM. Case history data on unilaterally hearing-impaired children. *Ear Hear* 1986; 7:14–19.
5. American Speech-Language-Hearing Association. Guidelines for the Audiologic assessment of children from birth through 36 months of age. *ASHA* 1991;33(suppl 5):37–43.
6. Chase PA, Hall JW III, Werkhaven JA. Medical and audiologic assessment and management of sensorineural hearing loss in children. In: Martin FN, Clark JG, eds. *Pediatric audiology.* New York: Allyn & Bacon (in press).
7. Kruger B, Ruben, AJ. The acoustic properties of the infant ear. *Acta Otolaryngol (Stockh)* 1987; 103:578–585.
8. Feigin JA, Kopun JG, Stelmachowicz PG, Gorga MP. Probe-tube microphone measures of ear canal sound pressure levels in infants and children. *Ear Hear* 1989;10:254–258.
9. Roush J, Gravel J. Acoustic amplification and sensory aids for infants and toddlers. In: Roush J, Matkin AND, eds. *Infants and toddlers with hearing loss: family-centered assessment and intervention.* Timonium, MD: York; 1994:65–79.
10. American Speech-Language-Hearing Association. Guidelines for fitting and monitoring FM systems. *ASHA* 1994;36(suppl 12):1–9.
11. Seewald RC. The desired sensation level method for fitting children: version 3.0. *Hear J* 1992; 45:36–41.
12. Seewald RC, Moodie KS, Sinclair ST, Corneliss LE. Traditional and theoretical approaches to selecting amplification for infants and young children. In: Bess FH, Gravel JS, Tharpe AM, eds. *Amplification for children with auditory deficits.* Nashville, TN: Bill Wilkerson Center Press (in press).
13. Kawell ME, Kopun JG, Stelmachowicz PG. Loudness discomfort levels in children. *Ear Hear* 1988;9:133–136.
14. Thibodeau LM. Counseling for pediatric amplification. In: Clark JG, Martin FN, eds. *Effective counseling in audiology—perspectives and practice.* Englewood Cliffs, NJ: Prentice-Hall; 1994: 147–183.
15. Matkin AND. Strategies for enhancing interdisciplinary collaboration. In: Roush J, Matkin AND, eds. *Infants and toddlers with hearing loss: family-centered assessment and intervention.* Timonium, MD: York; 1994:83–97.

HEARING AIDS: A MANUAL FOR CLINICIANS,
edited by Robert A. Goldenberg
Lippincott–Raven Publishers, Philadelphia © 1996

C H A P T E R ✦ *10* ✦

Cochlear Implants

Richard T. Miyamoto

Indiana University Medical School, Riley Hospital, Indianapolis, Indiana

Key Points

Description of a cochlear implant • special processing strategies • patient selection age considerations, and indications for use • audiologic and medical assessment • variables affecting performance for adults and children • importance of early implantation in children for speech and language production.

A cochlear implant is an electronic device consisting of an electrode array that is surgically implanted into the cochlea and an external unit consisting of a microphone that picks up sound energy and converts it to an electric signal and a signal processor that modifies the signal, depending on the processing scheme in use. The processed signal is amplified to an appropriate level and compressed to match the narrow electrical dynamic range of the ear. The typical response range of a deaf ear to electrical stimulation is on the order of only 10 to 20 dB, and even less in the high frequencies. Transmission of the electrical signal across the skin from the external unit to the implanted electrode array is most commonly accomplished by the use of electromagnetic induction or radiofrequency transmission. The various cochlear implant devices differ with respect to processing schemes (e.g., feature extraction or analog), placement of electrodes (e.g., intracochlear or extra-cochlear), stimulation configuration (e.g., monopolar or bipolar), and method of transmission of the signal through the skin (e.g., transcutaneous or percutaneous).

The critical residual neural elements stimulated appear to be the spiral ganglion cells or axons. Damaged or missing hair cells of the cochlea are bypassed. The current generation of multichannel, multielectrode cochlear implants use place coding to transfer high-frequency information in addition to accurately providing time and intensity information. The Nucleus 22-channel cochlear implant (Cochlear Corp.) has received U.S. Food and Drug Adminstration (FDA) approval for use in both adults and children and is currently the most commonly used multichannel system.

The implantable electrode array consists of platinum–iridium band electrodes placed in a silastic carrier (1). The Clarion device utilizes a radial bipolar configuration through electrodes positioned adjacent to the osseous spiral lamina in a 90-degree orientation. The radial bipolar orientation is theoretically more beneficial in achieving channel separation (2).

SPEECH PROCESSOR STRATEGIES

The most widely used speech processor for the Nucleus 22-channel cochlear implant (Figs. 10-1 and 10-2 is the Mini Speech Processor (MSP) (Cochlear Corp.). A speech feature-extraction strategy selects key features of speech to be presented to the central auditory system through the implanted electrode array. A later coding scheme builds on the F0F1F2 processor, which presented amplitude, voice pitch, and first- and second-format information via the implant. The MULTIPEAK scheme presents these acoustic features and additional information from three high-frequency spectral bands. The aim of the MULTIPEAK scheme is the presentation of additional consonant information, theoretically improving performance in moderate levels of noise. Recently, a new speech processor, the Spectra 22, and a new spectral peak (SPEAK) coding strategy have been introduced for use with the

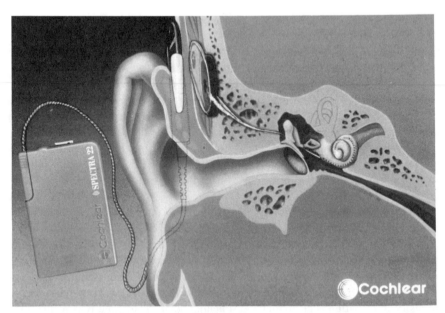

FIG. 10-1. Cochlear Spectra 22-channel implant (Cochlear Corp.) demonstrating speech processor, external coil on skin surface, internal coil implanted beneath skin, and 22-channel electrode array inserted in the cochlea.

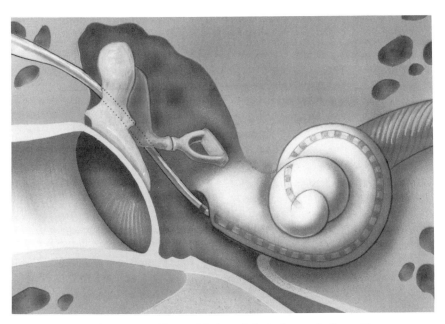

FIG. 10-2. Detail of Spectra 22-channel electrode array in the cochlea.

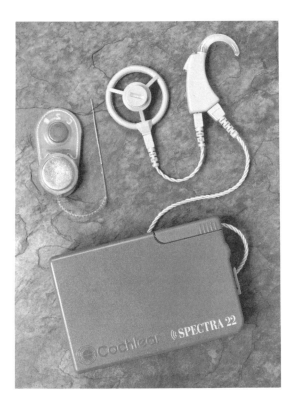

FIG. 10-3. Cochlear Spectra 22-channel signal processor, external coil, and internal coil with electrodes.

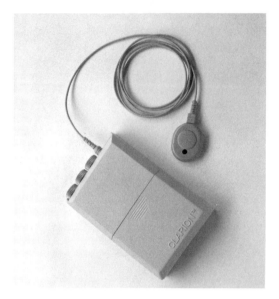

FIG. 10-4. Clarion speech processor, headpiece, and cable (Advanced Bionics Corp.).

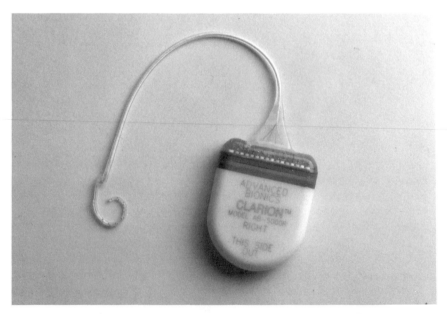

FIG. 10-5. Clarion intracochlear stimulator (Advanced Bionics Corp.).

Nucleus cochlear implant system. Rather than a feature extractor, the Spectral Maxima sound processor (SMSP) operates as a vocoder. The processor analyzes the acoustic input in terms of the relative amplitudes in 16 different filters. The processor scans the outputs of each of the filters and selects the six with the highest amplitudes for coding and transmission (Fig. 10-3).

The Advanced Bionics Clarion multistrategy cochlear implant is an extremely flexible device that allows programming in the digital or analog mode and can accommodate all strategies currently used by other cochlear implants. Advanced strategies termed continuous interleaved sampling (CIS) and compressed analog (CA) have been used with the eight-channel Clarion device (3) (Figs. 10-4 and 10-5).

PATIENT SELECTION

Profound hearing loss poses a monumental obstacle to the acquisition and maintenance of effective communication skills. The perception as well as the production of speech is highly dependent on the ability to process auditory information. Early identification of hearing loss is an important first step in managing the effects of hearing impairment. Once identified, the level of residual hearing, if any, must be determined and an appropriate sensory aid recommended. In most cases, conventional amplification is the initial procedure of choice. If little or no benefit is realized with hearing aids, cochlear implants become therapeutic options. This must be followed by the assessment of communication skills and needs, and the selection of a communication mode. Successful application of cochlear implant technology is highly dependent on a sophisticated multidisciplinary team approach that addresses the varied needs of the deaf recipient. The selection of cochlear implant candidates is a complex and ever-evolving process that requires careful consideration of many factors. Current selection criteria are as follows:

Age of ≥2 years
Profound bilateral sensorineural hearing loss (SNHL)
No appreciable benefit from hearing aids
No medical contraindications
High motivation and appropriate expectations
Enrollment in program that emphasizes development of auditory skills

AGE CONSIDERATIONS

A lower age limit of 2 years has been applied during the FDA clinical trials. However, because of the profound negative effect of early-onset deafness on the development of speech perception, speech production, and language competence, an even younger age limit would be advantageous if profound deafness can be substantiated and the inability to benefit from conventional hearing aids demonstrated. In addition, when the etiology of deafness is meningitis, progressive intracochlear ossification may occur, which can preclude standard electrode insertion.

A relatively short window of opportunity exists during which this advancing process can be circumvented. The feasibility of earlier implantation (earlier than the currently accepted age of 2 years) is substantiated by developmental anatomy. The cochlea is adult size at birth, and by 1 year of age the facial recess and mastoid antrum that provide access to the middle ear for electrode placement are adequately developed. For these reasons, extension of implant candidacy to the 1- to 2-year age group is feasible and in selected cases desirable. No upper age limit is applied as long as the patient's health status permits an elective surgical procedure. The age at implantation in the Indiana University Cochlear Implant Program spans the range from 16 months to 87 years at the time of this writing.

PEDIATRIC COCHLEAR IMPLANTATION

Pediatric cochlear implant recipients can be loosely divided into three main categories that significantly affect the anticipated outcomes when this technology is applied.

Postlingually Deafened Children

Children who become deaf at or after 5 years of age are generally classified as postlingually deafened. Even though these children have developed many aspects of spoken language before the onset of their deafness, they demonstrate rapid deterioration in the intelligibility of their speech once they lose access to auditory input and feedback. Early implantation can potentially ameloriate this rapid deterioration in speech production and perception abilities. However, a postlingual onset of deafness is an infrequent occurrence in the pediatric population. If this were to be the only category for which cochlear implants positively impacted deaf children, there would be limited applicability for this technology in children.

Congenitally or Early-Deafened Young Children

Congenital or early acquired deafness is the most frequently encountered type of profound sensorineural hearing loss. The acquisition of communication skills is a difficult process for these children. Whether sufficient acoustic input can be provided by cochlear implantation to perceive a speech signal linguistically is the focus of a comprehensive longitudinal study.

Congenitally or Early-Deafened Adolescents and Young Adults

When cochlear implantation is considered in adolescence or young adulthood for a patient who has had little or no experience with sound because of congenital or early onset deafness, caution must be exercised because this group has not demonstrated high levels of success with electrical stimulation of the auditory system.

ADULT COCHLEAR IMPLANTATION

Adult cochlear implantation has been focused primarily on postlinguistically deafened patients. Only rarely is implantation recommended on prelingually deafened adults.

Audiologic Assessment

The audiologic evaluation is the primary means of determining suitability for cochlear implantation. Both unaided and aided thresholds using conventional amplification are determined. A period of experience with a properly fitted hearing aid coupled with training in an appropriate aural rehabilitation program is necessary. Hearing aid performance can then be compared with normative cochlear implant performance. The children who have been the most obvious candidates for a cochlear implant are those who have demonstrated no response to warble tones in the sound field with appropriate hearing aids or responses suggestive of vibrotactile rather than auditory sensation, i.e., aided responses at levels of higher than 50 to 60 dB HL in the lower frequencies with no responses above 1,000 Hz.

Not all children with profound sensorineural hearing losses are implant candidates. Hearing aid performance data collected in our laboratory have shown that many children with pure-tone thresholds of 90 to 105 dB HL with residual hearing through at least 2,000 Hz demonstrate closed- and open-set speech recognition skills that are superior multichannel implant users. Sufficient receptive and expressive abilities to allow the child to learn to make a conditioned response assist in accurately estimating the child's auditory potential and, if accepted as an implant candidate, ultimately assist in device setting and permit the child to begin the extensive rehabilitation program.

Medical Assessment

The medical assessment includes the otologic history, physical examination, and radiologic evaluation of the cochlea (4). The precise etiology for the deafness is determined whenever possible. However, experience with cochlear implants has demonstrated that stimulatable auditory neural elements are nearly always present regardless of cause of deafness (5). Two exceptions are the Michel deformity, in which there is a congenital agenesis of the cochlea, and the small internal auditory canal syndrome, in which the cochlear nerve may be congenitally absent.

Routine otoscopic evaluation of the tympanic membrane is performed. An otologically stable condition should be present before considering implantation in children. The ear proposed for cochlear implantation must be free of infection, and the tympanic membrane must be intact. If these conditions are not met, medical and/or surgical treatment before implantation is required. Because children are more prone to otitis media than adults, justifiable concern has been expressed that a middle ear infection could cause an implanted device to become an infected foreign body requiring its removal. Of even greater concern is that infection might extend along the electrode into the inner ear, resulting in a serious otogenic complication such as meningitis or further degeneration of the central auditory system. To date, although the incidence of otitis media in children who have received cochlear implants parallels that seen in the general pediatric population, no serious complications have occurred in our patients.

PERFORMANCE RESULTS IN ADULTS

Evaluation Procedures

Implant benefit in adults is measured using a battery of audiological tests that assess sound and speech detection and reception of speech with the implant compared with the patient's preoperative performance with hearing aids. The least difficult tests are those that assess identification of environmental sounds and recognition of the prosodic characteristics of speech, such as temporal or intonation patterns. Speechreading enhancement is measured by comparing recognition of sentences or connected discourse with the implant turned off to performance with the implant turned on. Auditory word identification is assessed using a closed-set response format. In closed-set testing, the test (target) item is one of a limited number of choices, thus permitting guessing as in standard multiple-choice tests. The most difficult type of test is recognition of words or sentences in an open set. In open-set testing, the test (target) stimulus is one of a large number of possible stimuli, and the listener has no alternatives from which to select the answer. Thus, guessing becomes a negligible factor. The ability of patients to perform auditory-only speech recognition tasks using an open-set response format is the ultimate goal of cochlear implants.

Comparative studies by Gantz et al. (6) and a prospective randomized study funded by the Department of Veterans Affairs (7,8) demonstrated a performance advantage of multichannel devices over single-channel implants. However, a wide range of performance across subjects with various devices has been demonstrated. For any given implant system, scores on speech recognition tasks can vary from 0% to 100%. The reasons for the large difference in patient performance are not clearly understood, and for this reason implant benefit cannot be reliably predicted from preoperative measures (Fig. 10-6).

Variables Affecting Performance

Among the most important factors affecting performance is auditory nerve survival. However, preoperative tests for estimating the number and location of sur-

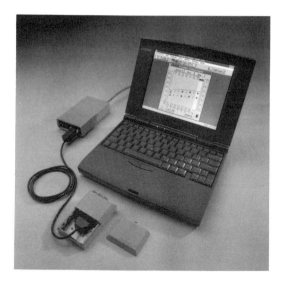

FIG. 10-6. Clarion fitting system (Advanced Bionics Corp.).

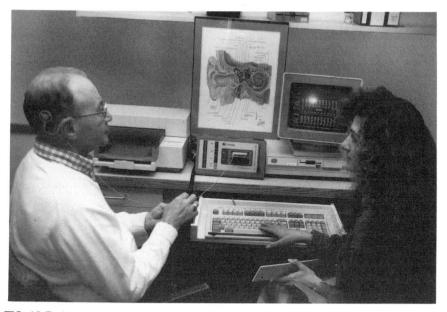

FIG. 10-7. Adult cochlear Spectra 22-channel implant recipient being programmed by audiologist.

viving auditory nerve fibers are lacking. To date, neither radiographic nor electro-physiological measures are able to determine the condition of the auditory nerve (9–11).

Postimplant speech recognition performance in adults has been moderately cor-related with electrical thresholds, dynamic ranges, and the number of electrodes in use (6,12). Moderate correlations between duration of profound deafness before implantation and speech recognition abilities also have been reported (6). Stan-dardized measures of intellectual ability have not been found to be predictive of implant outcome, but a measure of the patients' willingness to participate in their own health care was correlated significantly with speech understanding (13).

Initial results from the clinical trial with the Clarion device in adults revealed a median score of 65% on a test of open-set sentence recognition for the 61 patients tested after 6 months of device use. Roughly half of these patients obtained an open-set sentence recognition score higher than 70% with evidence of relatively rapid im-provements in speech recognition performance after implantation (Fig. 10-7).

PERFORMANCE RESULTS IN CHILDREN

Unlike postlingually deafened adults who use the information transmitted by an implant to compare with previously stored representations of spoken language, pe-diatric implant users must rely on the same information to first develop these rep-resentations. Because of this, perceptual skills develop over a relatively long time course in prelingually deafened children (14–16). Data suggest that substantial im-provements in closed-set word recognition usually did not occur in prelingually deafened children until after they had used their multichannel implants for more than 1 year, and improvements in open-set speech recognition occurred after an even longer period of device use.

Since pediatric implant work began, a number of new procedures have been de-veloped to evaluate children's pre- and postimplant performance. Similar to work with adults, procedures were developed to assess perception of the prosodic infor-mation, speechreading benefit, and closed- and open-set speech recognition.

Comparison Between Single- and Multichannel Implants

Relatively few comparative single- and multichannel implant studies have been conducted with children. Most investigations with children have reported on the performance of either single- or multichannel implant users, whereas relatively few implant investigations have conducted comparative device studies. A study conducted by Miyamoto et al. (15) compared the performance of matched groups of children who used either the 3M/House device or the Nucleus multichannel cochlear implant over time. The results showed that the performance of the Nu-cleus users was higher than that of the 3M/House users on every speech perception measure, even on those measures that assessed aspects of speech purportedly transmitted best by the single-channel device (i.e., prosodic information). Thus, the multichannel implant not only permitted better word recognition without speechreading, but it also conveyed better information about the time-intensity cues in speech. Even though some reports have shown that a small percentage of children demonstrated open-set speech recognition with the 3M/House implant (17), the highest level of performance achieved by the majority of single-channel users was the perception of stress pattern and syllable number in speech.

Performance with Multichannel Implants

The research design most commonly applied to evaluate implant benefit in children is a within-subjects design wherein the subject serves as his or her own control in the pre- and postimplant conditions. The largest studies of this nature have been conducted as part of the clinical trials of the Nucleus multichannel implant in children (18). After 12 months of multichannel implant use, Staller et al. (18) reported mean scores of 39% (n = 84) on a closed-set word identification test, 23% (n = 42) on a test of open-set sentence recognition, and 12% (n = 25) on a test of open-set, monosyllabic word recognition. Examination of individual data showed that 13% of the subjects demonstrated significantly above-chance closed-set word identification before implantation, whereas, postoperatively, 62% of the subjects achieved this level of performance. Preoperatively, the subjects showed no open-set speech recognition, but 12 months after implantation, 45% of the subjects recognized one or more words in sentences administered in an open set.

Pediatric implant performance also is reported in terms of clinically descriptive categories of benefit. Geers and Moog (19) developed a classification system that describes performance along a hierarchy of speech perception abilities: (category 1) no pattern perception, (category 2) consistent pattern perception, (category 3) inconsistent word identification, (category 4) consistent word identification, and (category 5) open-set word recognition. Staller et al. (20) reported that the percentage of children reaching category 3 and above (i.e., closed- or open-set word recognition) increased from 12% to 80% postoperatively, and roughly half of the subjects demonstrated open-set speech recognition and were assigned a category rating of 5. Osberger et al. (21) developed a similar classification scheme, modified to describe performance on the tests in their assessment battery, and reported that roughly half of the subjects demonstrated open-set speech recognition after they had used their implants for an average of 2 years.

Variables Affecting Performance with Multichannel Cochlear Implants

Large individual differences among implanted children have been documented on speech perception measures. Some children demonstrated relatively high levels of speech recognition, whereas others perceived primarily prosodic speech information from their devices (18,21). Age at onset of deafness, duration of deafness before implantation, and educational setting are the independent variables most often examined to explain such performance differences. Studies by Staller et al. (18,22) reported that two factors—age at onset of deafness and duration of deafness—were significantly related to speech perception performance in children who used the Nucleus multichannel cochlear implant. They found that subjects with later onset and shorter duration of deafness performed better on measures of speech perception than did subjects with early onset of deafness but relatively long duration of deafness at the time of implantation.

The effect of age at onset of deafness on speech perception skills was examined by Osberger et al. (23) in children who received a single- or multichannel cochlear implant. No significant differences were found in the mean postoperative speech perception scores as a function of age at onset of deafness unless the subjects were postlingually deafened (i.e., onset of deafness at ≥5 years of age). Subjects with postlingual deafness achieved significantly higher speech perception scores on all measures than did the subjects with prelingual deafness (i.e., congenital or acquired deafness). In a more recent study that included only children with multichannel implants (i.e., Nucleus device) with prelingual deafness who received their implants before 10 years of age, the results showed no significant difference between the speech perception scores of a group of subjects with congenital deafness and the mean scores of a second group of subjects with deafness acquired before 3 years of age (24). The general finding of similar performance between children with congenital and early acquired deafness is probably influenced by the secondary effects of meningitis (i.e., neurological problems and cochlear ossification) on the performance of the children with acquired deafness. These results indicate that children who are born deaf have the potential to derive the same benefit from multichannel implants as do children who had some exposure to spoken language before the onset of their deafness from meningitis.

The postimplant performance of children with postlingual deafness (i.e., onset of deafness at ≥5 years of age) differs from that of children with prelingual deafness in several important respects. Children with relatively late onset of deafness typically show rapid and marked improvement in speech perception abilities with an implant (14,23). As noted earlier, speech perception performance improves gradually in prelingually implanted children.

The results of several investigations have shown a significant relationship between the communication method used by the child and performance on speech perception measures. In these studies, more children who used oral communication achieved higher levels of implant performance than did children who used total communication (i.e., signs plus speaking and listening) (17,21). The relationship between communication mode and implant performance is less clear in other studies. For example, Miyamoto et al. (24) found that children who used oral communication obtained significantly higher scores on only two of the 13 speech perception measures in their study. Additional research is needed to clarify this issue.

Comparison of Cochlear Implants, Hearing Aids, and Tactile Aids

Children with profound hearing impairments demonstrate a wide range of auditory capabilities (25). A within-subjects research design is influenced by this variability confounding the evaluation of various sensory aids. Therefore, the establishment of a control group is desirable. Using the results of previous investigators as a guide, Osberger et al. (20) developed a descriptive system to classify the range of hearing levels in children with profound hearing impairments. Hearing aid users were divided into three groups based on the unaided better-ear pure-tone thresholds at 500, 1,000, and 2,000 Hz. Subjects classified as gold hearing aid users demonstrated pure-tone thresholds of 90 to 100 dB HL at two of the three frequencies (with none of the thresholds greater than 105 dB HL). Silver hearing aid users demonstrated hearing levels of 101 to 110 dB HL at two of the three frequencies, whereas bronze hearing aid users demonstrated two of three thresholds greater than 110 dB HL. Using this approach, the gold hearing aid users were viewed as setting the standard of performance for children with profound hearing impairments because children with this amount of residual hearing developed the most intelligible speech. At the other end of the continuum were bronze hearing aid users, who appeared to respond to auditory stimuli on the basis of vibrotactile sensation. To date, the majority of children who have received implants would be classified as Bronze hearing aid users. The unaided pure-tone thresholds of the silver hearing aid users were intermediate to those of the other two groups.

The benefits of multichannel cochlear implantation in prelingually deafened children can be demonstrated only by comprehensive longitudinal studies. Valid performance trends may not become apparent for 1 to 3 or even more years postoperatively. Studies in our laboratory have documented the ability of deaf children who were unable to even detect sound with conventional hearing aids preoperatively (bronze hearing aid users) to achieve scores with their multichannel implants that were comparable with those of the gold hearing aid users on most tests (except on a test of open-set speech recognition).

The intermediate group of children, classified as silver hearing aid users (i.e., pure-tone thresholds of 100–105 dB HL), clearly might derive more benefit from multichannel implants than from continued use of only hearing aids. Extension of implant candidacy to this group and even to selected gold hearing aid users is the target of future research. Improved implant technology and earlier implantation promise to widen the candidacy window.

An important issue in sensory aid research with profoundly deaf children has been determination of the benefits derived from noninvasive alternatives to cochlear implants, such as tactile aids. The results of a recent study by Miyamoto et al. (26) demonstrated that children who used multichannel implants derived substantially more speech perception benefit from their devices than did children who used multichannel tactile aids. Miyamoto et al. compared the performance of two groups of subjects who either received a Nucleus implant or a multichannel vibrotactile aid, the Tactaid 7. There were 10 subjects in each group, matched on the basis of age at onset of deafness, age fit with a multichannel device, and nonverbal intelligence. Subjects were tested on a battery of speech perception measures in the predevice interval and at one postdevice interval (i.e., after an average of roughly 1.5 years of device use). The results showed that the scores of the implant users improved significantly between the pre- and postdevice intervals on all measures. Moreover, the scores of the Nucleus users were significantly higher than those of the Tactaid users on all measures. In contrast, the scores of the tactile aid users showed negligible change over time, except on a test that evaluated open-set recognition of phrases with both auditory and visual cues. The results suggested that children learned to recognize words and understand speech without lip-reading with a multichannel implant, whereas children who used a multichannel tactile aid demonstrated evidence of speech recognition only if tactile cues were combined with visual ones (Fig. 10-8).

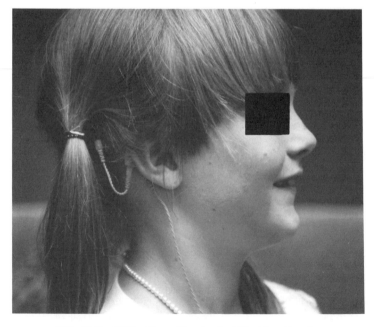

FIG. 10-8. Child with cochlear implant (Cochlear Corp.).

Speech Production

Although the primary role of a cochlear implant is to make speech sounds accessible auditorily, cochlear implants also serve as aids to speech production. Osberger et al. (27) have demonstrated that profoundly hearing impaired children's phonetic repertoires increase after receiving a multichannel cochlear implant. Improvements in the production of consonant and vowel features that are typically difficult for children with profound hearing losses to master have been documented (i.e., high vowels, diphthongs, alveolar consonants, and fricatives). Improvements in speech productions also have been documented by Tobey et al. (28). Children who are postlingually deafened or those who receive implants at an early age generally demonstrate large improvements in speech, whereas those with early onset of deafness who do not receive implants until adolescence typically show more limited improvements in speech production performance.

The scores for the implanted subjects showed gradual improvement over time. After 2.5 years of cochlear implant use, the average speech intelligibility of the implanted subjects began to exceed that of the silver hearing aid users. After 3.5 to 4 years of device use, the average intelligibility of the implant users was 40%, which is approximately 20% higher than that of the silver hearing aid users. The majority of the children in this study did not receive implants until they were 5 to 8 years of age. Further studies are underway to examine changes in speech intelligibility in children who were implanted at a younger age.

SUMMARY AND CONCLUSIONS

Cochlear implants are an appropriate alternative for selected deaf children and adults who do not benefit from conventional amplification. Improvements have been documented in both speech perception and speech production skills. However, the full impact of cochlear implantation will be determined only by detailed longitudinal studies. Multichannel systems that provide spectral information in addition to temporal and intensity cues have demonstrated performance advantages, and it is anticipated that continued improvements in signal coding and processing permit electrically transmitted information to even more effectively transcend the deafened peripheral auditory system. This requires refinements in assessing peripheral auditory neuronal survival and matching electrically transmitted signals to the future potential of the central auditory system in the deaf subjects.

REFERENCES

1. Clark G. The University of Melbourne Nucleus multi-electrode cochlear implant. *Adv Otol Rhinol Laryngol* 1987;38:189.
2. Schindler RA, Kessler DK, Rebscher SJ, Yanda JL, et al. The UCSF/Storz multichannel cochlear implant: patient results. *Laryngoscope* 1986;96:597.

3. Wilson BS, Finley CC, Lawson DT, et al. Better speech recognition with cochlear implants. *Nature* 1991;352:236.

4. Yune HY, Miyamoto RT, Yune ME. Medical imaging in cochlear implant candidates. *Am J Otol* 1991;12(suppl)11–17.

5. Hinojosa R, Marion M. Histopathology of profound sensorineural deafness. *Ann NY Acad Sci* 1983;405:459–484.

6. Gantz BJ, et al. Evaluation of five different cochlear implant designs: audiologic assessment and predictors of performance. *Laryngoscope* 1988;98:1100.

7. Cohen NL, Waltzman SB, Fisher SG. A prospective, randomized study of cochlear implants. *N Engl J Med* 1993;328:233.

8. Waltzman SB, Cohen NL, Fisher SG. An experimental comparison of cochlear implant systems. *Semin Hear* 1992;13;195.

9. Jackler RK. CT and MRI of the ear and temporal bone: current state of the art and future prospects. *Am J Otol* 1988;9:232.

10. Balkany TJ, Dreisback J. Workshop: surgical anatomy and radiographic imaging of cochlear implant surgery. *Am J Otol* 1987;8:195.

11. Stypulkowski P, Van den Honert C, Kvistad SD. Electrophysiologic evaluation of the cochlear implant patient. *Otolaryngol Clin North Am* 1986;19:249.

12. Kileny PR, Zimmerman-Phillips S, Kemink JL. Effects of active channel number and place of stimulation on performance with multichannel implant. *Am J Otol* 1992;13:117.

13. Knutson J, et al. Psychological predictors of audiological outcomes of multichannel cochlear implants: preliminary findings. *Ann Otol Rhinol Laryngol* 1991;100:817.

14. Fryauf-Bertschy H, Tyler RS, Kelsay DM, Gantz BJ. Performance over time of congenitally deaf and postlingually deafened children using a multichannel cochlear implants. *J Speech Hear Res* 1992;35:913.

15. Miyamoto RT, Osberger MJ, Robbins AM, et al. Longitudinal evaluation of communication skills of children with single- or multichannel cochlear implants. *Am J Otol* 1992;13:215.

16. Waltzman SB, Cohen NL, Gomolin R, et al. Long-term results of early cochlear implantation in congenitally and prelingually deafened children. *Am J Otol* 1994;14(suppl 2):9.

17. Berliner KI, Tonokawa LL, Dye LL, House WF. Open-set speech recognition in children with a single-channel cochlear implant. *Ear Hear* 1989;10:237.

18. Staller SJ, Dowell RC, Beiter AL, Brimacombe JA. Perceptual abilities of children with the Nucleus 22–channel cochlear implant. *Ear Hear* 1991;12(suppl):34.

19. Geers AE, Moog JS. *Early speech perception test*. St. Louis: Central Institute for the Deaf, 1990.

20. Osberger MJ, Maso M, Sam L. Speech intelligibility of children with cochlear implants, tactile aids, or hearing aids. *J Speech Hear Res* 1993;36:186.

21. Osberger MJ, Miyamoto RT, Zimmerman-Phillips S, et al. Independent evaluation of the speech perception abilities of children with the Nucleus 22–channel cochlear implant system. *Ear Hear* 1991;12(suppl):66.

22. Staller SJ, Beiter AL, Brimacombe JA, et al. Pediatric performance with the Nucleus 22–channel cochlear implant system. *Am J Otol* 1991;12(suppl):126.

23. Osberger MJ, Todd SL, Berry SW, et al. Effect of age at onset of deafness on children's speech perception abilities with a cochlear implant. *Ann Otol Rhinol Larnygol* 1991;100:883.

24. Miyamoto RT, Osberger MJ, Robbins AM, et al. Prelingually deafened children's performance with the Nucleus multichannel cochlear implant. *Am J Otol* 1993;14:437.

25. Boothroyd A. Auditory perception of speech contrasts by subjects with sensorineural hearing loss. *J Speech Hear Res* 1984;27:134.

26. Miyamoto RT, Robbins AM, Osberger MJ, et al. Comparison of tactile aids and cochlear implants in children with profound hearing impairments. *Am J Otol* (in press).

27. Osberger MJ, et al. Analysis of the spontaneous speech samples of children using a cochlear implant or tactile aid. *Am J Otol* 1991;12(suppl):151–164.

28. Tobey EA, et al. Speech production performance in children with multi-channel cochlear implants. *Am J Otol* 1991;12(suppl):165–173.

HEARING AIDS: A MANUAL FOR CLINICIANS,
edited by Robert A. Goldenberg
Lippincott–Raven Publishers, Philadelphia © 1996

C H A P T E R ✦ *11* ✦

Assistive Technology for the Hearing Impaired

Daniel J. Orchik

Department of Audiology, Shea Clinic, and Hearing Services of Memphis, Memphis, Tennessee

Key Points

Definition of assistive listening technology • supplement of hearing aids • review of representative types of devices • description of common devices and their use.

For the purpose of this chapter, assistive technology is defined as any device, other than a hearing aid, that enhances the hearing-impaired individual's ability to hear and understand speech or be made aware of environmental signals. By definition then, assistive technology for the hearing impaired includes not only devices that provide auditory information, but systems that generate visual and tactile signals as well.

The typical patient uses assistive technology either in lieu of a hearing aid or in addition to a hearing aid. Many are not ready to accept a hearing aid, although their families are concerned (or even annoyed and irritated) over the patient's hearing problems. Assistive technology allows the clinician to provide solutions to specific problems, which often leads to acceptance of a hearing aid by patients who need them.

Then there is the group of patients that wear hearing aids, but the degree of hearing loss or poor speech understanding renders the patient unable to understand anything but face-to-face conversation in a quiet listening environment. Fortunately, these patients are typically unconcerned with cosmetics (1). They only want to hear.

The available technology for both of these groups literally fills catalogues. It is impossible to review all of the available technology in a single chapter, nor is it necessary for clinicians to be familiar with all of the technology or have it available in their practices. In the pages to follow are reviewed the general types of assistive systems to provide a familiarity with current technology. Then the typical problems presented by patients in the two groups mentioned above are reviewed and possible solutions provided.

AVAILABLE ASSISTIVE TECHNOLOGY

For purposes of discussion within this chapter, assistive technology is divided into three categories: auditory assistive devices, telecommunication devices, and alerting devices. These categorizations are made with the understanding that a certain amount of overlap may be found among the three classifications.

Auditory Assistive Devices

This category includes infrared (IR) systems, frequency-modulated (FM) systems, induction loop systems, and self-contained amplification (hard-wired) systems. The primary purpose for use of any of these systems is to enhance the signal-to-noise ratio that has been diminished either by increased background noise or increased distance between the listener and the sound source. Although all of the above-mentioned auditory assistive devices are available in wide-area systems as well as personal systems, this chapter is directed toward individual patient use of assistive technology; thus, wide-area systems are not covered.

As the name implies, IR listening systems use modulated IR light to transmit an auditory signal. A small transmitter converts an audio signal to IR light and sends the IR signal across the room. The audio signal is frequency modulated around a carrier light frequency, typically 95 kHz (2), and transmitted to the receiver. The patient wears an IR receiver that picks up the IR signal and decodes it into a high-fidelity audio signal. The IR system is a wireless system; thus, the individual can sit anywhere within the coverage area of the system. A typical personal IR system is illustrated in Fig. 11-1. The most common uses of the personal IR system include listening to television, radio, or tape recordings.

FM systems transmit auditory signals using radio waves. As shown in Fig. 11-2, a personal FM system consists of a transmitter that picks up the desired audio signal and sends it to a receiver worn by the listener. The audio signal is frequency modulated around a carrier frequency that is transmitted to the receiver, where it is demodulated and delivered to the ear of the listener. The Federal Communications Commission (FCC) has allocated a range of radio frequencies between 72 and 76 MHZ for use in FM auditory assistive devices (3). The FM transmitter may use a microphone or may be coupled directly to the output of a television, radio, or tape recorder.

Induction loop systems have been used for decades in classrooms of the hearing impaired. They operate on the principle of magnetic induction. When an electrical current is amplified and passed through a coil of wire, a magnetic field is generated around the wire that varies in intensity and frequency according to the strength and

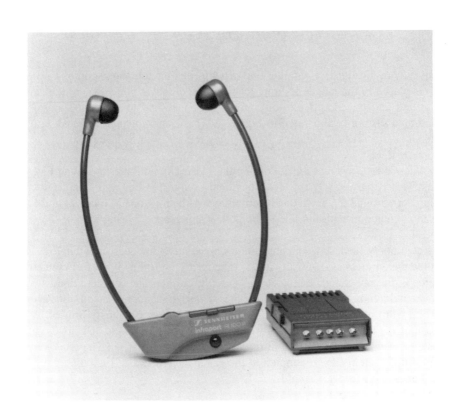

FIG. 11-1. A personal IR system (courtesy Sennheiser Electronics).

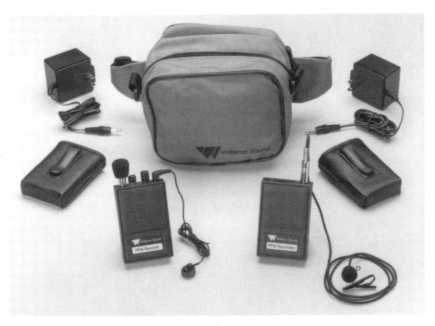

FIG. 11-2. A personal FM system (courtesy Williams Sound Corp.).

frequency of the signal. If another coil of wire (i.e., the telephone coil of a hearing aid) is placed in the magnetic field, an electrical signal is generated which can be amplified and transduced into an audio signal identical to the sound source. A small-area system is illustrated in Fig. 11-3. This system is also wireless, and the listener can receive the signal as long as they remain within close proximity to the magnetic field.

Induction loop systems are not as popular in the United States as IR and FM systems. This is particularly true with personal systems, although a small induction loop, worn around the neck, can be combined with an IR or FM receiver and operate in conjunction with the telephone coil of a personal hearing aid, as shown in Fig. 11-4

A commonly used, self-contained, auditory assistive device is shown in Fig. 11-5. Unlike the wireless systems previously discussed, the audio signal from the sound source is directly connected (electrically) to the patient. The self-contained system shown in the figure uses a microphone that is electrically connected to the receiver portion worn by the patient. The range of this system is obviously limited by the length of the microphone cord; however, its operation is simple and the device is less expensive than the other auditory devices described earlier. The receiver portion of this system can be coupled to the ear in several ways, including ear buds, earphones, and custom earmolds.

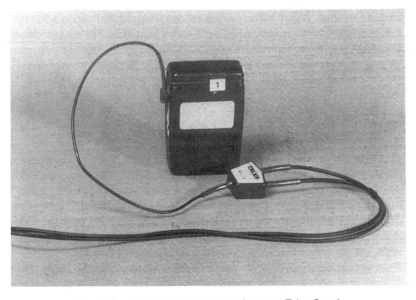

FIG. 11-3. An induction loop system (courtesy Telex Corp.).

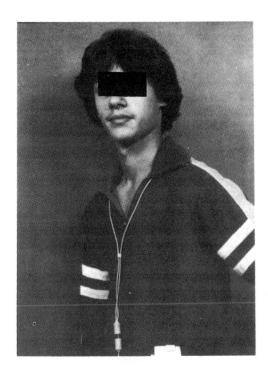

FIG. 11-4. Personal FM system with neck loop (courtesy Phonic Ear, Inc.).

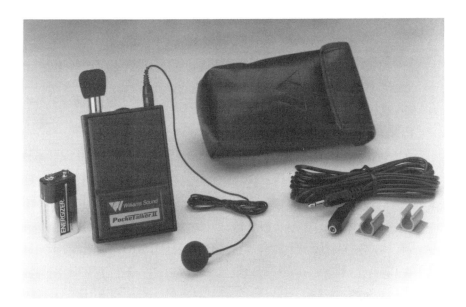

FIG. 11-5. The pocket talker. A self-contained assistive device (courtesy Williams Sound Corp.).

Telecommunication Devices

For most of us, the telephone is our link to the outside world. The telephone is used to communicate with friends and family, to conduct business, to seek medical care, and for a host of other reasons. Imagine what a typical day would be like without the use of a telephone. It is easy to see what a hardship it is for the hearing-impaired individual who cannot hear or understand conversation over the telephone.

A wide variety of assistive technology to aid the hearing impaired with telephone use is available. However, the compatibility of the assistive device with the telephone of the hearing-impaired individual can be a problem. With the divestiture of AT&T came the proliferation of telephone products without any standard of performance. The result is that performance among telephones varies widely, and thus so does the performance of telephone assistive devices. For an analysis of the

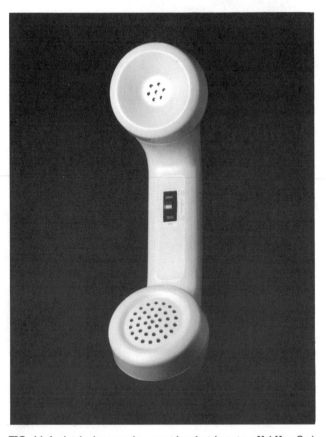

FIG. 11-6. A telephone replacement handset (courtesy Hal-Hen Co.).

problems related to individual telephone performance, the reader is referred to the excellent review of Slager (4). The reader should be advised that the performance of a telephone amplifier will be influenced by the performance characteristics of the telephone to which it is attached.

If a telephone has a detachable receiver, the simplest way of providing amplification to the telephone is to replace the handset. A typical replacement handset is shown in Fig. 11-6. The volume is controlled by using a rotary dial on the handset. Some handsets have a touch control for volume adjustment that automatically resets to normal volume upon hanging up the telephone. This is a useful feature when a number of people use the same telephone, especially if some have normal hearing. As mentioned above, the performance of replaceable handsets will be affected by the characteristics of the telephone to which they are attached. A number of newer electronic telephones do not have enough power coming to the handset to drive the amplifier of the assistive device.

Instead of replacing the handset, one can acquire an amplified telephone, as shown in Fig. 11-7. Although more expensive than a replacement handset, the amplified telephone offers certain advantages. One model allows for the adjustment of high frequencies independently. This is particularly helpful for individuals with high-frequency hearing loss whose requirements are improved clarity more than increased volume. Another model of replacement telephone allows for 40 to 50 dB of gain and is suitable for moderate to severe hearing losses.

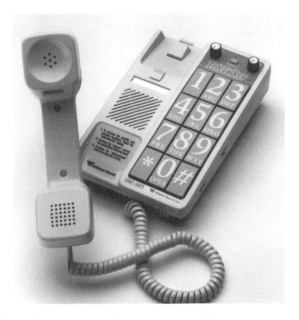

FIG. 11-7. An amplified telephone (courtesy Williams Sound Corp.).

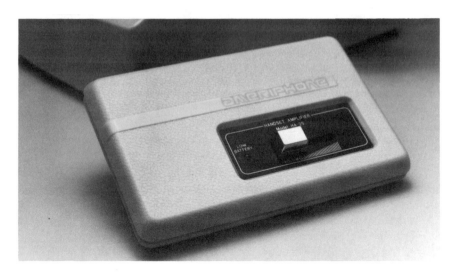

FIG. 11-8. In-line telephone amplifier (courtesy Ameriphone, Inc.).

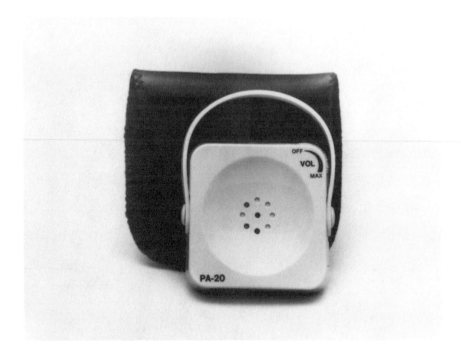

FIG. 11-9. A portable telephone amplifier (courtesy Ameriphone, Inc.).

Figure 11-8 shows an in-line telephone amplifier. This particular model is battery powered and works with any telephone except those with the dial in the handset. In the author's experience, this device works when replacement handsets do not because of compatibility issues. This type of telephone amplifier is also available with a plug-in transformer power supply, obviating the need to replace batteries.

A portable telephone amplifier is also available and is shown in Fig. 11-9. This device has its own microphone, enabling an acoustic coupling to the telephone receiver. This device works on any telephone and provides in excess of 20 dB of gain. Thus, this amplifier can be used by individuals with up to moderate hearing losses without need of a hearing aid.

For those individuals whose degree of hearing loss or reduced speech discrimination precludes understanding the spoken word over the telephone, regardless of the amount of amplification provided, the telephone device for the deaf (TDD) provides a visual signal to enable telephone communication. A typical TDD is shown in Fig. 11-10. Such a device requires that both parties to the conversation have a TDD or that a telephone relay service be used. In the relay service, the call

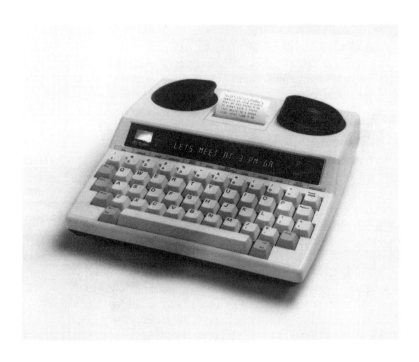

FIG. 11-10. A TDD (courtesy Ultratrec, Inc.).

is relayed back and forth by a third party. This individual reads what the TDD user types, and types what the voice telephone user speaks. Title IV of the Americans with Disabilities Act required all telephone companies to provide intra- and interstate relay services nationwide beginning July 2, 1993 (5).

Television for the Hearing Impaired

The television has become the major source of information for most individuals. The television provides news, both locally and from around the world. It is a primary source of entertainment for many. For the hearing impaired, the audio signal from the television is often not sufficient to provide understanding. In some cases, turning up the volume helps, but at the inconvenience of normal-hearing friends and family members. Fortunately, a number of assistive devices are available to aid the hearing impaired and their families in enjoying television. In the author's experience, the personal IR system, illustrated in Fig. 11-1, has been the most popular device for enhanced television viewing. It is portable, easily moved from room to room for use with other televisions, and provides complete freedom of movement for the user because there is no direct connection between television and receiver. The system can be taken on trips and used in motel rooms. In addition, because almost all wide-area IR systems transmit on the same frequency, the hearing-impaired person who owns a personal IR system can use the receiver at theaters and auditoriums that have an IR installation (1).

A personal FM system is also easily adapted for television viewing. One need only place the transmitter and microphone at the loudspeaker of the television and the hearing-impaired person wears the FM receiver in the normal manner. An FM system also allows freedom of movement because there is no direct connection between the television and FM receiver. However, the typical personal FM system is more expensive than a personal IR system.

The self-contained auditory assistive device shown in Fig. 11-5 also can be adapted for use with television. Although a less expensive solution to the problem of television than the IR and FM systems, this device does limit the movement of the listener to the length of the microphone cord.

Finally, one should keep in mind closed captioning as an enhancement to television viewing. As shown in Fig. 11-11, closed captioning provides a visual message to accompany the audio signal. Most top-rated television shows are closed captioned. In addition, local and national news casts are closed captioned. In the past, a closed-caption decoder (Fig. 11-12) was required to read the incoming signal and display it on the television screen (6). Thanks to the Television Decoder Circuitry Act (TDCA), a closed-caption decoder is no longer necessary (5).

The TDCA was signed into law in October 1990. Under the TDCA, all television sets with screens 13 inches or larger that are manufactured in or imported to the United States must have the ability to display closed-captioned television transmissions without the need for external equipment. Also, under the TDCA, the FCC

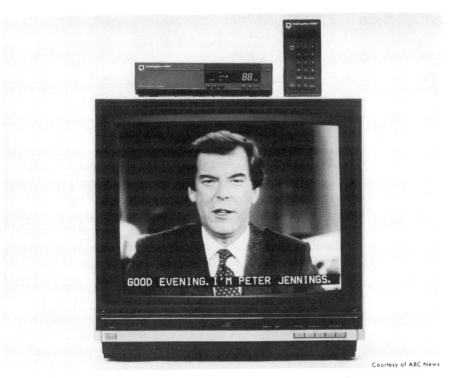

Courtesy of ABC News

FIG. 11-11. An example of closed captioning (courtesy National Captioning Institute).

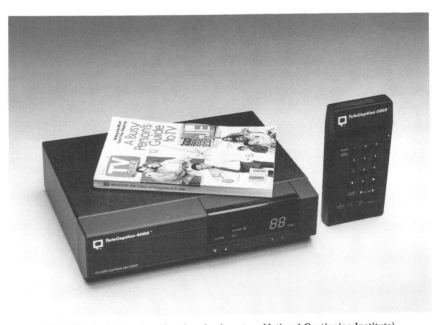

FIG. 11-12. A closed caption decoder (courtesy National Captioning Institute).

has adopted standards of performance and display for built-in decoder circuitry. Thus, closed captioning is available on any television manufactured after October 1990 (7).

Alerting Devices

Occasionally the needs of the hearing impaired include recognition of a number of environmental auditory signals. These include the ring of the telephone, the doorbell, and smoke alarms, among others. In determining the need for an alerting device, several factors must be taken into account. These include the type of sound to be monitored, the environment in which it is located, and the mode of transmission the alerting device should use (8). For example, does the hearing-impaired individual need to be alerted to the doorbell or door knock at their home, or

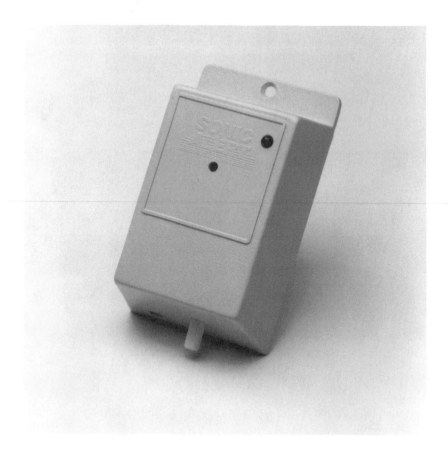

FIG. 11-13. A sound-activated transmitter (courtesy Sonic Alert Corp.).

is the main concern hearing the telephone or smoke alarm in a hotel room while traveling.

The most commonly requested alerting devices in our practice are those that signal an alarm clock and smoke alarm. In addition, requests for signalers for the doorbell and telephone are fairly common. The primary reason is that most hearing aid users do not sleep in their hearing aids, and a wake-up alarm and smoke alarm are very important for obvious reasons. When they are awake and wearing a hearing aid, most, but not all, of our patients are able to hear the doorbell and telephone.

The applications mentioned above can all be handled by using a system that uses a sound-activated pickup, as shown in Fig. 11-13, paired with a corresponding receiver, as shown in Fig. 11-14. The receiver can have a lamp plugged into it to provide a visual signal, or a vibrator to provide a tactile signal. The receiver and transmitter may be combined in a single unit as shown in Fig. 11-15. One must keep in mind that there are exceptions to most rules, and in individual cases, more elaborate measures may be required. This is especially true if an individual requires multiple devices. The reader is referred to the superior review by Larson et al. (8) regarding various options in signaling devices.

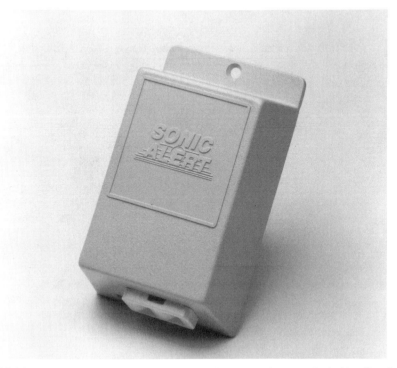

FIG. 11-14. An example of a receiver used in a signaling system (courtesy Sonic Alert Corp.).

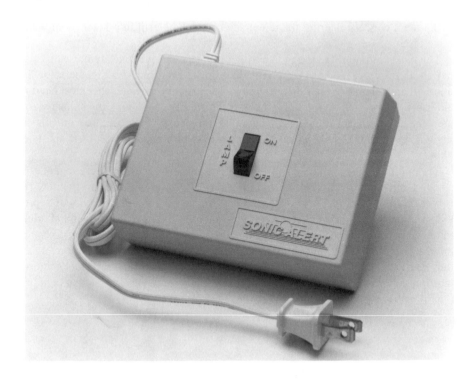

FIG. 11-15. A combination receiver–signaler (courtesy Sonic Alert Corp.).

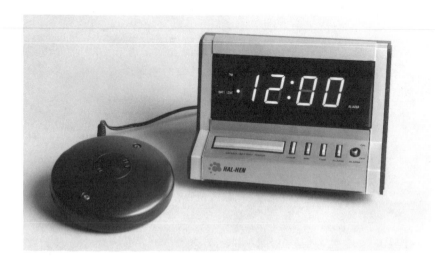

FIG. 11-16. A self-contained alarm clock for the hearing impaired (courtesy Hal-Hen Co.).

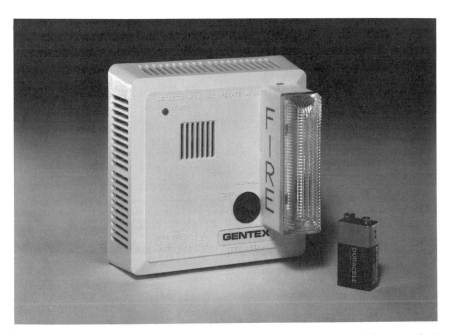

FIG. 11-17. A smoke alarm with strobe designed for the hearing impaired (courtesy Gentex Corp.).

Some devices are available that combine the typical function, such as an alarm clock or smoke detector, with a signaling device for the hearing impaired. Hearing-impaired individuals find these devices simple and uncomplicated. Examples of a dedicated alarm clock and smoke detector for the hearing impaired are shown in Figs. 11-16 and 11-17.

ASSISTIVE TECHNOLOGY IN THE MEDICAL OFFICE

Solving Problems with Assistive Technology in Lieu of a Hearing Aid

As mentioned earlier in this chapter, the typical patient uses assistive technology either in lieu of a hearing aid or in addition to a hearing aid. The patient who may use an assistive device instead of a hearing aid usually presents to the otolaryngologist, or family physician, with a mild hearing loss, sometimes confined to the high frequencies. Often a family member is responsible for the initial office visit. The family member is concerned about the safety of the patient or a perceived change in the patient's quality of life.

Patients with mild hearing loss may project their problem to the environment (9). Comments such as "people mumble" or "if they speak clearly, I can hear fine" are commonplace. They may state straightforwardly, "I'm only here because my daughter (son) insisted." Audiometrically this patient might well benefit from a hearing aid; however, emotionally they are just not ready to accept amplification.

The problems presented by this type of patient typically center around use of the television, telephone, and the ability to hear certain signals around the home. A family member may notice that the television volume is set too high, or the family member may be concerned that the patient cannot hear the ring of the telephone, doorbell, or smoke alarm.

To the clinician, this patient presents a challenge. How this patient is advised may influence attitudes about hearing aids and the need and availability of help for years to come. The patient with a mild hearing loss should not be told "your hearing's okay" or "your hearing's normal for your age." This patient should be told to what degree hearing is impaired. Moreover, the benefits of assistive technology as a matter of personal safety and improved quality of life should be discussed. The use of assistive technology can be a first step to acceptance of a hearing aid if needed.

The audiogram displayed in Fig. 11-18 illustrates the type of hearing loss this first group of patients may present. This particular individual is a 51-year-old, re-tired state highway patrolman who visited our center primarily at the request of his wife. Her primary complaint was the volume level at which her husband had to have the television in order to understand it. Although the patient and his wife both

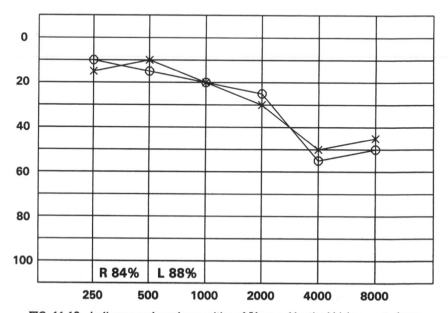

FIG. 11-18. Audiogram and word recognition of 51-year-old retired highway patrolman.

acknowledged that he had occasional difficulty understanding his wife and young grandchildren, neither felt he was ready for a hearing aid. Both the patient and his wife were counseled about the ramifications of his predominantly high-frequency hearing loss; however, no effort was made to "talk him into" a hearing aid. A personal IR system was demonstrated in the office, and the patient was impressed with the ease with which he could understand the television; his wife was pleased with the reduction in volume of the television. Although one might argue that this individual could benefit from a hearing aid, his lack of motivation for amplification made him a poor candidate. He and his wife left with an understanding of his hearing loss and a solution to a problem affecting family harmony.

Figure 11-19 illustrates the audiogram of a 43-year-old man with a family history of hearing loss as well as a long history of recreational noise exposure. He is an accountant and came to our center at the urging of his wife. Her primary complaint was also the level of television volume. This gentleman obviously has a greater hearing impairment than the patient in case 1 because of the significant hearing loss detected at 1,500 and 2,000 Hz. However, he was no less reluctant to consider a hearing aid. In addition to discussing the benefits of amplification, an IR system was demonstrated to the patient and his wife. Although his wife supported his use of a hearing aid, she also supported his decision to "think about" a hearing aid for a while; an IR system, on the other hand, was considered a must. As so often happens in cases like this, this gentleman was fitted with bilateral hearing

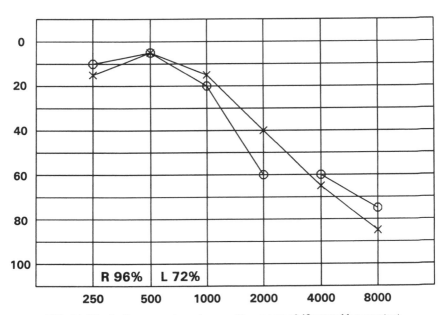

FIG. 11-19. Audiogram and word recognition scores of 43-year-old accountant.

aids approximately 6 months later. Although he was not ready to pursue amplification at the time of his initial office visit, he left well informed and with an answer to one of his family's major hearing concerns. The patient and his wife were left with a positive image of our center and viewed it as a facility that offered solutions.

Solving Problems with Assistive Technology in Addition to a Hearing Aid

Then there is that group of patients who are successful hearing aid users but have hearing difficulty in certain situations that are not solved by a traditional hearing aid. Individuals in this group are typically open to any technology that enables improved hearing in difficult listening environments. Cosmetics are almost never an issue. Shown in Fig. 11-20 is the audiogram of a 75-year-old retired government worker. As can be seen, he has little or no usable hearing above 1,500 Hz. He wears binaural, postauricular, programmable hearing aids with good success in face-to-face conversation. Since his retirement, he and his wife have traveled extensively in their motor home. However, his severely reduced speech discrimination made it difficult, if not impossible, for him to understand his wife while he drove the motor home. For this gentleman, a personal FM system provided the so-

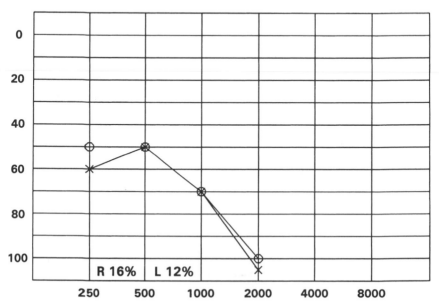

FIG. 11-20. Audiogram and word recognition scores of 75-year-old retired government worker.

lution. Now as they travel, his wife wears the FM transmitter and he wears the FM receiver in his right ear, continuing to wear a hearing aid in his left ear. The use of the FM system increased significantly their travel enjoyment by facilitating their communicative interaction. Moreover, they came to appreciate the FM system in other situations as well. They routinely use it in noisy restaurants, and he will wear the receiver when he is working in the yard when they are at home, thus allowing his wife to communicate with him from inside the house or the back porch.

The audiogram in Fig. 11-21 is that of an active and energetic 82-year-old retired executive with a large grocery chain. During most of his daily activities he wears binaural, postauricular, programmable hearing aids. However, he too enjoys the use of a personal, postauricular FM system in restaurants and at cocktail parties. At a noisy restaurant, he places the FM transmitter in a glass in the center of the table so that he may converse with all those at his table. At a cocktail party, he keeps the small FM transmitter in the breast pocket of his sports coat or suit jacket, and finds he is able to mingle and converse quite effectively despite the constant din of background conversations. At home he uses an IR receiver for television viewing, and he is able to use his IR receiver at the community theater, which has an IR system. He also uses an amplified telephone handset and a vibrating alarm clock. To say this gentleman is aggressive in his efforts to not let hearing loss diminish his active life-style is an understatement.

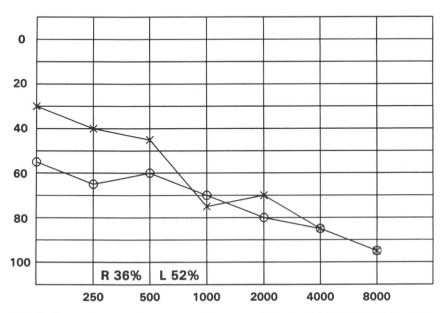

FIG. 11-21. Audiogram and word recognition scores of 82-year-old retired business executive.

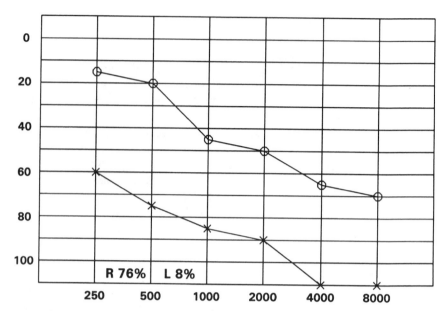

FIG. 11-22. Audiogram and word recognition scores of 72-year-old business owner.

The gentleman whose audiogram is illustrated in Fig. 11-22 is 72 years of age and actively runs his own business. He also wears a postauricular, programmable hearing aid in each ear. This gentleman feels strongly that the auditory information he receives in the left ear enhances his benefit from a hearing aid in the right ear. However, he, too, finds hearing aids to be inadequate in certain situations. In restaurants and meetings he uses a postauricular FM system in the right ear. He also enjoys a personal IR system, the receiver of which he uses at the theater and cinema. He uses a vibrating alarm clock, has an amplified handset on his office and home telephones, and carries a portable telephone amplifier with him at all times. Another aggressive hearing impaired person who refuses to let hearing loss change his life-style? Yes, and there are many more like him. You see them in your own practice, but perhaps they are not recognized. They must be made aware of available technology and its application in their particular case. If they are told by their physician that the only alternative is to use a hearing aid, then, in all probability, that will be as far as they will go.

SUMMARY

It has been the intent of this chapter to acquaint the clinician with the wide variety of assistive technology available for the hearing-impaired patient. All of the available technology cannot be reviewed in a single chapter. Moreover, systems are being improved and new devices added on a regular basis. Nonetheless, it is hoped that the clinician has an appreciation that no matter the degree of hearing loss or listening problem presented, there is technology available to help. By making assistive technology available, either directly in the office or indirectly through referral to appropriate agencies, the clinician will promote a positive image for his or her practice and receive the gratitude of patients and their families.

REFERENCES

1. Pruitt JB. Assistive listening device versus conventional hearing aid in an elderly patient: case report. *J Amer Acad Audiol* 1990;1:41–41.
2. Beaulac DA, Pehringer JL, Shough LF. Assistive listening devices: available options. *Semin Hear* 1989;10:11–30.
3. Hammond LB. *FM auditory trainers.* Minneapolis: Gopher State Litho Corp; 1991:1–5.
4. Slager RD. Romancing the phone: the adventure continues. *Semin Hear* 1989;10:42–56.
5. Dubow S, Geer S. *Legal rights: the guide for deaf and hard of hearing people.* Washington, DC: Gallaudet University Press; 1992:203–216.
6. Jensema CJ, Compton CL. Television for the hearing impaired. *Semin Hear* 1989;10:57–65.
7. Dubow S, Geer S. *Legal rights: the guide for deaf and hard of hearing people.* Washington, DC: Gallaudet University Press; 1992:191–202.
8. Larose GM, Evans MP, Larose RW. Alerting devices: available options. *Semin Hear* 1989;10:66–77.
9. Orlans H. Adjustment to adult hearing loss. San Diego, CA: College-Hill; 1985:102–110.

HEARING AIDS: A MANUAL FOR CLINICIANS,
edited by Robert A. Goldenberg
Lippincott–Raven Publishers, Philadelphia © 1996

C H A P T E R ✦ *12* ✦

The Problem Patient

Patricia K. Lambert

Division of Audiology, University ENT Specialists, Cincinnati, Ohio

Key Points

Identification of the problem patient • challenging patterns of hearing loss • recruitment and reduced dynamic range • anatomical abnormalities • unilateral hearing loss • feedback • unacceptable cosmetics • overamplification.

Among the many patients encountered in a busy otolaryngology practice, there is a fairly high percentage who will seek advice regarding amplification. In nearly all cases, it is safe to say that hearing aids will benefit the patients who demonstrate hearing loss. Typically, there are certain audiometric patterns that elicit concern about the value of amplification as a rehabilitative solution. In almost all cases it is appropriate to recommend a trial period with amplification. There are groups of patients who pose more of a challenge than others to the dispensing audiologist. Among the most challenging group are those with one or more of the following characteristics:

Steeply sloping high-frequency sensorineural hearing loss
Low-frequency sensorineural hearing loss
Poor speech discrimination ability in one or both ears
Hearing aid acceptance problems related to recruitment
Reduced dynamic range
Anatomical abnormalities of the external ear
Unilateral hearing loss

Patient complaints among these groups regarding amplification usually include one or more of the following:

Feedback
Occlusion effect
Overamplification of background noise
Lack of benefit for word recognition

Unacceptable cosmetic appeal
Overamplification of sound
Retention problems
Distorted sound

In this chapter, some of these problems are discussed, and possible solutions are provided. Case studies have been included when applicable. It should be noted that there is not one single answer for any given problem. What is a satisfactory solution for one patient may not apply to the next patient with an identical audiogram.

Technological advances in the hearing aid industry in the past few years have made this an exciting and enjoyable time to be serving the hearing-impaired population. It was not until recently that patients have consistently volunteered positive comments about their new hearing devices. There will undoubtedly be further improvements in hearing aid design and circuitry, and the solutions proposed in this chapter subsequently may become obsolete in the near future. The suggestions presented in this chapter are not all inclusive but are meant to be general guidelines for the practicing otolaryngologist.

THE SLOPING HIGH-FREQUENCY SENSORINEURAL HEARING LOSS

The patient with normal or near-normal hearing through the low and midfrequency range (250–1,000 or 2,000 Hz) presents several problems during the hearing aid fitting process. There are limitations on the amount of high-frequency gain or amplification that the user can receive before feedback occurs. There is the additional problem of unwanted amplification of the low frequencies. Even if there is success in reducing the amount of gain in the low and midfrequencies, this is no guarantee that the patient will accept the resulting sound quality. In addition, there are inherent limitations on the amount of gain provided by many hearing aids in the region above 3,000 Hz. It logically follows that individuals with a steeply sloping high-frequency hearing loss may report a lack of benefit from the use of amplification. In some cases, depending on the configuration of their audiogram, users may report increased difficulty in precisely the same situations that prompted them to seek help (e.g., noisy restaurants, group settings, etc.).

Another situation often encountered when fitting an individual with normal hearing in the low frequencies is the occlusion effect. The occlusion effect is essentially an enhancement of low-frequency sound pressure in the ear canal in response to one's own voice when the ear is occluded by an earmold or hearing aid. Patients who experience the occlusion effect typically report that they sound as if they are in a barrel or that their own voice sounds hollow. Comments concerning the quality of their own voice are often the first responses the new user provides when questioned about the sound of their hearing aid. Historically, the solution to the occlusion effect has been to increase the vent size of the earmold or hearing aid (1). Unfortunately, this action is often counterproductive because the larger vent can introduce feedback problems. The solutions for the various problems encountered in fitting for the high-frequency loss are dependent on the type of hearing aid selected and the slope of the hearing loss.

Behind-the-Ear Hearing Aids and High-Frequency Hearing Loss

When traditional behind-the-ear (BTE) hearing aids are fitted, many of the solutions arise from tubing, earmold, and earhook modifications. Each of these parts can potentially alter the frequency response characteristics of the hearing aid. In addition, most BTE hearing aids offer tone and output controls that allow for an increase or decrease in the amount of low- and/or high-frequency gain provided by the hearing aid. In cases of programmable hearing aids, the variety of adjustments is substantially greater than in traditional nonprogrammable aids. This situation is analogous to a comparison between an inexpensive stereo system that offers only a bass/treble dial versus a more costly system that features an equalizer, allowing the user to discretely boost certain frequencies. Some of the programmable systems allow users to modify their own hearing aids, whereas other systems give the audiologist many options while minimizing the manual adjustments accessible to users.

Although many programmable instruments do not offer new circuitry for processing speech signals, some do offer new compression technology that is not available in nonprogrammable instruments (2).

It has been suggested that the earmold style and features (vent size, material, size of the sound bore, and tubing type) should vary with the degree and slope of the loss (3). In general, a long canal length on the earmold should be used to assist in delivering high-frequency gain. Martin (4) also recommends an extra-long canal for fitting high-frequency losses in order to avoid feedback. He suggests that a wide-band frequency response is an important characteristic for optimizing amplification at 4,000 to 6,000 Hz. The wide-band aids have an extended high-frequency response that allows a greater percentage of speech cues to be passed onto the hearing aid user. Until recently, narrow-band hearing aids were most commonly dispensed because of unresolved problems with amplifier distortion (5).

Case Study: Programmable BTE Hearing Amplication for High-Frequency Sensorineural Hearing Loss

Figure 12-1 depicts the aided results with binaural programmable wide-band full dynamic range compression BTE hearing aids. The patient had previously worn a vented canal hearing aid in his right ear. He was not able to increase the volume on the hearing aid to achieve optimal results without experiencing feedback. He reported very little benefit from amplification.

His new hearing aids are coupled to vented earmolds with horned tubing. After three postfitting visits for program modifications, he is able to wear his hearing

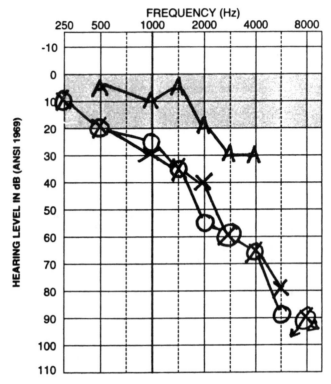

FIG. 12-1. Bilateral high-frequency sensorineural hearing loss and programmable BTE wide-band full dynamic range compression hearing aid fitting.

aids at the desired volume level without feedback. He does not express annoyance with loud sounds, and his spouse reports that he no longer withdraws from group conversations.

In-the-Ear Hearing Aids and High-Frequency Hearing Loss

There are several in-the-ear (ITE) styles of hearing aids from which to choose for the high-frequency hearing loss. A full-shell ITE aid may be modified by venting and customized for a high-frequency response. The shell may be made progressively smaller, as in the half-shell and canal hearing aids. Venting options become more limited with these smaller instruments because of the increased likelihood of feedback. Fewer frequency response and circuit choices are available from most manufacturers for the smaller ITE styles. When K-AMP circuitry is selected, there is evidence that there may be a reduction in the amount of low-frequency amplification in a canal aid fitting (6). This should result in a more favorable self-perception of the user's voice.

Completely-in-the-Canal Hearing Aids and High-Frequency Hearing Loss

In a completely-in-the-canal (CIC) hearing aid, the visible end of the hearing aid is 1 to 2 mm inside the entrance of the ear canal. The CIC hearing aid is designed to be inconspicuous in the ear canal. In most, but not all, cases a CIC hearing aid has a deeply sealed eartip that extends into the bony portion of the ear canal. A CIC aid that terminates within approximately 5 mm of the superior portion of the tympanic membrane (TM) is referred to as a deep-canal or peritympanic hearing aid. There is an increase in output of approximately 9 to 13 dB when a deep-canal fitting is used. This increase in output is due to the decreased residual volume in the ear canal between the end of the hearing aid and the TM. As the volume is decreased, the resulting sound pressure is increased.

When a CIC hearing aid is not classified as a deep-canal aid, the acoustic advantages may be limited to the concha and pinna effects. The concha is not occluded with a CIC, and the natural acoustical properties of the concha may be used to advantage in the fitting process. When the concha is not occluded, there is a 6- to 8-dB enhancement of the signal in the region of 4,000 to 5,000 Hz before it enters the microphone of the hearing aid due to resonance in the concha. The pinna effect is an increase in the high-frequency sound energy starting at approximately 2,000 Hz. The effect increases steadily in the higher frequencies. The pinna effect may account for as much as an 8-dB increase (4) in the input for the high frequencies because of the location of the hearing aid's microphone. A CIC hearing aid fitting, if deep enough, should reduce the occlusion effect (7).

Case Study: CIC Hearing Aids and High-Frequency Sensorineural Hearing Loss

Figure 12-2 depicts the sound-field test results in the aided and unaided condition for a bilaterally symmetrical moderate mid/high-frequency sensorineural hearing loss. The user had previously worn "standard" or linear BTE aids with limited benefit. He previously reported great difficulty hearing in the presence of background noise. The aided speech discrimination scores in the presence of background noise (0 dB signal-to-noise ratio) suggest significant benefit from this fitting.

UPWARD SLOPING SENSORINEURAL HEARING LOSS

For the individual with an upward sloping sensorineural hearing loss, the difficulties encountered usually relate to selection of the appropriate circuitry among the many hundreds of choices. Use of the appropriate earmold style for a BTE hearing aid or selection of the shell style for ITE amplification are also variables

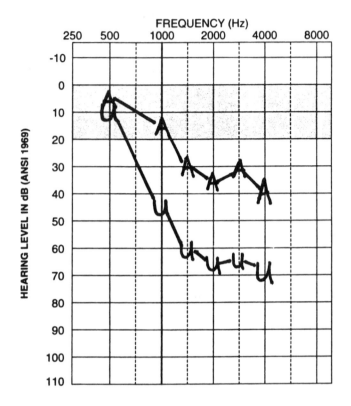

SOUNDFIELD		UNAIDED	AIDED		
			Bin	Left	Right
SRT		**25** dB HTL	**15** dB HTL	dB HTL	dB HTL
Discrimination In Quiet Test Stimuli	Speech Level	**50** dB HTL	**50** dB HTL	dB HTL	dB HTL
	Score	**80** %	**92** %	%	%
Discrimination In Noise	Speech Level	**50** dB HTL	**50** dB HTL	dB HTL	dB HTL
	Noise Level	**50** dB HTL	**50** dB HTL	dB HTL	dB HTL
	Score	**48** %	**88** %	%	%

FIG. 12-2. Bilateral high-frequency sensorineural loss and CIC fitting.

that will affect the amount of gain that the patient receives in the low-frequency region. These choices will determine how much hearing in the mid/high-frequency region will be acoustically altered. Certain earmold and ITE shell styles can significantly alter the normal resonance of the ear canal.

The upward sloping or reverse slope hearing loss is relatively uncommon. Most hearing aid manufacturers do not gear their marketing literature or new product developments for this pattern of hearing loss. Patients with normal or near normal hearing above 1,500 to 2,000 Hz usually function remarkably well when given the appropriate amplification. Patients with hearing loss in the low frequencies do not usually battle feedback and they typically have excellent aided speech discrimination scores in quiet and in noise.

Case Study: Congenital Upward Sloping Sensorineural Hearing Loss

Figure 12-3 shows the audiometric profile of a young teen-ager with a bilateral upward sloping sensorineural hearing loss of a severe degree in the lower and middle frequencies. Her thresholds increase into the normal range at 8,000 Hz. This patient has worn binaural BTE aids for 10 years. She receives excellent grades in advanced placement classes at school. Her aided speech discrimination scores are 100% in quiet and with competing background noise. Her hearing aids are moderate-gain instruments with automatic gain control amplification. The aids were selected with audio input capability. Audio input capability allows her to use her own hearing aids in conjunction with an FM system in the classroom.

Case Study: Endolymphatic Hydrops with Fluctuating Upward Sloping Sensorineural Hearing Loss

Figure 12-4 This patient exhibits a bilateral upward sloping hearing loss that fluctuates in the middle and lower frequency regions. He was originally fit with programmable BTE hearing aids, which allowed him to switch among four different programs. The four programs were set with various frequency response parameters and gain limits in anticipation of fluctuating hearing thresholds. In addition, he drove a noisy truck, was a woodshop enthusiast, and operated his own business involving one-to-one conversations with clients. He quickly became dissatisfied with the constant adjustments required with these hearing aids.

The next fitting involved binaural BTE K-AMP hearing aids. The goal was to have hearing aids that would adjust automatically to the various noise environments. After several fitting sessions, these aids were returned and he requested a trial period with CIC amplification.

The aided thresholds were obtained with CIC K-AMP hearing aids. The user is able to make his own screwdriver adjustments to the volume control when he feels

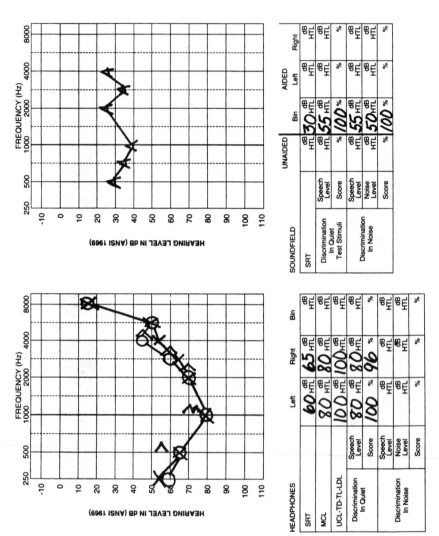

FIG. 12-3. Upward sloping sensorineural hearing loss (left). Sound-field test results with binaural BTE hearing aids (right).

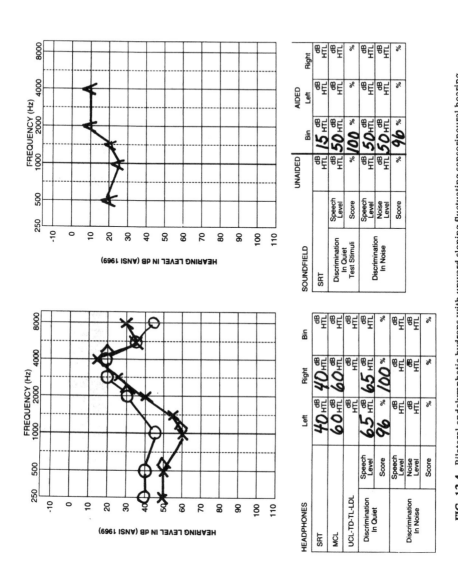

FIG. 12-4. Bilateral endolymphatic hydrops with upward sloping fluctuating sensorineural hearing loss (left). Aided test results with binaural CIC K-AMP hearing aids (right).

a change in his hearing levels. He reports superior sound quality with these aids. Additional benefits include the ability to use the telephone without feedback.

PATIENT WITH POOR SPEECH DISCRIMINATION ABILITY

Patients showing word discrimination scores at or below approximately 50% are considered to have poor speech discrimination ability and probably have difficulty following conversation. There are many factors that contribute to a reduced word discrimination score. Not only does the degree of hearing loss play a role, but the slope of the hearing loss affects the amount of available speech information in the test material. As the available amount of high-frequency information is reduced, there is a progressive decrease in the ability to discriminate syllables. Low-frequency information below 500 Hz does not appear to contribute substantially to syllable discrimination ability.

Other variables, such as type of test material, mode of presentation (live voice vs. taped), presentation intensity level, and acoustic environment can have an enormous effect on the resulting speech discrimination score. The age of onset of hearing impairment plays a role in determining how well an individual can discriminate speech. For example, a person who acquired hearing loss many years after normal speech and language development has occurred has a distinct advantage over those who acquire hearing loss before speech and language development. Educational and psychosocial factors also influence speech discrimination ability. Figure 12-5 shows the audiometric findings on a patient with a congenital severe/profound sensorineural hearing loss. This patient has no measurable speech discrimination ability. He relies primarily on manual communication with the addition of limited oral language. He uses amplification on an irregular basis for awareness of environmental sounds and to monitor his own voice.

Central lesions (brain stem–cortex) may produce poor word discrimination scores. An example of this is the stroke patient with an auditory processing disorder. Prognosis for benefit from amplification is guarded in patients with this type of communication problem. Test scores may have to be interpreted with caution because of cognitive and/or language deficits from the cerebrovascular accident. Conventional amplification may be recommended on a trial basis once the patient's condition has stabilized. In the period immediately after the infarct, the use of a simple remote microphone assistive listening device may prove to be beneficial. This is a relatively inexpensive option. Some hospitals and long-term care facilities keep such devices in stock, specifically for this purpose. Careful patient and family counseling are recommended because expectations for improvement through the use of amplification may be unrealistic. In addition, disorders at the peripheral level (e.g., endolymphatic hydrops, sudden sensorineural loss) may result in reduced and/or variable word discrimination scores.

The presence or absence of visual cues certainly has an effect on one's ability to discriminate speech. There is a wide range among the hearing impaired population in their ability to integrate auditory and visual information.

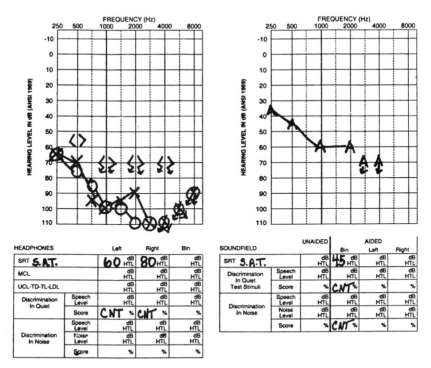

FIG. 12-5. Bilateral severe–profound sensorineural hearing loss with no measurable speech discrimination ability (left). Aided sound-field test results with BTE amplification (right).

Case Study

In Fig. 12-6 the speech discrimination scores have been obtained with and without the addition of visual cues. The scores increased dramatically with the addition of visual cues. The poor scores obtained without visual cues are not predictive of this patient's performance with amplification. This patient wears two wide-band programmable hearing aids with multiband compression. It is clear that the patient is gaining significant benefit from the use of amplification. The aided speech discrimination scores even without visual cues are far better than the speech discrimination test scores obtained under earphones without visual cues.

Some evidence suggests that speech discrimination ability can be influenced by hearing aid use. A study by Silman et al. (8) showed a decrease in word recognition scores for the unaided ears of a group of patients with bilaterally symmetrical sensorineural hearing loss. Silverman and Silman later completed a retrospective study to investigate the effects of binaural amplification on the apparent auditory deprivation from monaural amplification (9). Although his study consisted of only two subjects, the criteria for inclusion in his study were stringent and the subjects were followed over long periods of time (6–11 years). In both cases, the decrement

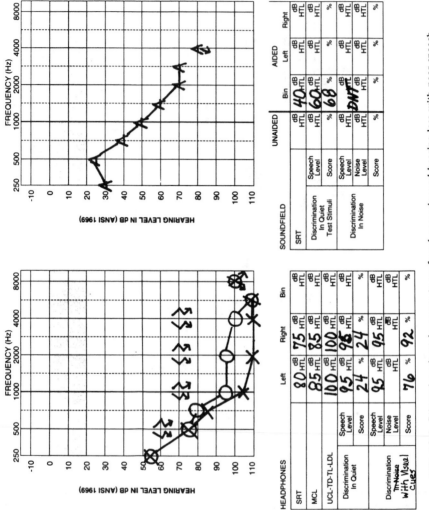

FIG. 12-6. Bilateral moderately severe to profound sensorineural hearing loss with poor speech discrimination ability (left). Aided sound-field test results with binaural wide-band full dynamic range compression programmable hearing aids (right).

Headphones graph (left)

FREQUENCY (Hz): 250, 500, 1000, 2000, 4000, 8000
HEARING LEVEL IN dB (ANSI 1969)

HEADPHONES		Left	Right	Bin
SRT		80 dB HTL	75 dB HTL	dB HTL
MCL		85 dB HTL	85 dB HTL	dB HTL
UCL-TD-TL-LDL		100 dB HTL	100 dB HTL	dB HTL
Discrimination In Quiet	Speech Level	95 dB HTL	95 dB HTL	dB HTL
	Score	24 %	24 %	%
Discrimination In Noise With Visual Cues	Speech Level	95 dB HTL	95 dB HTL	dB HTL
	Noise Level	dB HTL	dB HTL	dB HTL
	Score	76 %	92 %	%

Soundfield graph (right)

FREQUENCY (Hz): 250, 500, 1000, 2000, 4000, 8000
HEARING LEVEL IN dB (ANSI 1969)

SOUNDFIELD		UNAIDED		AIDED	
			Bin	Left	Right
SRT		dB HTL	40 dB HTL	dB HTL	dB HTL
Discrimination In Quiet Test Stimuli	Speech Level	dB HTL	60 dB HTL	dB HTL	dB HTL
	Score	%	68 %	%	%
Discrimination In Noise	Speech Level	dB HTL	DNT dB HTL	dB HTL	dB HTL
	Noise Level	dB HTL	dB HTL	dB HTL	dB HTL
	Score	%	%	%	%

in suprathreshold scores that were observed after the monaural use of amplification were at least partially reversed. The reversals occurred within 2½ years after binaural hearing aid fitting.

ANATOMICAL FACTORS OF THE EXTERNAL CANAL

Reaching a targeted goal based on the degree of hearing loss is one of the greatest concerns when fitting hearing aids. In patients with abnormal external ears, however, the overriding concern is with the physical coupling of the hearing instrument to the ear. There are numerous congenital disorders that result in anatomical abnormalities of the outer ear. These abnormalities can make it extremely difficult or impossible to provide ear level amplification. There are also many surgical procedures that significantly alter the size and shape of the external ear. The existing hearing losses are most often conductive or mixed in nature. The degree of loss may be mild to severe and usually require greater amounts of gain than would be expected with a sensorineural hearing loss. Because of the lack of recruitment among those with conductive hearing loss, the output of the hearing aid may reach fairly high levels before the patient experiences discomfort.

Surgically Altered Ear Canals

One of the biggest problems associated with fitting surgically altered ear canals is obtaining an accurate impression of the ear. Another major problem is the delivery of adequate gain without feedback.

Ear Impression Problems

Unlike the unaltered ear canal, the surgically altered canal tends to widen the further down the canal you extend. This can pose a problem when it comes time to remove the ear impression from the ear. Impression material is in a thick liquid state as it is shot into the ear canal. It hardens quickly (3–10 minutes) to provide us with a solid model for production of either an ITE aid or an earmold for a BTE aid. If the impression material has been injected into the largest part of the ear canal it cannot be expected to compress and emerge through the narrower diameter opening of the surgically altered ear canal. It is therefore imperative that some type of block be used to ensure that the impression material does not leak into the wider medial portion of the ear canal.

Cotton blocks with waxed removal strings are recommended for a more accurate ear impression (10). Foam blocks are available, but they may not hold the shape of the ear impression as well. In addition, cotton blocks can be shaped by flattening or fraying the cotton. Flattened cotton blocks may help prevent leakage of the impression material behind the block. Multiple blocks may be necessary in extremely large cavities such as those present after radical mastoidectomies.

The type of material used for the impression also makes a difference in ease of removal and overall accuracy of the impression. Silicone impression material is recommended over the powder and liquid type for a few reasons. The silicone material is not subject to shrinking, warping, or distorting with high temperatures. Most silicone materials can be removed easily from the ear without danger of breaking off in the ear canal.

Feedback Issues

The choice between BTE and ITE amplification for the patient with a surgically altered ear canal is dependent on the degree of hearing loss, the size of the air–bone gap, and the most comfortable listening level and uncomfortable listening level (UCL) values obtained. The venting requirements also must be taken into account when deciding which styles of amplification are appropriate. If a large vent is required and the patient's audiometric profile suggests that he or she will require a fair amount of gain from the instrument, an ITE fitting would probably result in feedback problems. It is easier to resolve feedback problems with BTE aids because of the greater distance between the microphone and the receiver opening. There are also many choices of earmold styles designed to reduce or eliminate feedback.

CASE STUDY: Unilateral Hearing Loss with Predominant Conductive Component

This patient had a long history of chronic middle ear disease (Fig. 12-7). His recent middle ear surgery left him with a rather large mastoid cavity. He insisted on ITE amplification. His physician requested a vented hearing aid or earmold. After several unsuccessful attempts to provide ITE amplification (at least three different manufacturers were tried), it was suggested that he evaluate BTE amplification. The lack of success was due to persistent feedback when the volume was adjusted to the level that provided noticeable benefit for the patient. The patient did not follow the recommendation for BTE amplification and went elsewhere. Two years later, he returned for a BTE fitting. He has since successfully been fit with a moderate-gain (45–50 dB) instrument. After one remake on his earmold, he is able to set the hearing aid to comfortable levels without feedback.

Congenital Abnormalities of the External Ear

Examples of congenital conditions that can adversely affect hearing aid fittings include microtia, atresia, and stenosis of the canal. These abnormalities may be associated with other craniofacial anomalies. It is problematic to fit instruments to these ears because of difficulty in physically coupling the instrument to the ear. Unless surgical intervention is advised, bone conduction aids are usually recom-

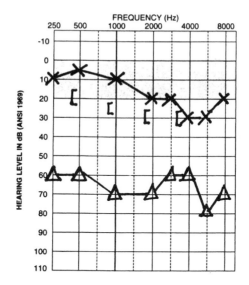

FIG. 12-7. Moderate unilateral conductive hearing loss.

mended for atretic ears (11). Depending on the auricular malformation, ear level amplification may be possible in some cases of microtia. Surgical intervention may facilitate placement of an ITE on some ears that could not retain BTE amplification. As is the case with surgically altered ears of patients with chronic middle ear disease, a large conductive hearing loss requires increased gain. Feedback may be a nuisance with ITE fittings on these surgically reconstructed ears.

In cases with stenotic ear canals, surgical enlargement of the ear canal should allow the options for amplification to include either ITE or BTE amplification. The patient should be advised that cerumen build-up in the hearing aid or earmold can cause instrument malfunction.

Cerumen problems are the number one reason for ITE hearing aid repairs. In a very narrow ear canal, cerumen may tend to build up more rapidly in the hearing aid. In a BTE fitting this is not a problem because it is a simple matter to clean the earmold. If the patient is advised of the potential repair problems associated with cerumen in the hearing aid, the decision regarding whether to purchase ITE or BTE amplification can be left to the user.

THE PATIENT WITH REDUCED DYNAMIC RANGE

The dynamic range is the arithmetic difference between the patient's threshold and UCL. For example, a patient with a pure-tone threshold of 55 dB and a UCL of 95 dB has a dynamic range of 40 dB. There is a correlation between reduction of the dynamic range and hearing threshold levels (12). Individuals with sensorineural hearing loss can have a reduced dynamic range because of recruitment. Recruitment refers to an abnormally rapid growth of loudness as intensity is increased. In other words, the intensity difference between what is audible and what is judged to be loud is smaller in ears with sensorineural hearing loss. The intensity levels that are judged to be loud by the hearing-impaired individual often occur at the same intensity levels judged to be loud by the person with normal hearing. In some cases (with severe/profound hearing loss) the levels that are just audible are also judged to be too loud. This can easily be observed in the test booth. The patient will respond at threshold level with a strained look and quite often describe the sound as painful.

Many unsuccessful hearing aid fittings can be attributed to the fact that the hearing aid produced signals in the patient's ears that exceeded their upper intensity limits of comfort. Even when some type of output limiting is used to keep the amplified sound from exceeding the tolerance level of the user, the results can be less than desirable due to the introduction of distortion. Many of the newer compression circuit designs successfully address the issue of output limiting with minimal distortion. There are a variety of hearing aids available that have compression characteristics. Some of these aids are digitally programmable and others do not require any sophisticated programming equipment. The additional expense involved in fitting the newer instruments has not been an issue for most patients once they are able to hear the difference in sound quality. Some of these hearing aids, such as those with K-AMP chips, solve the problem of overamplification by not amplifying loud sounds. Hearing aids with this circuitry only amplify quiet sounds.

FITTING THE UNAIDABLE EAR

An ear with a profound hearing loss and no measurable speech discrimination ability is not usually considered to be a candidate for amplification. An ear with a lesser degree of hearing loss and very poor speech discrimination ability is likewise not a candidate for a traditional hearing aid. It is often useful for these individuals to have the incoming signals to their poor ear routed to the better hearing ear. Contralateral routing of signals (CROS) hearing aids are designed to meet the needs of the person with one unaidable ear. The options for CROS amplification are described as follows:

Wired CROS ITE or BTE. In the wired system a cord links the microphone on the poor ear to the receiver on the good ear. The wire goes around the back of the neck at the hairline.

Wireless CROS BTE. For this system, a BTE microphone unit is coupled to the poor ear and a BTE receiver is coupled to the good ear. The receiver on the good ear can deliver the routed signal to the good ear via a nonoccluding earmold or through a preshaped tube that extends into the ear canal.

Wireless CROS system with an ITE unit in the better ear and a BTE unit on the poor ear. This system is essentially the same as the BTE wireless system except that the good ear is fitted with an ITE unit with a very large vent.

Transcranial CROS. For a transcranial CROS fitting, a high-power BTE or ITE aid is used in the poor ear. The aid should be set for the broadest frequency response and the highest tolerable output. The signal crosses over to the good ear via bone conduction to stimulate the cochlea of the better ear.

Each of these systems has advantages and disadvantages. The wired systems may be undesirable because of the visibility of the cord and inconvenience during hair styling, etc. The wired and wireless systems reportedly produce an unnatural sound, and they both involve occlusion of the better ear. Most patients with only

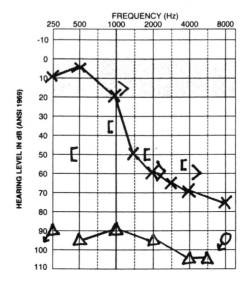

HEADPHONES		Left	Right	Bin
SRT		25 dB HTL	85 dB HTL	dB HTL
MCL		60 dB HTL	95 dB HTL	dB HTL
UCL-TD-TL-LDL		95 dB HTL	100 dB HTL	dB HTL
Discrimination In Quiet	Speech Level	dB HTL	dB HTL	dB HTL
	Score	84 %	CNT %	%

FIG. 12-8. Bilateral hearing loss with no measurable speech discrimination ability in one ear.

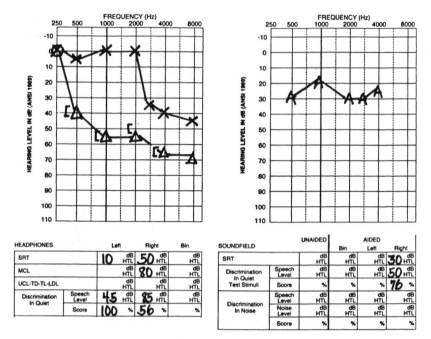

FIG. 12-9. Bilateral asymmetrical sensorineural hearing loss with poor speech discrimination in one ear.

one usable ear are not comfortable blocking the sound to that ear in any manner. Telephone use becomes a problem when the good ear is even partially occluded.

The transcranial CROS aid offers the advantage of keeping the good ear unoccluded. The primary problem encountered with this option is providing enough usable gain in a wide-band response without feedback.

When one ear is unaidable and the better ear also has a hearing loss, a bi-CROS aid not only routes the signal from the poor ear to the good ear but also provides amplification to the incoming signal on the good side.

Case Study

Figure 12-8 shows the audiometric profile of a patient with a high-frequency sensorineural hearing loss in the better ear and a mixed profound hearing loss in the poor ear. This patient had previously worn traditional amplification on the left ear only. He still reported significant communication difficulties. He also tried a programmable BTE hearing aid with an open earmold on the better ear. He finally chose a trial period with bi-CROS amplification. His results are still not optimal (he complains about the sound of his own voice), but he is receiving additional speech cues from the right side that help him in group situations.

Finally, there are some cases of unilateral hearing loss that are not of the profound degree that show poor speech discrimination ability. Some of these losses may respond well to traditional amplification instead of a CROS system.

Case Study

Figure 12-9 shows the test results of a patient with a long-standing history of high-frequency hearing loss for the left ear and a sudden sensorineural hearing loss on the right side. His otoneurologic workup was negative for retrocochlear pathology. He was recently fitted with a CIC hearing aid in the right ear. His aided test results (obtained using earphones) show significant improvement for pure tone and speech tests. He was originally told that amplification would not benefit the right ear because of the poor speech discrimination score for that side.

REFERENCES

1. Agnew J. Acoustic advantage of deep canal hearing aid fittings. *Hear Instrum* 1994;45: 22–25.
2. Mueller HG, Hawkins DB, Northern JL, eds. *Probe microphone measurements*. San Diego: Singular Publishing Group; 1992.
3. Schlaegel N, Jelonek S. Selecting the right earmold for a high-frequency fitting. *Hear J* 1991;44:15–18.
4. Martin RL. Reader asks how to optimize gain at high frequencies. *Hear J* 1995;48:47.
5. Killion MC. The K-AMP hearing aid: an attempt to present high fidelity for persons with impaired hearing. *Am J Audiol* 1993;2:52–74.
6. Painton SW. Objective measure of low frequency amplification reduction in canal hearing aids with adaptive circuitry. *J Am Acad Audiol* 1993;4:152–156.
7. Mueller HG. CIC hearing aids: what is their impact on the occlusion effect? *Hear J* 1994; 47:29–35.
8. Silman S, Gelfand SA, Silverman CA. Effects of monaural versus binaural hearing aids. *J Acoust Soc Am* 1984;76:1357–1362.
9. Silverman CA, Silman S. Apparent auditory deprivation from monaural amplification and recovery with binaural amplification: two case studies. *J Am Acad Audiol* 1990;1:175–180.
10. Staab WJ, Martin RL. Taking ear impressions for deep canal hearing aid fittings. *Hear J* 1994;47:19–28.
11. Jahrsdoerfer RA, Jacobson JT. Treacher Collins syndrome: otologic and auditory management. *J Am Acad Audiol* 1995;5:93–102.
12. Pascoe DP. Hearing aid selection based on equalizing abnormal/normal MCLs. *Hear Instrum* 1994;45:9–15.

Glossary

Americans with Disabilities Act (ADA)   Enacted in 1992, the ADA provides for equal access for all citizens. The ADA provides legal requirements for removing communication barriers to the deaf and hard of hearing.

Articulation Index (AI)   A rating of how much of the speech signal is available to a listener. AI scores range from 0.00 (no speech sounds are audible) to 1.00 (all speech sounds are audible). In general, the higher the AI, the greater a person's ability will be to understand speech.

Air Conduction   Stimuli presented to the outer ear via headphones or insertion molds.

Analog Hearing Aid Circuit   Sound pressure waves are received at the microphone, amplified and modified by the circuitry, and the enhanced signal is transmitted to the listener receiver.

Analog–Digital Hearing Aid Circuit   A combination of a conventional analog system and a digital system.

ANSI   American National Standards Institute.

Assistive Listening Device   Any device, other than a hearing aid, that enhances the hearing-impaired individual's ability to hear and understand speech or be made aware of environmental signals.

Audiogram   A graph depicting hearing threshold level (HTL) at various discrete frequencies.

Automatic Gain Control (AGC)   The means by which gain is automatically controlled by the level of the signal being amplified.

Automatic Signal Processing (ASP)   Monitors incoming sound then electronically changes or alters sound in frequency and intensity.

Binaural Fusion   Input from both ears is necessary to process sounds as a composite.

Binaural Summation   An increase of 3 to 6 dB in hearing ability when the signal is presented to both ears rather than to just one ear.

Bone Conduction   Stimuli presented directly to the inner ear (cochlea) via a bone conduction oscillator.

BTE   Behind-the-ear.

Compression   A type of automatic gain control (AGC) whereby the amount of gain produced by a hearing instrument varies depending on the input level of the signal entering the hearing instrument.

Compression (Amplifiers)   Nonlinear amplification for which the amount of gain applied to the signal varies automatically depending on the input to the system.

Compression Ratio   Ratio of the change in output level produced by a hearing instrument when compression is active as compared with when compression is not active. For example, a hearing instrument with a 2:1 compression ratio will amplify a sound increase of 10 dB by only 5 dB.

Conductive Hearing Loss   Type of hearing impairment caused by an obstruction in the outer ear, middle ear, or both. The inner ear functions within normal limits, whereas the stimuli presented by air conduction are 15 dB or poorer than the bone conduction.

CORFIG   Coupler response for flat insertion gain or CORrection FIGure. The values added to a prescribed real-ear insertion response to obtain a prescribed 2-cm^3 coupler response. CORFIG is the arithmetic inverse of GIFROC.

Coupler   A device for acoustic measurement of a hearing aid for testing purposes.

Damper   A mechanical device that decreases the magnitude of amplified signals in a hearing instrument. Also referred to as acoustic filters.

Deep Canal Hearing Aid   A completely-in-the-canal (CIC) hearing aid that terminates within approximately 5 mm of the superior portion of the tympanic membrane.

Degradation Effect   Occurs when a word recognition score is poorer in a binaural listening situation than in a monaural listening situation.

Digital Hearing Aid Circuit   Sound pressure received by the microphone is converted to a digital (binary) signal, amplified, modified, and converted back to sound pressure through the receiver, and transmitted to the user

Dynamic Range   The arithmetic difference between the patient's threshold for hearing and the intensity level at which sounds produce discomfort (in decibels).

Effective Masking Level (EML)   The amount of masking noise necessary to appropriately "cover up" the better ear from responding for the poor ear.

Electroacoustic Measure   Referring to a physical measurement of a hearing instrument output in which no behavioral response is required from the hearing instrument wearer being evaluated. ANSI 2-cm^3 coupler gain measurements are an example of electroacoustic measurements.

False-Negative Response   The patient does not respond when a response was audible to the hearing mechanism.

False-Positive Response   The patient responds when no stimuli was presented.

Feedback   The oscillation (whistling sound) a hearing instrument makes when the amplified receiver enters back into the microphone and is reamplified.

FM System   Frequency modulation system. An amplification system that uses radio waves to transmit auditory information. It is a wireless system with a transmitter worn by the talker and a receiver worn by the hearing-impaired person.

Frequency Response   Usually plotted as a curved line, this is a charting of the hearing frequencies amplified.

Functional Gain   The difference between aided and unaided thresholds typically determined by sound-field measurements.

Gain   The amount (expressed in decibels) by which a hearing instrument increases the volume of a signal above the level of the signal that entered the hearing instrument.

GIFROC   The values added to a 2-cm³ coupler response to predict the real-ear insertion response. GIFROC is the arithmetic inverse of CORFIG.

Hard-Wired Amplification System   In this system the sound source is coupled directly to the listener using a cord or wire. An example would be plug-in headphones for use with a television.

Headroom   The difference in sound-pressure level (SPL) between the level a sound is amplified, at user settings, to the level at which the signal intensity exceeds the maximum output of the hearing instrument. As an illustration, when a patient has the hearing instrument set to a comfortable level for conversational speech and someone starts speaking loudly, if the hearing instrument has little headroom, the peaks of the loud speech could saturate the hearing instrument and cause distortion. The greater the amount of headroom a hearing instrument has, the less chance the aid will go into saturation.

Hearing Level (HL)   The level of a signal relative to 0 dB on an audiogram.

Hearing Threshold Level (HTL)   The softest level at which a listener can hear a signal 50% of the time relative to 0 dB on an audiogram.

In-Line Telephone Amplifier   A telephone amplifier that is connected between the handset and body of the telephone. Can be line powered or powered by transformer or batteries. This type of amplifier works with almost all telephones.

Induction Loop   System that operates on the principle of electromagnetic induction. In this case the induction typically involves the passage of an electrical signal from the loop to the telephone coil of a hearing aid.

Infrared System   Assistive device that uses infrared light waves to transmit auditory signals. One of the most popular types of assistive technology.

Input   Signal (dB SPL) of sound entering the microphone of a hearing aid.

Insertion Gain   The difference between aided and unaided sound pressure in the ear canal determined by probe-microphone measurements.

Integrated Circuit   A miniaturization of components in a hearing aid amplifying system.

Interaural Attenuation (IA)   IA indicates the amount of energy necessary for sound to cross from one side of the skull to the opposite side. Using standard headphones, IA is generally 40 dB for air conduction, whereas bone conduction IA is 0 dB.

ITE   In-the-ear.

K-AMP Circuit   A specific amplifier circuit that provides a high-frequency boost for quiet sounds and gradually reduces the gain for loud sounds. This circuit has a wide-band frequency response with low distortion levels.

Lipreading (Speechreading)   The ability to gain understanding of what is being said by watching the lips as well as watching the face, expressions, and gestures. The term "speechreading" is now recognized as more descriptive because it includes watching the facial expressions.

Loudness Balancing A process of balancing the loudness of sound in one ear with the perceived loudness in the second ear.

Masking The process by which the threshold of audibility for one sound is raised by the presence of another sound or sounds (R).

Matrix Method of selecting electroacoustic characteristics for manufacturing a hearing aid.

Maximum Output Refers to the limit of amplification available in a specific aid.

Maximum Tolerance The critical point where amplified sound becomes uncomfortably loud to the user. The aid must be set within the maximum tolerance limits of the user.

Mixed Hearing Loss Type of hearing impairment resulting from loss of both inner and outer/middle ear function. Air and bone conduction thresholds are both below normal limits with a 15 dB or more difference between the air and bone conduction thresholds.

Most Comfortable Loudness (MCL) A level at which speech or continuous discourse is comfortable to the listener. Speech discrimination tests are often evaluated at the MCL.

Occlusion Effect An increase in bone conduction thresholds in frequencies below 1,000 Hz due to the earphone being placed over the contralateral ear.

Octave The exact doubling of a lower frequency to a higher frequency.

Output Signal (dB SPL) delivered into a patient.

Output Limiting A method of controlling or varying the upper limits of amplification.

Phonetically Balanced (PB) Monosyllabic words representative of the English language presented for speech discrimination or word recognition tests.

Presbycusis A sensorineural loss of hearing sensitivity due to changes in the cochlear and retrocochlear systems as a result of increasing age.

Probe Microphone A specialized microphone assembly that measures sound-pressure levels generated in the ear canal in reference to an established input signal.

Programmable Hearing Aid A hearing aid that can be digitally programmed by the dispenser in order to modify the gain, output, frequency response characteristics, and/or other features of the hearing aid.

Psychoacoustic Measure Referring to a behavioral measure requiring a response from the hearing instrument wearer being evaluated. An example of a psychoacoustic measurement is functional gain.

Pure Tone Average (PTA) An average of the obtained thresholds at 500, 1,000, and 2,000 Hz.

Pure Tone Thresholds The softest level at which a pure tone can be heard 50% of the time.

Real-Ear Aided Response (REAR) The difference, in decibels, between the sound-pressure level at a reference point just outside the ear as compared with a point in the ear canal with a hearing instrument in place and turned on.

Real Ear–to–Coupler Difference (RECD) The difference between the sound-pressure level developed in an actual ear canal versus a metal 2-cm^3 coupler.

Recruitment An abnormally rapid growth of loudness as intensity is increased.

Real-Ear Insertion Response (REIR) The difference in sound-pressure level measured in the ear canal with a hearing instrument in place and turned on as compared with no hearing aid in place.

Real-Ear Measurement (REM) Measurement of the effects of sound as they actually occur at the tympanic membrane, rather than as estimated by an artificial ear.

Real-Ear Occlusion Response (REOR) The difference in decibels between the pressure level at a reference point just outside the ear as compared with a point in the ear canal with a hearing instrument in place and turned off.

Real-Ear Unaided Response (REUR) The difference, in decibels, between the pressure level at a reference point just outside the ear as compared with a point in the open ear canal.

Sensation Level (SL) Audiogram scores referenced to decibels sensation level (SL) indicate the decibel level above the patient's threshold speech stimuli.

Sensorineural Hearing Loss Type of hearing impairment caused by damage to the inner ear. Both air and bone conduction results are within 10 dB of each other and are below the normal range of hearing.

Signal-to-Noise Ratio Speech stimuli presented at a level different from the noise presented to the same ear. For example, a +10 signal-to-noise ratio indicates that the speech signal is 10 dB louder than noise presented to the same ear.

Slope Difference between amplification at 500 Hz and the highest point on the gain curve.

Sound Field An area or room in which sound waves originating from a loudspeaker are contained.

Speech Discrimination A list of 25 to 50 phonetically balanced words are given in quiet or noise to a patient. From this is determined a percentage of word recognition.

Speech Reception Threshold (SRT) The lowest level at which spondee words are repeated correctly 50% of the time.

Sound-Pressure Level (SPL) A logarithmic ratio of a measured sound pressure to a reference pressure, usually 0.0002 dynes/cm. Can be thought of as a measure of the intensity of sound.

Spondee A two-syllable word with equal emphasis on each syllable, such as "baseball" or "toothbrush."

Standing Wave When a sound hits a reflective surface, it bounces back. In certain areas the peaks and valleys of the sound hitting the reflective surface collide with those bouncing off the wall and cancel each other out. This produces reduced areas of sound. In other areas the waves of sound may add to each other, resulting in areas of increased volume.

Suprathreshold Above threshold.

Television Decoder Circuitry Act (TDCA) Enacted in 1990, the TDCA requires all television sets manufactured or imported into the United States with screens 13 inches or larger to have the technology to display closed captions without the need for external equipment.

Telephone Device for the Deaf (TDD) Based on teletypewriter technology, the TDD allows the individual to transmit and receive information over telephone lines. Both parties to the conversation must use a TDD, or a relay service must be used.

Telecoil A magnetic induction coil mounted in a hearing aid. Enables more efficient use of the telephone for the hearing aid wearer. Also allows the hearing aid to be used with induction loop systems.

Threshold This level is determined by the lowest level a signal is audible to the hearing mechanism.

Uncomfortable Loudness Level (UCL) The minimum level of sound intensity that will produce a sensation of discomfort.

Upward Spread of Masking When loud, low-frequency sounds mask out softer, higher frequency sounds.

Voice Awareness Level (VAL) The lowest level at which speech is just barely audible (but not necessarily understood) to the listener.

Warble Tone A frequency-modulated pure tone.

SUBJECT INDEX

ISBN 0-397-51687-8